Pediatric
Physical
Examination

EDITION 4

An Illustrated Handbook

KAREN G. DUDERSTADT, PHD, RN, CPNP-PC, PCNS, FAAN
Clinical Professor Emerita
Department of Family Health Care Nursing
School of Nursing
University of California, San Francisco
San Francisco, California

VICTORIA F. KEETON, PHD, RN, CPNP-PC, CNS
Assistant Professor
Betty Irene Moore School of Nursing
University of California, Davis
Sacramento, California

ELSEVIER

Elsevier
3251 Riverport Lane
St. Louis, Missouri 63043

PEDIATRIC PHYSICAL EXAMINATION –
AN ILLUSTRATED HANDBOOK, FOURTH EDITION

978-0-323-83155-0

Notice

Practitioners and researchers must always rely on their own experience and knowledge in evaluating and using any information, methods, compounds or experiments described herein. Because of rapid advances in the medical sciences, in particular, independent verification of diagnoses and drug dosages should be made. To the fullest extent of the law, no responsibility is assumed by Elsevier, authors, editors or contributors for any injury and/or damage to persons or property as a matter of products liability, negligence or otherwise, or from any use or operation of any methods, products, instructions, or ideas contained in the material herein.

Previous editions copyrighted 2019, 2014, and 2006.

Senior Content Strategist: Sandra Clark
Senior Content Development Specialist: Rishabh Gupta
Publishing Services Manager: Deepthi Unni
Project Manager: Thoufiq Mohammed
Design Direction: Brian Salisbury

Printed in India

Working together
to grow libraries in
developing countries

www.elsevier.com • www.bookaid.org

Last digit is the print number: 9   8   7   6   5   4   3   2   1

To the children and families who have trusted me with their care or made valuable
contributions to family health through participation in my research;
To the students, colleagues, and mentors who have inspired and fueled my passion for
teaching and learning; and
To my husband, Mike, and children, Benjamin and Juliet, for their love, patience, and
support.
~ Victoria Keeton

To all the students who have shaped my work as a teacher, mentor, and author;
To all the Nurse Practitioner Faculty who have continue to support & encourage use
of this text; and
To Chris, my constantly caring & patient husband, who has supported my life's work.
~ Karen Duderstadt

Abbey Alkon, RN, PNP, MPH, PhD
Professor
Department of Family Health Care Nursing
University of California, San Francisco
School of Nursing
San Francisco, California

Annette Carley, DNP, MS, RN, NNP-BC
  PPCNP-BC
Clinical Professor
Department of Family Health Care Nursing
University of California, San Francisco
School of Nursing
San Francisco, California

Carrie T. Chan, MS, MPH, RN, CPNP-PC
Associate Clinical Professor
Department of Family Health Care Nursing
University of California, San Francisco
School of Nursing
Pediatric Nurse Practitioner
Children's Orthopedic and Sports Medicine Center
Stanford Medicine Children's Health
Stanford, California

Laura C. Cooke, CPNP, MSN, RN
Pediatric Nurse Practitioner
Pediatric Gastroenterology
University of California, San Francisco
Benioff Children's Hospital
San Francisco, California

Karen G. Duderstadt, PhD, RN, CPNP-PC, PCNS,
  FAAN
Clinical Professor Emerita
Department of Family Health Care Nursing
University of California, San Francisco
School of Nursing
San Francisco, California

Julianne Evangelista, DNP, APRN, CPNP
Pediatric Nurse Practitioner
The Benderson Family Heart Center
Boston Children's Hospital
Boston, Massachusetts

Keely E. Giss, MS, RN, CPNP-PC
Pediatric Nurse Practitioner
Children's Orthopedic and Sports Medicine Center
Stanford Medicine Children's Health
Stanford, California

Bridget Ward Gramkowski, MS, RN, CNS, PHN,
  CPNP-PC
Associate Clinical Professor
Department of Family Health Care Nursing
University of California, San Francisco
School of Nursing
San Francisco, California
Pediatric Nurse Practitioner
Children's Health Center
Zuckerberg San Francisco General
San Francisco, California

Victoria F. Keeton, PhD, RN, CPNP-PC, CNS
Assistant Professor
Betty Irene Moore School of Nursing
University of California, Davis
Sacramento, California

Michelle Klosterman, MSN, MS, NP, RD, RN
Pediatric Nurse Practitioner
Pediatric Gastroenterology, Hepatology,
  Pancreatology and Nutrition
University of California, San Francisco
Benioff Children's Hospital
San Francisco, California

Angel C. Kuo, EdD, MSN, RN, CPNP-PC
Clinical Professor and Vice Chair
Department of Family Health Care Nursing
University of California, San Francisco
School of Nursing
Pediatric Nurse Practitioner
Pediatric Urology
Zuckerberg San Francisco General
San Francisco, California

Adam J. Leonard, MS, MPH, CPNP-PC, PMHS
Assistant Clinical Professor
Department of Community Health Systems
University of California, San Francisco
School of Nursing
San Francisco, California

Janis Mandac-Dy, MS, RN, CPNP-PC, PMHS
Clinic Director
Multi-Disciplinary Assessment Center
Zuckerberg San Francisco General
Assistant Clinical Professor
Department of Family Health Care Nursing
University of California, San Francisco
School of Nursing
San Francisco, California

Renee P. McLeod, PhD, APRN, CPNP, FAANP
Owner and Pediatric Nurse Practitioner
Pacific Integrative Pediatric Health
San Diego, California
Adjunct Professor
School of Nursing and Health Professions
Chaminade University of Honolulu
Honolulu, Hawaii

Patricia O'Brien, MSN, CPNP-AC, FAHA
Nurse Practitioner (Retired)
Department of Nursing/Patient Services
Cardiology Program
Boston Children's Hospital
Boston, Massachusetts

Adebola M. Olarewaju, PhD, MS
Pediatric Nurse Practitioner
Otolaryngology—Head & Neck Surgery
University of California Davis Health
Sacramento, California

Naomi Ann Schapiro, PhD, RN, CPNP-PC
Clinical Professor Emerita
Department of Family Health Care Nursing
University of California, San Francisco
School of Nursing
San Francisco, California

Linda M. Stephan, MSN, MSc, RN, CPNP-PC
Associate Clinical Professor
Department of Family Health Care Nursing
University of California, San Francisco
School of Nursing
San Francisco, California

Angela R. B. Todd, PhD, RN, FNP-BC
Assistant Professor
Director of Curriculum and Assessment
Masters of Science Physician Assistant Studies
Dominican University of California
San Rafael, California

Concettina (Tina) Tolomeo, DNP, MBA, APRN,
   FNP-BC, AE-C
Senior Director
Patient Access
Nurse Practitioner
Pediatric Pulmonary, Allergy, Immunology, & Sleep
   Medicine
Yale University School of Medicine
New Haven, Connecticut

Alison Bennett, DNP, CPNP-AC/PC, CNS, RN
Pediatric Nurse Practitioner
South University
High Point, Colorado

Chelsea Elyse Buchanan, MSN, APRN, CPNP-PC
Texas Pediatric Specialists and Family Sleep
Center
San Antonio, Texas

Sheri Carson, DNP, RN, CPN, CPNP-PC
Clinical Assistant Professor
College of Nursing
University of Arizona
Pediatric Nurse Practitioner
Northwest Urgent Care
Tucson, Arizona

Carol Clark, DNP, APRN, FNP-BC
Clinical Assistant Professor
Indiana University School of Nursing
Indianapolis, Indiana

Tamika Dowling, DNP, FNP-c, PCCN
Assistant Professor and Nurse Practitioner
Norfolk State University
Ocoee, Florida

Sharyn Renee Flippo, DNP, APRN, CPNP-PC
Clinical Associate Professor
Louise Herrington School of Nursing
Baylor University
Dallas, Texas

**Charity Markham Gates, MSN, APRN, CPN,
  CPNP-PC**
Certified Pediatric Nurse Practitioner
Nursing Faculty
Child Plus Pediatrics, PA
Saginaw, Texas
Harris College of Nursing
Texas Christian University
Fort Worth, Texas

Anjali Johnson, RN, BSN
School of Nursing
University of Minnesota
Minneapolis, Minnesota

Angela Kehrley, DNP, CNP, FNP-BC
Nurse Practitioner
Lenoir-Rhyne University
Hickory, North Carolina

Ann Sheehan, DNP, CPNP-PC, FAANP
Assistant Professor Health Professions
College of Nursing
Michigan State University
East Lansing, Michigan

Kari Varner, DNP, FNP-C
Associate Professor of Graduate Nursing
Morningside College
Sioux City, Iowa

This is the fourth edition of the *Pediatric Physical Examination: An Illustrated Handbook* for students, educators, and pediatric health care providers dedicated to mastering the art and technique of the comprehensive physical examination of infants, children, and adolescents. Facing increasing time pressures, primary health care providers need astute assessment skills combined with quick references to assist them in caring for children, youth, and families. This fourth edition of *Pediatric Physical Examination: An Illustrated Handbook* will provide the novice or experienced provider with pediatric content from experts in the field, useful examination techniques from birth through adolescence, and pediatric clinical pearls not covered in other texts on health assessment across the life span.

This fourth edition contains enhancements that reflect key ways in which health care has evolved in recent years, in response to advances in health technology and a deeper understanding of the influence of social and structural factors on health. Chapters now include a section dedicated to telehealth, with tips for providers on safe and evidence-based approaches to adapting physical assessment to virtual modalities. Also threaded throughout the text are concepts related to health inequities and social factors that may influence disparities in health conditions or variations in findings encountered during physical examination. Language throughout the text has also been updated using person-first and inclusive terms to celebrate the diversity of patients encountered in pediatric health care settings. There are also many new photos and illustrations of important physical assessment findings and with greater representation of diverse populations.

The initial chapters of this handbook begin with an overview of the developmental approach to information gathering and assessment of children from birth through adolescence. Chapter 3 focuses on developmental and mental health surveillance, including expanded coverage of pediatric emotional health assessment, and presents evidence on reliable and valid developmental, emotional, and behavioral screening tools. Chapter 4 presents comprehensive information on history taking in infants, children, and adolescents, grounded in principles of trauma-informed care and cultural humility. Chapter 5 reviews the unique vulnerability of children to environmental hazards and focuses on the importance of the environmental health history in identifying and reducing environmental risk factors that have an impact on child health.

Chapter 6 features a head-to-toe assessment of the term newborn and reviews pertinent health history and common newborn conditions. Chapter 7 presents assessment of the skin, hair, and nails, with enhanced content related to common dermatologic findings in children with varying amounts of skin pigmentation. The chapters that follow are organized in the pediatric-oriented "quiet-to-active" approach to physical examination. Pediatric experts consider this to be the most effective approach to assessing young children. This format begins with the quieter parts of the exam—cardiac and respiratory—that require astute listening skills and less active participation of the young child. Then, Chapters 10 through 13 cover assessment of the eyes, ears, nose, throat, neck, and lymphatic system, which require more active participation from the child and are better performed after the quiet parts of the physical examination. Chapter 14 reviews abdominal and rectal assessment from birth to adolescence.

A unique feature of the fourth edition text remains the developmental approach to examination of the genitalia and the developing breast from infancy through adolescence, presented in Chapters 15 through 17. Chapter 18 includes a comprehensive assessment of the child and adolescent athlete for sports participation. Finally, Chapter 19 presents the head and neurological assessment from a pediatric developmental perspective, including the recent guidelines on assessment for concussion.

Working with children and families is a hopeful endeavor, and health in childhood builds the foundation for health promotion and health protection throughout life. Through astute physical assessment, providers build trust with children and families and preserve the provider/patient relationship, ultimately improving health outcomes and decreasing health care costs. This handbook assists the pediatric health care provider with this most important undertaking: protecting and promoting the health of the next generation.

I would like to first acknowledge Sandra Clark, Senior Content Strategist, who has supported me and loyally carried my vision for this text through four editions to make it a wonderful resource for students and educators. I would also like to acknowledge my wonderful co-editor on this fourth edition, Dr. Victoria Keeton. As my former student and faculty colleague, she graciously agreed to work with me and has made significant contributions in all the new features in this fourth edition.

We are grateful to Shweta Pant and Rishabh Gupta, the Senior Content Developmental Specialists, who kept us on track and patiently ensured that all components of the text came together seamlessly. Lastly, we acknowledge Ellen Wurm-Cutter, Director of Content Development, for her communication and oversight, and Thoufiq Mohammed, for his assistance as the Project Manager for this text during the final stages of publication.

This fourth edition has several new contributors—Carrie Chan, Laura Cooke, Keely Giss, Bridget Gramkowski, Michelle Klosterman, Adam Leonard, Janis Mandac-Dy, Adebola Olarewaju, Linda Stephan, and Angela Todd. Each of them brought unique expertise in pediatric primary care, adolescent health care, or pediatric specialty care that greatly enhanced this edition of the text. We are thankful for their invaluable contributions during a particularly challenging time, as the global pandemic continued to impact the work of clinicians and educators. We would like to acknowledge previous chapter contributors—Pat Jackson Allen (Ears, Nose, Mouth, and Throat) and Erica Monasterio (Breast and Genitalia) and Renee McLeod for her previous contribution to the newborn chapter—for providing foundational content that was retained or updated for this edition. Naomi Schapiro was willing to return as a key adolescent health contributor during a very busy time for her research work. All of these pediatric colleagues made excellent contributions and were instrumental to the publication of this fourth edition. We are also grateful to Tiffany Lambright, PNP, for contributing personal photos to the text.

Finally, we would like to acknowledge our husbands and families. Without their constant patience, love, and support, this fourth edition would not have happened. Our hope is that the knowledge in this text will help to shape the next generation of pediatric health care providers who advocate for and promote optimum health for children, adolescents, and families.

CHAPTER 1

APPROACH TO CARE AND ASSESSMENT OF CHILDREN AND ADOLESCENTS

Victoria F. Keeton; Karen G. Duderstadt

UNIQUE ROLE OF THE PEDIATRIC PROVIDER

Pediatric health care providers have a unique role in the development of a child's health over a lifetime. Health is an interactive, dynamic process shaped by genetics, exposures, human experiences, and individual choice.[1] From a life course perspective, early experiences can "program" a child's health and development. Protective factors, such as a nurturing family and safe neighborhood, improve health and contribute to healthy development, whereas risk factors, such as limited access to quality health care and social services, have a negative effect on a child's development and ability to reach his or her full developmental potential.[1]

Physical, cognitive, and social-emotional health are established in the early years of life. A significant body of literature indicates that many chronic conditions in adulthood and inequities in adult health have their origins during childhood and increase over time.[2,3] Pediatric health care providers are charged with identifying developmental concerns early and focusing on interventions that promote the health and well-being of children and families and limit the adverse effects of toxic stress on brain development.[3] Toxic stress, in contrast

to tolerable stress, is defined as prolonged activation of the physiologic stress response system that is not buffered by environmental protections or by stable, responsive caregiver relationships.[3] Early investments in health promotion can empower healthy choices for both child and family, greatly improve child health outcomes, alter the life course, and decrease the cost of health care services.

ESTABLISHING A CARING RELATIONSHIP

Children have unique needs because of their long period of dependency and development, which presents a unique challenge to the pediatric health care provider. Children's health and well-being depend greatly on the care received from their family units and the environment in which they live. Addressing the needs of the caregiver while caring for the child and fostering a healthy relationship in the family unit is among the most important and challenging tasks in pediatrics.

Care is best provided in a *patient-centered medical or health care home*, which promotes holistic care of the child and family. The patient-centered health care home allows the provider to create a trusting partnership, to limit the effects of psychosocial adversity in

1

childhood, and to improve the quality of care through empowerment and support of the family unit.[4] Children, adolescents, and families benefit from motivational and anticipatory guidance in health promotion. Care provided over time by the same provider is associated with higher odds of receiving multiple preventive services, particularly for adolescents.[5] The caring relationship established by the primary care provider reinforces positive caregiving and provides medical and behavioral consultation to the child, adolescent, and family at critical periods of development.

CAREGIVER AND CHILD INTERACTION

One of the most important aspects of the health interview is observing and eliciting interactions between the caregiver and child or adolescent. Analyzing verbal responses and interactions during the encounter gives the health care provider an idea of how the caregiver relationship fosters child development and child self-esteem. It also gives the health care provider a window into the child's world. Interactions between the caregiver, family members, and the health care provider may reveal family dynamics, family connectedness, family authority, and the approach to problem solving.

Nonverbal cues provide the most revealing picture of the child's demeanor and of the caregiver-child relationship and give the health care provider additional understanding of the context in which the child lives. Stop and observe these cues and verbalize your concerns to the caregiver and child: "You look sad today. Can you tell me about how you are feeling?" Ask yourself the following: Is the caregiver disengaged with the child or infant during the encounter? Does the caregiver appear depressed or angry? Does the data from the health interview fit with the demeanor of the child during the encounter? It is important to observe the caregiver-child relationship with compassion and empathy, avoid judgment, and provide care in the context of family cultural differences in communication and interaction.

A child who is withdrawn, refuses to make eye contact, or is consistently stressed when communicating with a caregiver is exhibiting signs of strain in their environment. This should alert the health care provider to communicate concern to the family and provide support, counseling, and referral when indicated. Children often mirror the emotions of the adults around them. Families involved in conflict, who have experienced violence, or who are under stress often cannot see their own interactions clearly or the effect that their interactions have on the child.[6] Pediatric health care providers should assess caregiving behaviors by asking open-ended questions,[7] such as "What do you do when your child is acting out?" or "How do you negotiate limiting screen time?" By fostering and supporting effective caregiving in early childhood and providing problem-based counseling, the pediatric health care provider offers a service that is critical to the healthy psychosocial development of the child.[7]

Temperament

Assessment of *temperament* is a key part of comprehensive health assessment in infants, children, and adolescents. Temperament is the inborn tendency to react to one's environment in certain ways and is thought to be generally constant and at least partially genetically determined. The personality of an individual child reflects the interaction between the child's temperament and environment. Temperament can be assessed by report, clinical observation, or by a formal assessment tool. The term *goodness of fit* describes the concept of how well the child's temperament meets the expectations of his or her parents and caregivers. *Goodness of fit* promotes healthy development in the family unit through adaptation to the infant's personality, and it has a critical influence on a child's emotional well-being and behavior. Table 1.1 identifies the nine characteristics of temperament. Certain temperamental characteristics may be associated with resiliency in children, whereas other characteristics may signal emotional difficulties. Characteristics

TABLE 1.1	TEMPERAMENT CHARACTERISTICS
Characteristics	**Description**
Activity	Amount of motor activity and proportion of active to inactive periods
Intensity	Amount of emotional energy released with responses
Sensitivity	Amount of sensory stimuli required to produce response
Approach/withdrawal	Nature of initial response to new stimuli
Adaptability	Ease of accepting new situation after initial response
Frustration tolerance	Length of time activity is pursued
Mood	Amount of pleasant versus unpleasant behavior child exhibits
Distractibility	Effectiveness of extraneous stimuli in altering direction of ongoing behavior
Regularity	Predictability of physiological functions such as hunger, sleep, elimination

of frustration tolerance and intensity may be specific indicators of emotional dysregulation in some children and may indicate an underlying dysfunction in affective processes that significantly increases risk for mood disorders in later childhood or in adulthood.[8] An easy temperament with strong characteristics of regularity and adaptability acts as a protective factor for social-emotional development and could be related to resilience in children living in an adverse social environment.[9]

An understanding of temperamental characteristics removes judgment and blame and helps parents to recognize that all rules do not work equally well with all children. Setting limits and time out is more difficult with some children, and some children are more difficult to discipline and require more parental ingenuity. Temperament theory objectifies these differences. A comprehensive approach to assessing development includes assessing and understanding temperament and sharing this information with parents and caregivers. A temperament assessment tool for parents may be accessed online at http://www.preventiveoz.org.

A CHILD'S PERSPECTIVE

The view of the parent or caregiver may differ quite remarkably from the view of the child, and this difference can affect health care decisions and treatment outcomes. Promoting opportunities for children and adolescents to contribute to health care decisions creates a child-centered approach to care that empowers and enables the child or adolescent within the family unit.

A child's participation in the health history should be facilitated within a framework for communication that is attentive, sensitive, and values the child's perspective while capturing the shared responsibility of families, health care professionals, and health care organizations.[10] An exemplary model[10] provides a child-centered approach to health care while considering the needs and views of the family unit:

- The child's voice is heard irrespective of their age.
- The child is supported in expressing their views.
- The child's views are considered.
- The child is involved in the decision-making process.
- The child can share power and responsibility in decision making.

CULTURAL HUMILITY

Increasing global migration offers health care professionals continuous opportunities to work with diverse populations.[11] An understanding of diversity includes knowledge about a family's culture and also respect and tailoring communication to embrace and value diversity. Cultural beliefs may affect care-seeking behavior and the delivery of clinical care by health care providers. Effective models of care incorporate sensitivity to cultural variations and enhance the protective factors of cultural practices within families. Embracing and valuing cultural diversity in the health care encounter builds honesty and trust in the caring relationship.[11] *Cultural humility* is an essential component of responsible health care services for multicultural populations. *The practice of cultural humility* requires a life-long commitment to engage in self-assessment, acquire cultural knowledge and skills consistent with the practice setting, and value diversity within the health care team.[12] *Cultural humility* also involves a change in overall perspective around diversity and increasing awareness of power imbalances in the provider-patient relationship.[12]

It is important for providers to acknowledge cultural differences, understand their own background and culture, and recognize how that influences the care they deliver. The attitudes and behaviors of health care providers have been identified among many factors contributing to health inequities for diverse populations.[13] Providers may carry implicit biases related to their patients' race, ethnicity, socioeconomic status, gender identity or expression, or several other characteristics. Implicit biases can influence behavior and clinical decision making without the provider's awareness. The perception of bias in clinical encounters undermines the caring relationship between provider and patient.[13] Health care providers must make conscious efforts to overcome bias in their actions and care of patients.

Ideally, delivery of health care services should occur in the first language of the patient and caregiver. When this is not possible, access to and effective use of professional interpreter services are essential to providing equitable care. A model approach for the encounter between the health care provider, child, and family should include the following:
- Recognizing language barriers and effectively using interpreters

- Exploring family beliefs and their impact on the child
- Building on family strengths
- Recognizing and exploring the use of cultural beliefs and alternative therapies, how they influence child health, and the effect on clinical care
- Understanding how your values and beliefs as a health care provider influence your care delivery and affect health outcomes
- Altering care practices to eliminate inequities in health care delivery will help to mitigate the impact of structural racism in health care settings

INTERVIEWING CHILDREN

Children are accepting of many different styles of interaction and will adapt to the health care provider who is at ease communicating and engages the child. Engaging children in the interview process can reveal their understanding of health, allow their participation in the health care encounter, and provide insight into their social-emotional world. Eye-level encounters are the most effective with young children and make the health care provider appear more approachable. The skilled pediatric health care provider learns to make eye contact when a child is interested and to avoid eye contact when a child is fearful. Initially directing attention to the parent or caretaker allows the infant or young child time to adjust to the environment.

Children are comfortable when they know what to expect in an environment. Explaining clearly to the young child or adolescent exactly what you are going to assess during the physical exam will decrease anxiety and build trust. With each part of the exam, explain or "talk through" the assessment and the findings. Reassure the child or adolescent of your findings when normal and explain abnormal findings as appropriate for the child's age. Talking through every step of the encounter decreases anxiety in the child and adolescent. Even busy practitioners in time-pressured environments will find the child or adolescent to be a more willing participant when this *talk-through* approach is added to the health care encounter.

Many young children are effective communicators and can respond to questions about their dietary habits, daily activities, school or childcare, and relationships with school friends. It is important to engage children early in gathering health information. Health education can easily follow when this interview technique is used, and the child's responses create a dialogue that establishes a supportive provider-patient relationship.

Children 6 to 11 years old can be directly interviewed and can be participants in their health care. Health care providers can be role models for parents as they engage the child in the health interview and teach aspects of health and safety education. This approach teaches children from a young age to understand and care about their health and establishes the importance of building healthy habits for life.

Adolescents should always be interviewed separately from the parent. It is important to prepare the parent for this transition to a more independent role for the adolescent during the health care encounter. Allowing time to engage the adolescent independently will provide the best opening for discussion of personal or sensitive concerns that need to be voiced and for discussion of any conflicts in the home or school environment that are affecting the adolescent's well-being.

Use of the following clear communication techniques when interviewing will build a caring, trusting relationship with children/adolescents and their families:

- **Question indirectly** to encourage children and adolescents who are reluctant to discuss feelings. Engage the young child with, "I am going to tell you a story about a 5-year-old who lost his favorite pet. How do you think he feels?" or the adolescent with, "Some 15-year-olds have tried vaping or smoke marijuana. Do you have any friends who smoke?"
- **Pose scenarios** to the child or adolescent. "What would you do if…?" is appropriate for

the young child, in contrast to, "How would you feel if…?" which is appropriate for the older school-age child and adolescent.
- **Begin with less threatening topics** and move slowly to more sensitive topics for the child or adolescent. "Tell me how things are going at school this year," in contrast to, "Has anyone ever hurt you?" or directed to the adolescent, "Has anyone forced you to have sex without your consent?"
- **State your expectations clearly**. Say to the child, "I need you to be very quiet now so I can listen to…" Or to the adolescent, "To take care of you, I need you to tell me…"
- **Do not offer a choice** to the child or adolescent when in reality there is no choice.
- **Use "I"** when speaking to the child or adolescent. "I need to ask you this question because I want to help you…" in contrast to, "You need to tell me what is going on." Avoid using the word *you*, which creates a defensive atmosphere when interviewing children or adolescents. This will provide positive role modeling for parents and also build the caring relationship between the health care provider, the child, and the parent.
- **Ask the young child to draw a picture or draw his or her family**. This captures the child's attention and establishes your interest in the child's abilities. Children often reveal feelings or communicate important issues through their art.[14]

THE IMPORTANCE OF PHYSICAL EXAMINATION

Imaging and technology play an increasingly important role in the diagnosis of health conditions, but the physical exam remains an important diagnostic tool. When applied by skilled hands, physical examination can yield important diagnostic information and decrease the need for unnecessary imaging.[15] The physical exam helps providers to ask better questions of the diagnostic tests they order. Further, performing the physical examination provides important psychosocial benefits to the patient and can relieve stress and provide reassurance. Diagnostic evidence is important, but it is most valuable when decisions about diagnostic testing and imaging are made after completing a thorough health history and performing a thorough physical examination.[15]

The physical examination also facilitates the meaningful encounter between the patient and provider.[15] Recent studies have indicated that the trusting relationship between the provider and the family is the most influential factor in assisting families in making sound decisions about the care of their child. This provider-patient relationship is an important part of the therapeutic effect when working with families. It is crucial for pediatric health care providers to master the skills of history taking and physical examination to decrease or prevent medical errors and to increase efficiency in ordering diagnostic testing and treating patients and families, which decreases overall health care costs.

"QUIET TO ACTIVE" APPROACH TO THE PHYSICAL EXAMINATION

"Quiet to active" is an important mantra that should be adopted by the health care provider who will be caring for infants and young children. It refers to the approach of beginning with the parts of the physical examination that require the child to be quiet or silent for the health care provider to differentiate physical findings, rather than following a traditional "head to toe" order of assessment. The "quiet" parts of the physical examination in infants and young children include pulse and respiratory rate, auscultation of cardiac sounds and respiratory sounds, and auscultation and assessment of the abdomen. Respiratory and cardiac sounds are subtle, and accurate assessment requires a relatively cooperative child. Therefore, approaching these areas first during the physical examination produces the best results. The "active" parts of the exam include those that require the child's cooperation, such as the otoscopic, musculoskeletal,

or neurological assessments. Leaving the more invasive or uncomfortable assessments for the end of the examination, such as the ears and mouth, maximizes the likelihood that the child will be cooperative for the majority of the encounter. Varying the sequence of the physical examination to fit the temperament and activity level of the child is an essential part of pediatrics. Omitting an aspect of the physical examination does not serve the health care needs of the child and risks a diagnosis made on the basis of an incomplete assessment.

DEVELOPMENTAL APPROACH TO ASSESSMENT

Newborn Infants up to 1 Month of Age

In the clinical setting, it is important to begin the physical assessment with the infant initially swaddled on the examining table or in the parent's arms to maintain body temperature. In this manner, auscultation of the cardiac and respiratory sounds can be accomplished before disturbing a sleeping infant or cooling the infant significantly. After the "quiet" parts of the examination are completed, transfer the infant to the examining table if in the parent's arms and begin a complete assessment with the infant wearing only a diaper. Observing the movements of the newborn for symmetry, strength, and coordination must be observed with the infant undressed. Assessment of overall appearance, skin color, breathing pattern, and degree of alertness or responsiveness should be noted. The health care provider should remain flexible in regard to the order of the exam throughout the encounter as often the physical examination is performed between the feeding and sleep cycles of the newborn.

Infants up to 6 Months of Age

Until 6 months of age, infants are most effectively assessed on the examination table. It provides a firm surface to support the infant's head during the physical exam and provides a stable surface for the examination techniques required during a complete physical assessment. A calm, gentle approach works well and avoids possibly frightening the infant. The "quiet" parts of the exam may be accomplished with the infant in the parent's arms, but other parts are difficult to accomplish effectively in that position. Remember never to leave a young infant unattended on the examining table.

Children 6 Months to 2 Years of Age

The inspection of infants and young children necessitates a completely different social approach than with any other age groups. In establishing a therapeutic relationship with an adult, etiquette requires immediate eye contact. With infants 7 to 9 months of age, a progressive approach to eye contact is required because of the developmental phenomenon of stranger anxiety. First, observe the infant or young child covertly while speaking with the caregiver in order to allow the child to adjust to your presence in the environment. If the young child is looking at you and listening, then make glancing eye contact. If you are not rejected, then speak to the young child and, finally, reach out to touch the child. This approach will produce the best results in establishing the caring relationship. By offering puppets or small, washable toys to the child or using dolls to demonstrate parts of the physical examination, you will also often provide a calming effect at the beginning of the encounter.

Once the infant can sit stably, normally around 6 to 8 months of age, the examination can proceed with the child in the parent's lap, to decrease fear and stranger anxiety. Clothing should be removed gradually as the physical examination progresses from "quiet" to "active." Optimal examination of the abdomen and genitalia occurs with the child on the examination table, but in the fearful child, the exam may proceed with the child still in the parent's lap and with the examiner seated at the same level as the parent in a knee-to-knee position to create a surface for the child to lie on (Fig. 1.1). With the young child's head and shoulder on the parent or caretaker's lap, the examiner proceeds

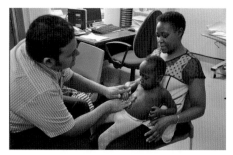

FIGURE 1.1 Knee-to-knee position for examining abdomen in infancy and early childhood. (From Glynn M, Drake, WM, eds. *Hutchison's Clinical Methods: An Integrated Approach to Clinical Practice.* 25th ed. Elsevier; 2023.)

with assessment of the abdomen, genitalia, and hips, thereby avoiding the need to place the child on the examination table, which may elicit anxiety. When the infant is old enough to begin walking, it is important to observe the infant toddling in only a diaper to evaluate gait and musculoskeletal coordination.

Young Children

By 3 years of age, most children, though still apprehensive, are able to make eye contact and separate briefly from the parent. Observe their ability to be comforted, evaluate their response to the environment, their level of social interaction, and their relationships with parents or caregivers and siblings if present. How appropriate is their behavior in the setting? What is the quality and variety of their verbal responses? What is their level of activity and attention span? Young children generally respond best to a slow, even, steady voice. Give the young child time to warm to the situation before undressing him or her. The confident young child should be able to be examined sitting on the examination table. The "quiet" to "active" approach is still advisable with this age group, that is, beginning with the cardiac and respiratory examination and then proceeding head to toe. Give children 3 to 5 years of age clear directions, allow them to respond, and praise success. Young children particularly enjoy games, drawing, and role playing the physical examination with dolls

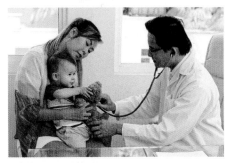

FIGURE 1.2 Use of play to decrease anxiety in a young child. (From Freepik.com)

or stuffed animals (Fig. 1.2). Modesty sets in during the preschool years, and health care providers need to be respectful and mindful of this developmental stage.

Children 6 to 11 Years of Age

Children 6 to 11 years old benefit most from the "talk-through" approach to the physical exam. They are interested in learning about their bodies and are forming a body image of themselves. They are becoming more independent from their parents. School-age children gain the most from education about good health habits. Learning more about their bodies helps them connect their health with their health habits. Allow the child to participate in all aspects of the physical exam and respect his or her modesty. A "head-to-toe" assessment with the child on the examining table is most effective during middle childhood.

Adolescents

The approach to the health care encounter should be based on the child's developmental stage rather than their chronological age. This is true for all children but particularly those in adolescence. Development during early, middle, and late adolescence proceeds unevenly and can vary widely among 11- to 18-year-olds. Respect and confidentiality are essential components of developing a trusting relationship with the adolescent. Parental input is important during the health encounter, but adolescents should be interviewed and examined separately from the parent or peers. Avoid power struggles and give the adolescent control whenever possible. Involve adolescents in planning their health care and in establishing realistic goals and health habits. Chapter 4 further discusses assessment and evidence-based practice for the care of children from infancy through adolescence, and the system-based chapters to follow address further details of the physical examination at different ages and stages.

TELEHEALTH ASSESSMENT

Pediatric telemedicine or telehealth services have increased over the last several years. Benefits of telehealth include increased access to resources and care for patients in areas with few healthcare providers, reduced health care costs, or increased patient satisfaction due to convenience and efficiency of care.[16] Telehealth may also optimize disease management and monitoring of health conditions with the goal of improving the patient's health and outcomes. Potential disadvantages of telehealth are limitations to performing the physical exam, inequities in access to proper technology across diverse populations, and concerns related to security and confidentiality.[16] Barriers to telehealth at the provider and patient level include adequate internet connection, software capabilities, and equipment. When these challenges are resolved, telehealth improves access to care by allowing providers and patients to conduct clinic visit remotely.

Best practices in telehealth include considerations for technology, setting, and provider interaction.[17,18] The telehealth visit can be conducted by video or phone; however, video is the preferred method because it supports patient-provider engagement and a similar office visit experience. If video conferencing is used, it must be on a trusted HIPPA-compliant platform, with a reliable connection, and the name and title of the examiner should be clearly displayed. The setting for telehealth should include a neutral and well-lit background, with privacy ensured by location and headphone use. Continuing a patient-centered approach remains key during these visits. The provider should have professional dress, badge visibility, and be making eye contact and appropriate facial expressions at the welcome and throughout the visit. Exercise clinical judgment when determining what medical conditions can reasonably be addressed using telehealth. If the chief complaint cannot be properly visualized and/or the caregiver cannot provide an adequate history of the present illness, schedule the patient for an office visit.

The systems-based chapters in this text provide tips on performing various parts of the history and physical examination via telehealth.

REFERENCES

1. Halfon N, Larson K, Lu M, Tullis E, Russ S. Lifecourse health development: past, present and future. *Matern Child Health J.* 2014;18:344–365.
2. Williams TC, Drake AJ. What a general paediatrician needs to know about early life programming. *Arch Dis Child.* 2015;100:1058–1063.
3. Shonkoff JP. Capitalizing on advances in science to reduce the health consequences of early childhood adversity. *JAMA Pediatr.* 2016;170:1003–1007.
4. Bair-Merritt MH, Mandal M, Garg A, Cheng TL. Addressing psychosocial adversity within the patient-centered medical home: Expert-created measurable standards. *J Prim Prev.* 2015;36:213–225.
5. Garcia-Huidobro D, Shippee N, Joseph-DiCaprio J, O'Brien JM, Svetaz MV. Effect of patient-centered medical home on preventive services for adolescents and young adults. *Pediatrics.* 2016;137:e20153813.
6. Waters SF, Karnilowicz HR, West TV, Mendes WB. Keep it to yourself? Parent emotion suppression influences physiological linkage and interaction behavior. *J Fam Psychol.* 2020;34:784–793.
7. O'Connell LK, Davis MM, Bauer NS. Assessing parenting behaviors to improve child outcomes. *Pediatrics.* 2015;135:e286–288.
8. Calkins SD, Dollar JM, Wideman L. Temperamental vulnerability to emotion dysregulation and risk for mental and physical health challenges. *Dev Psychopathol.* 2019;31:957–970.
9. Derauf C, LaGasse L, Smith L, et al. Infant temperament and high-risk environment relate to behavior problems and language in toddlers. *J Dev Behav Pediatr.* 2011;32:125–135.
10. Shier H. Pathways to participation: Openings, opportunities and obligations. *Child Soc.* 2001;15:107–117.
11. Dell'Aversana G, Bruno A. Different and similar at the same time. Cultural competence through the leans of healthcare providers. *Front Psychol.* 2017;8:1426.
12. Foronda C. A theory of cultural humility. *J Transcult Nurs.* 2020;31:7–12.
13. Hall WJ, Chapman MV, Lee KM, et al. Implicit racial/ethnic bias among health care professionals and its influence on health care outcomes: A systematic review. *Am J Public Health.* 2015;105:e60–76.
14. Davies D, Troy MF. *Child Development. A Practitioner's Guide.* Guilford Publications; 2020. 4th ed.
15. Committee on Diagnostic Error in Health Care; Board on Health Care Services; Institute of Medicine; The National Academies of Sciences, Engineering, and Medicine. Improving diagnosis in health care. In: Balogh EP, Miller BT, Ball JR, eds. National Academies Press (US) 2015.
16. Gajarawala SN, Pelkowski JN. Telehealth benefits and barriers. *J Nurse Pract.* 2021;17:218–221.
17. Daniel H, Snyder Sulmasy L, et al. Policy recommendations to guide the use of telemedicine in primary care settings: An American College of Physicians position paper. *Ann Intern Med.* 2015;163:787–789.
18. Ansary AM, Martinez JN, Scott JD. The virtual physical exam in the 21st century. *J Telemed Telecare.* 2021;27:382–392.

ASSESSMENT OF GROWTH AND VITAL SIGNS

Linda M. Stephan

GROWTH

Growth is a key indicator of health in childhood and typically proceeds in a predictable pattern from *cephalocaudal* (head to tail) and *proximodistal* (near to far). The anthropomorphic measurements used to evaluate growth in children are height (length), weight, and head circumference. Table 2.1 presents average weight, height (length), and head circumference gains from infancy through middle childhood and adolescence. Abnormalities of weight, height/length, or head circumference parameters may be the first indicator to the health care provider of an abnormality. As such, accurate evaluation of these parameters begins in the newborn period and continues throughout childhood and adolescence.

MEASUREMENT AND INTERPRETATION OF GROWTH

Growth measurements should be taken at every well visit in childhood. It is important to use the correct technique when gathering measurements as incorrect technique can result in an inaccurate measurement and ultimately may lead to an inaccurate diagnosis. Box 2.1 presents a summary of recommendations for accurate measurement in different age groups.

Growth Charts

Growth patterns are interpreted using anthropomorphic measurement data plotted on a growth chart that depicts normative growth for the population being measured. The growth chart used in this analysis can either be based upon a dataset that is a *growth reference* or a *growth standard*. The Centers for Disease Control and Prevention (CDC) growth charts include normative values for children raised in a variety of nutritional conditions in the United States prior to the year 2000 and are therefore considered a *growth reference*.[1] The World Health Organization (WHO) growth charts are considered a *growth standard* because they include ideal normative values for the growth of healthy children in multiple countries living with optimal nutritional and environmental conditions. Fig. 2.1 presents examples of the CDC and WHO charts for young children. The CDC recommends using WHO growth charts for full-term infants from 0 to 2 years old and recommends using the CDC growth charts for children >2 years old.[1] CDC and WHO growth charts are accessible at: https://www.cdc.gov/growthcharts/who_charts.htm.

WHO growth charts follow the 2nd, 5th, 10th, 25th, 50th, 75th, 90th, 95th, 98th percentiles; CDC growth charts follow the 5th, 10th, 25th, 50th, 75th, 90th, 95th percentiles. The middle line on each growth chart is the 50th percentile, and this represents the mean value for individuals of that age and sex. Therefore, an individual with a weight value that plots at the 50th percentile on a growth chart is considered to have a weight that is more than about half of individuals of the same sex and age in the *reference population* and less than about half of the individuals in that *reference population*.

Typical growth is considered to be any value that falls within 2 standard deviations (SD)

TABLE 2.1	AVERAGE WEIGHT, HEIGHT, AND HEAD CIRCUMFERENCE GAINS IN INFANCY THROUGH ADOLESCENCE			
	WEIGHT	**HEIGHT**	**HEAD CIRCUMFERENCE**	
Age	**Average Weekly Gain**	**Average Monthly Gain**	**Average Monthly Gain**	**Comments**
0–3 months	210 g (8 oz)	3.5 cm	2.0 cm	Regain or exceed birth weight by 2 weeks Birth weight doubles in 4–6 months
3–6 months	140 g (5 oz)	2.0 cm	1.0 cm	—
6–12 months	85–105 g (3–4 oz)	1.2–1.5 cm	0.5 cm	—
	Average Yearly Gain	**Average Yearly Gain**	**Average Yearly Gain**	
1–3 years	2–13 kg (4.4–6.6 lb)	12 cm	3.0 cm	Height at 2 years, approximately half of adult height
3–6 years	2 kg (4.5 lb)	3–7 cm	1.0 cm	—
6–12 years	3–3.5 kg (7 lb)	6–7 cm	2–3 cm during middle childhood	Growth occurs in spurts lasting about 8 weeks, occurring 3–6 times per year
	Average Total Gain	**Average Yearly Gain**		
Females 9.7–13.5 years	17.7 kg (39 lb)	8–14 cm/year	—	95% of growth achieved by onset of menarche
Males 11.7–15.3 years	22.2 kg (50 lb)	8–14 cm/year	—	95% of growth achieved by 15 years; weight gain follows linear growth and is delayed by several months

Adapted from data in Kliegman R, Nelson WE, Stanton B, et al. *Nelson Textbook of Pediatrics.* Elsevier; 2019.

from the mean for age and sex on the growth chart.[1] On the CDC growth charts, the normal range (+/− 2 SD from the mean) is from the 5th to 95th percentiles, while the normal range for WHO growth charts (+/− 2 SD from the mean) is between the 2nd to 98th percentiles. A single data point is not always enough to evaluate pediatric growth. It is important to also

evaluate trends over time as a single value may fall within the normal range, but there may be a trend of either increasing or decreasing percentiles that is significant enough to require further evaluation. Values that fall more than 2 SD above or below the mean, or plotted growth measurements that either increase or decrease by more than two major percentile

---

BOX 2.1   ACCURATE MEASUREMENT OF HEIGHT AND WEIGHT

Height

Birth–24 Months
- Infant's head must be held firm on flat surface against top of measuring device.
- Push knees, with legs extended, gently toward table. Bottom of foot is placed directly against footboard of measuring device.

24–36 Months
- Transitioning to a stadiometer at 24 months of age is most accurate to assess linear growth; use of a measuring device for fearful children from 24 to 30 months can be used with child lying on a flat surface or examination table.

36 Months Through School Age
- Child should be standing erect with buttocks and back against stadiometer or wall.
- For accurate height measurement in the young child, maintain the head erect by placing slight upward pressure under the chin.

Weight

Birth–12 Months
- Infant should be undressed and weighed consistently with clean, dry diaper or without diaper when placed on infant balance scale.
- *Safety* is of primary concern. Examiner cannot leave infant unattended at any time.

12–24 Months
- Before 2 years of age, weight is measured most accurately on infant balance scale with dry diaper. Exceptions: when child is very large or more cooperative/stable, a standing scale may be used.

2–6 Years
- At 2 years, when child is cooperative, weight can be measured accurately on a standing balance scale in clothing without shoes.

---

lines between well-child visits, are concerning for atypical patterns of growth and require further evaluation by the health care provider.

Normative growth data is available for healthy term infants, children, and adolescents, but historically has been limited for preterm infants. Currently, high-quality neonatal growth charts have been developed to better estimate growth patterns in preterm infants.[2] A thorough prenatal and birth history is required to determine the correct gestational age for a newborn in order to use these charts. Growth charts have also been developed to present normative standards of growth for children and adolescents with a variety of conditions associated with altered patterns of growth, such as Down syndrome, Turner syndrome, Williams syndrome, achondroplasia, and Prader-Willi syndrome.

The best way to evaluate growth of the pediatric population with special conditions that impact growth is to use the correct corresponding growth chart based on the most up-to-date evidence-based guidelines. For example, growth charts for children in the United States with Down syndrome can be accessed on the CDC website at: https://www.cdc.gov/ncbddd/birth-defects/downsyndrome/growth-charts.html.

EVIDENCE-BASED PRACTICE TIP

A growth parameter that falls outside of the accepted 2 standard deviations (SDs) above or below the mean may be normal when the parental stature is considered.

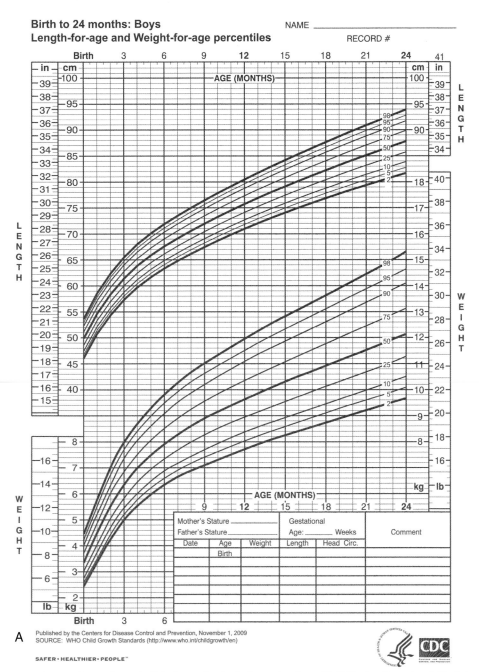

FIGURE 2.1 Comparison of clinical growth charts for males from (A) WHO: length and weight, 0 to 24 months; and

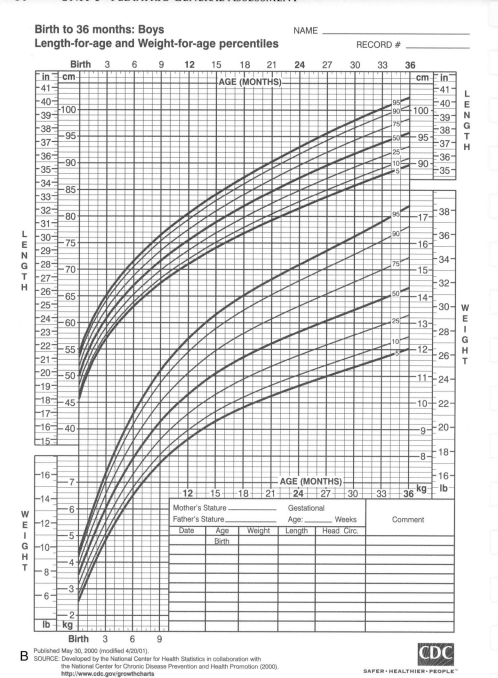

FIGURE 2.1, CONT'D (B) CDC: length and weight, 0 to 36 months. (Reprinted with permission. Available at: https://www.cdc.gov/growthcharts/who_charts.htm)

Head Circumference

Measurement of *head circumference* is a routine part of growth assessment in the first 2 years of life. An accurate measurement of the head is taken with the measuring tape placed around the head at the point of greatest circumference from the occipital protuberance above the base of the skull to the midforehead or point of greatest bossing of the frontal bone (Fig. 2.2). The *head circumference* measurement is plotted on the growth chart at each well-child visit to determine if the growth pattern is normal. If the initial head measurement is plotted on the growth chart and indicates a concerning pattern of growth, it is important to remeasure the head to ensure accuracy of the measurement.

A *head circumference* value that is 2 SD below the mean on the growth chart, or that has a trend of decreasing by more than 2 major percentile lines over time, is concerning for *microcephaly*. *Microcephaly* may be indicative of various genetic anomalies, prenatal or postnatal brain injury, premature closure of the cranial sutures, termed *craniosynostosis*, or may be idiopathic. A *head circumference* value that is 2 SD above the mean on the growth chart or that has a trend of increasing by more than 2 major percentile lines over time is concerning for *macrocephaly*. *Macrocephaly* may indicate increased brain parenchyma, hydrocephalus, increased bone or blood, a mass or lesion,

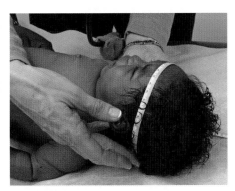

FIGURE 2.2 Accurate measurement of head circumference.

benign enlargement of the subarachnoid space, or may be idiopathic. Consistent and accurate assessment of the *head circumference* is a critical part of the evaluation of normal growth and development in the first 2 years of life.

Chest Circumference

Chest circumference is measured along the nipple line during the newborn exam. It is typically only measured when other abnormal physical findings are present, but not generally a part of routine well-child assessment. The *head circumference* is normally 1 to 2 cm greater than the *chest circumference* for the first 18 months of life. With the progression of growth, the *chest circumference* becomes larger than the head circumference at about 2 years of age and continues to grow more rapidly during childhood.

Height/Length

Height/length is the most stable measurement of growth and maturation in childhood. Linear growth is genetically predetermined, and therefore adult height generally occurs within a predictable range if accurate family history is available. Linear growth often occurs in spurts followed by long quiescent periods in which no growth occurs. Infants and young children may demonstrate an increase in appetite before a growth spurt, followed by an increased need for sleep.

Height refers to how tall an individual is while standing, while length refers to how long an individual is while lying down. Due to gravity, an individuals' length is usually just slightly greater than their height. It is most appropriate to measure length in infants and for young children who are not yet standing well on their own and height in children who are able to stand independently. When plotting length and height on a growth chart is important to consider the measurement type to have accurate interpretation of the growth. WHO growth charts indicated for children <2 years old utilize length measurements, and CDC growth charts indicated for individuals 2 to 20 years old utilize height measurements. Always compare height/length measurements with previous growth trends to assure accuracy.

Although infant measurement is often taken on the examination table by marking the position of the top of the head and the bottom of the foot on table paper and then determining length with a measuring tape, this method can result in inaccurate measurements. To measure length in an infant or toddler, place them supine on a flat surface or examination table equipped with a *measuring device* or *length board* (Fig. 2.3). Accurate measurement requires the infant's legs to be flat against the measuring device with the foot in the level position and head held erect against the measuring device. After 2 years of age, measurement of standing height is appropriate; however, recumbent length with a measuring device is often easier to obtain in the first part of the second year if the child is fearful. Standing height should be taken using a wall-mounted or portable *stadiometer* for accuracy (Fig. 2.4). Accurate measurement requires a cooperative child to stand erect with head level, feet flat, and heels against the measuring surface. Measurement is recorded without shoes to the nearest 0.1 cm or 0.25 inches.

Term newborns typically vary in length between 45 to 55 cm (18 and 22 inches) at birth. Length increases by approximately 2.54 cm (1 inch) per month over the first few months of life, with an overall increase by approximately 50% of the birth length in the first year. The

increase is primarily in truncal lengthening. Doubling the height at 2 years of age can give an estimate of adult height.[3] Height increases by an average of 3 inches (7.5 cm) over the second and third years. From the end of the third year until the onset of puberty, height increases an average of 3 to 7 cm (2 to 3 inches) per year. Height potential for adolescents assigned female at birth is generally realized by 16 years of age, whereas males' growth potential continues until 18 years of age. Linear growth ceases when the maturation of the skeleton is complete (see Chapters 15 and 17 for discussions of growth and sexual maturity rating).

A height/length measurement that is 2 SD below the mean on the growth chart, or that has a trend of decreasing by more than 2 major percentile lines over time, is concerning for *short stature*. *Short stature* can be caused by a variety of endocrine or genetic causes, nutritional causes, or chronic illnesses. However, as much as 90% of short stature is a result of nonpathological causes, such as familial short stature. In *familial short stature*, growth follows

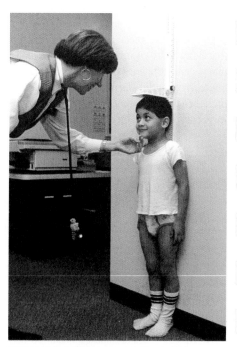

FIGURE 2.4 Measuring standing height.

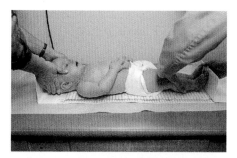

FIGURE 2.3 Recumbent measurement of infant length using a length board (Hockenberry MJ, Wilson D, Rodgers CC. *Wong's Essentials of Pediatric Nursing*. Elsevier Health Sciences; 2021.)

a curve below the normal growth curves, and both biological parents and the infant are short.[1] A *height/length measurement* that is 2 SD above the mean on the growth chart, or that has a trend of increasing by more than 2 major percentile lines over time, is concerning for *tall stature*. *Tall stature* can be caused by fetal overgrowth syndromes, postnatal overgrowth syndromes, or can be idiopathic.

PEDIATRIC PEARLS

Height at 2 years of age is approximately 50% of adult height. To estimate adult height, double the height at 2 years of age.[4]

Arm Span

Arm span is the distance between the tips of the middle fingers when the arms are raised to a horizontal position. A typical arm span for a child less than 10 to 12 years old is approximately 2.5 cm less than height/length and for a child greater than 10 to 12 years old may be up to 10 cm greater than height. Arm span is not a measurement typically taken at a well-child visit; however, a pediatric patient with a finding of tall stature should have an *arm span* measurement. *Marfan syndrome* is a genetic syndrome that causes tall stature, and arm span that exceeds the height can be associated with cardiac anomalies.

Weight

The average birth weight in healthy term infants is 3175 to 3400 g (7 to 7.5 lb) and can range from 2500 to 4000 g (5 lb 8 oz to 8 lb 13 oz). Infants may lose up to 10% of their birth weight in the first week of life and normally regain it by the end of the second week.[4] *Poor weight gain* in early infancy may be caused by challenges in feeding, malnutrition, neglect, cardiac or renal disease, chronic infection, or chromosomal and congenital anomalies.

Infants can be accurately weighed while lying on an infant balance scale without a diaper or wearing a dry diaper if the scale is zeroed first with a dry diaper on the scale. Infants should be weighed in the sitting position only with extreme caution and only after they are able to sit well without support. Weight is recorded to the nearest 0.5 oz or 0.01 kg (10 g). After 2 years of age, standing weight should be recorded to the nearest 0.25 lb or 0.1 kg (100 g). If a young child is very fearful or irritable, the caregiver and child can be weighed together on a standing scale, and the caregiver's weight is subtracted from the total weight to obtain an *estimate* of the child's weight. For children with special health care needs or disabilities, accommodations for wheelchair scales or special purpose scales should be made available in the clinical setting.

A weight measurement that is 2 SD below the mean on the growth chart, or that has a trend of decreasing by more than 2 major percentile lines over time, is concerning for *poor weight gain*. *Poor weight gain* may be caused by acute illness, chronic illness, difficulty with activities of daily living, an energy imbalance, psychosocial stress, or it may be idiopathic or nonpathologic.

Body Mass Index

Body mass index (BMI) is an *anthropometric index* of weight and height. The formula for determining BMI is weight in kilograms divided by height in meters squared (BMI = weight [kg]/height squared [m^2]). BMI is not a diagnostic tool, rather it is used as a screening tool to identify children at risk for *underweight* (BMI less than the 5th percentile for age and sex), *overweight* (BMI between the 85th and 94th percentiles for age and sex), or *obesity* (BMI at the 95th percentile or greater for age and sex).[5] The American Academy of Pediatrics (AAP) recommends calculating and plotting BMI on a growth chart during the routine health visit for all children 2 to 20 years old,[3,6] primarily to screen for *overweight* or *obesity*. A BMI greater than the 85th percentile requires further evaluation as it may be a result of a genetic or endocrine disorder, energy imbalance, or have an idiopathic or nonpathologic cause.

Adipocytes, or fat cells, are a repository of energy in the body, and *obesity* is defined as an excess of *adiposity*.[7] Many studies have found an association between high levels of *adiposity* and poor health, including hypertension, stroke, type 2 diabetes, cardiovascular disease, and some forms of cancer.[8] BMI percentile is a population measure and not a direct measure of individual body fat; however, it may have value as a proxy measure to screen for excess *adiposity* in children.[7] In a typical pattern of growth and development in children, BMI declines in later infancy and then rebounds in middle childhood; this is sometimes referred to as the *adiposity rebound*.[9] Lack of this expected rebound pattern, or a rebound that occurs earlier than middle childhood, is a risk factor for *obesity*. A high ratio of *waist circumference* to height may be another indicator of risk of obesity and related conditions in adolescents. Some research has found that a high ratio of *waist circumference to height* is more strongly associated with adverse risk factors than a high BMI for age or skinfold thickness.[10] BMI or *waist circumference* cannot be used alone to determine an individual's risk for metabolic disease—the etiology of *metabolically unhealthy obesity*[11] is multifactorial, including genetics, environment, behavior, and psychosocial stress.[7] Thorough evaluation of BMI or *waist circumference* requires a thoughtful and comprehensive history and physical exam to develop an accurate assessment and effective plan of care.

It is important for the pediatric provider to approach the assessment of weight and BMI through a lens of *body positivity*. Weight *stigma* and shaming of individuals with elevated BMI is associated with negative physical and mental health outcomes and can be particularly harmful if perpetuated in the clinical setting.[12] Measurement of weight and review of growth charts during the clinical visit should be performed with sensitivity and using empathetic and empowering counseling techniques. Conversations with families around lifestyle behaviors should be centered around concepts of health and wellness rather than weight. Other strategies for a *body positive* approach to care include using nonbiased language in visits and documentation and creating a clinical environment that is more inclusive of body diversity.[12]

VITAL SIGNS

Temperature

Currently there are a range of methods available for measuring temperature in the infant and young child, including rectal, axillary, oral, infrared measurement of tympanic membrane or temporal artery, and smartphone or wearable devices. Rectal temperature remains the standard and most reliable method for detecting core body temperature in infants and young children. Most studies establishing the risk for serious infections in febrile infants have relied on rectal temperatures. However, there can be a time lag between a change in core body temperature and a change in temperature in the rectal vault.[13] Oral temperature is typically 0.6° C (1.0° F) lower than rectal temperature because of air cooling via mouth breathing. Axillary temperature is also consistently lower than rectal temperature, but the absolute difference varies too widely for a standard conversion.[13]

Peripheral thermometers such as infrared tympanic membrane and temporal artery thermometers do not have sufficient agreement with established methods of core temperature measurement, and studies show that they are more reliable for confirming a fever (specificity: 94%–96%) than for ruling one out (sensitivity: 64%–72%).[13,14] To date there has not been sufficient research to establish the accuracy of smartphone or wearable thermometers either. For this reason, these types of thermometers cannot be used in situations where detection of a fever has clinical implications for diagnosis and treatment (i.e., evaluation of a febrile infant), and their use in the clinical setting cannot be recommended at this time. Anticipatory guidance for caregivers using peripheral thermometers at home should include counseling regarding their limited sensitivity for detecting fever.

Rectal temperature is most accurately measured in infants up to 8 or 9 months by placing the infant in the supine position on the examining table with knees flexed toward the abdomen. The infant can see the practitioner and be secured more easily in this position. Proper positioning prevents injury. A child from 9 months to 2 years of age can be placed in the caregiver's arms or laid supine on the caregiver's lap. Insert the lubricated tip of thermometer approximately 0.5 to 1 inch into the anal opening of the rectum. *Oral temperature* can be taken by placing the thermometer under the individual's tongue. Recent ingestion of either hot or cold liquids may impact the accuracy of the measurement. *Axillary temperature* is often taken in newborns by placing the thermometer under the arm at the base of the axilla for 3 to 5 minutes and holding the arm firmly against the side of the body with swaddling.

Infrared tympanic membrane thermometers measure the amount of heat produced by the tympanic membrane. These thermometers are used by placing the probe inside the ear canal for a few seconds to obtain a reading. Infrared contact and noncontact *temporal artery or forehead thermometers* measure the amount of heat being produced by the temporal artery. Contact forehead temporal artery thermometers are used by making contact between the thermometer and forehead for a few seconds and noncontact temporal artery thermometers by holding the thermometer close to the forehead for a few seconds. *Smartphone thermometers* measure temperature via an external sensor that communicates with the smartphone.

Mean body temperature is approximately 37.0 degrees Celsius (98.6 degrees Fahrenheit), and normal body temperature ranges between 35.5–37.7 degrees Celsius (96–100 degrees

Fahrenheit).[4] Body temperature fluctuates throughout the day, with the lowest point in the morning and the highest in the early evening. Fever is defined as a rectal temperature of 38.0 degrees Celsius (100.4 degrees Fahrenheit).[4]

Pulse

Although pulse is most often monitored electronically, pulses should also be assessed by the provider for the quality of rate, rhythm, volume, or strength, and differences between the upper and lower extremities. Children under 2 years of age require apical pulse (AP) measurements. Readings should be taken when the child is quiet. AP measurements are taken with the stethoscope placed over the heart below the nipple at the ape x. For children over 2 years of age, the radial pulse is a satisfactory measurement. In infants and young children, the pulse should be counted for a full minute to account for irregularities in rhythm. Fig. 2.5 illustrates the location of the pulses. The radial and femoral pulses should be evaluated and compared for strength and quality. Detecting the femoral pulse in newborns and young infants requires focus and concentration by the examiner. The

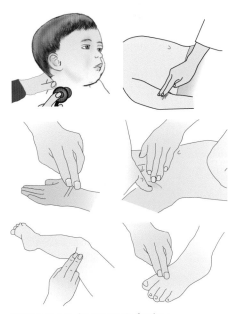

FIGURE 2.5 Assessment of pulses.

femoral pulse is located in the midinguinal area over the head of the femur. In children with more adipose tissue, locating the femoral pulse is challenging and requires deeper palpation to determine the presence and strength of the pulse. An absent or weak pulse in the lower extremities compared with the upper extremities is a red flag for *coarctation of the aorta* (*see* Chapter 8). Table 2.2 presents the grading of pulses used to evaluate strength and quality. The expected range for heart rate depends on the age of the child.[4] Table 2.3 shows the typical range of pediatric heart rates.

Respirations

Respirations should be assessed for rate and pattern. They should be taken when the child is quiet to accurately assess the rate and quality of breathing. In infants and young children, observe the abdominal movements when you are evaluating respiratory rate. An infant's breathing is primarily diaphragmatic. Also evaluate the use of any accessory muscles in the upper chest or any difficulty breathing. Respirations should be assessed for a full minute, because the typical respiratory rate is irregular in the newborn and very young infant. The expected range for respiratory rate depends on the age of the child.[4] Table 2.3 shows the typical range of pediatric respiratory rates.

Oxygen Saturation

Pulse oximetry is a noninvasive method of measuring the percentage of saturated hemoglobin in the capillary bed (SpO_2). The AAP recommends checking oxygen saturation (SpO2) in the first 24 hours of life to screen newborn infants for critical heart disease. The AAP recommends checking oxygen saturation (SpO_2) in the first 24 hours of life to screen newborn infants for critical heart disease.[3] *Pulse oximetry* alone may detect cyanotic heart disease in the asymptomatic newborn, preventing morbidity and delayed diagnosis of cardiac disease. Outside of the neonatal period, measurement of oxygen saturation is not typically measured for routine well-child care; however, it

TABLE 2.3	EXPECTED RANGES OF PEDIATRIC RESPIRATORY RATE AND HEART RATE	
Age	Respiratory Rate (breaths/ minute)	Heart Rate (beats/ minute)
0–3 months	34–57	123–164
3–6 months	33–55	120–159
6–9 months	31–52	114–152
9–12 months	30–50	109–145
12–18 months	28–46	103–140
18–24 months	25–40	98–135
2–3 years	22–34	92–128
3–4 years	21–29	86–123
4–5 years	20–27	81–117
6–8 years	18–24	74–111
8–12 years	16–22	67–103
12–15 years	15–21	62–96
15–18 years	13–19	58–92

Data from Fleming S, Thompson M, Stevens R, et al. Normal ranges of heart rate and respiratory rate in children from birth to 18 years of age: A systematic review of observational studies. *Lancet.* 2011 377:1011.

TABLE 2.2	STRENGTH AND QUALITY OF PULSES
Strength	Quality
0	Not palpable
1+	Difficult to palpate, thready, obliterated by pressure
2+	Weak, difficult to palpate, may be obliterated by pressure
3+	Palpable, normal strength
4+	Strong, bounding, not affected by pressure

has become a standard in most clinical settings for respiratory assessment in the pediatric patient presenting with acute respiratory symptoms. *Pulse oximetry* should be part of the criteria for evaluating any infant for cardiovascular defects or any child presenting with wheezing or respiratory distress, as it assists the practitioner in clinical decision-making when the need for prolonged observation or hospital admission is being determined. A SpO$_2$ of 95% to 96% is adequate, and 97% is generally considered to be within the expected range. A SpO$_2$ ≤92% is considered *hypoxemic*.

Blood Pressure

Blood pressure should be assessed at all routine well-child visits beginning at 3 years of age and more frequently and/or earlier in life for individuals identified as being at risk for hypertension.[3,15] The size of the blood pressure cuff is critical to obtaining an accurate measurement. The blood pressure cuff should cover about two-thirds of the upper arm and should encircle the arm once. A cuff that is too large will result in a low blood pressure reading. If the cuff is too small, the blood pressure reading may be too high. For larger children and adolescents, an extra-large adult cuff may be needed to obtain an accurate measurement. Blood pressure readings can increase in children who are crying and in children and adolescents who are feeling anxious. Normal ranges for blood pressure in children under 13 years of age vary by age, assigned sex, and height percentile and must be interpreted using established normative tables.[15] See Table 2.4 for blood pressure values that require further evaluation.

Pain

An accurate assessment of pain response in infants, children, and adolescents requires strategies specific to the developmental level of the child as research has shown that caregivers' assessments of a pediatric patient's pain do not always correlate with their self-assessment of pain. Adolescents can rate their pain on a numerical scale (1–10) without the use of a pain

TABLE 2.4	SCREENING BP VALUES REQUIRING FURTHER EVALUATION			
	BP, mm Hg			
	Males		**Females**	
Age (years)	Systolic	Diastolic	Systolic	Diastolic
1	98	52	98	54
2	100	55	101	58
3	101	58	102	60
4	102	60	103	62
5	103	63	104	64
6	105	66	105	67
7	106	68	106	68
8	107	68	107	69
9	107	70	108	71
10	108	72	109	72
11	110	74	111	74
12	113	75	114	75
>12	120	80	120	80

Data from Flynn JT, Kaelber DC, Baker-Smith CM, et al. Clinical practice guideline for screening and management of high blood pressure in children and adolescents. *Pediatrics.* 2017; 140: e20171904.

assessment tool. Children 8 to 11 years old can typically rate their pain using a visual analog tool, such as the FACES pain scale,[16,17] that allows them to convert an image the child identifies with into a numerical value on a scale. Fig. 2.6 presents the FACES pain rating scale used across most pediatric clinical settings. For infants and younger children, observation tools such as the Face, Legs, Activity, Cry, Consolability (FLACC) Behavioral Scale[18] can be used (see Table 2.5).

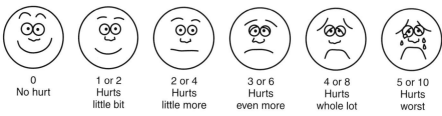

| 0
No hurt | 1 or 2
Hurts
little bit | 2 or 4
Hurts
little more | 3 or 6
Hurts
even more | 4 or 8
Hurts
whole lot | 5 or 10
Hurts
worst |

FIGURE 2.6 FACES pain rating scale. *Brief word instructions:* Point to each face using the words to describe the pain intensity. Ask the child to choose the face that best describes its own pain and record the appropriate number. *Note*: Use of these instructions is recommended. A rating scale can be used with children 3 years of age and older. *Original instructions:* Explain to the child that each face is for a person who feels happy because he has no pain (hurt) or sad because he has some or a lot of pain. FACE 0 is very happy because he doesn't hurt at all. FACE 1 hurts just a little bit. FACE 2 hurts a little more. FACE 3 hurts even more. FACE 4 hurts a whole lot. FACE 5 hurts as much as you can imagine, although you don't have to be crying to feel this bad. Ask the child to choose face that best describes how much hurt he has. Record the number under the chosen face on the pain assessment record. (From Hockenberry MJ, Wilson D, Rodgers CC. *Wong's Essentials of Pediatric Nursing.* Elsevier Health Sciences; 2021. Reprinted with permission.)

TABLE 2.5	FACE, LEGS, ACTIVITY, CRY, CONSOLABILITY (FLACC) BEHAVIORAL SCALE		
	SCORING		
Categories	**0**	**1**	**2**
Face	No particular expression or smile	Occasional grimace or frown, withdrawn or disinterested	Frequent to constant frown, clenched jaw, quivering chin
Legs	Normal position or relaxed	Uneasy, restless, or tense	Kicking, or legs drawn up
Activity	Lying quietly, normal position, moves easily	Squirming, shifting back and forth, or tense	Arched, rigid, or jerking
Cry	No cry	Moans, whimpers, or occasional complaint	Crying steadily, screams or sobs, frequent complaints
Consolability	Content, relaxed	Reassured by occasional touching, hugging, or being talked to; distractible	Difficult to console or comfort

Each of the 5 categories is scored from 0 to 2: (F) Face; (L) Legs; (A) Activity; (C) Cry; (C) Consolability. The total score will be between 0 and 10. For pediatric/preverbal children (validated 2 months to 7 years). Not valid for children with developmental delay.
Adapted from American Academy of Pediatrics. *Reference Range Values for Pediatric Care.* Soghier L, Fratantoni K, Reyes C, Mullins K, eds. American Academy of Pediatrics; 2019.

PHYSICAL ASSESSMENT TECHNIQUES

Inspection

Inspection is about *looking*. *Inspection* is a skill acquired by developing detailed and meticulous observation of children and learning to see the whole as well as the parts. It involves not only the sense of sight but also the senses of hearing and smell. Inspection requires good room lighting and complete visibility of the body part to be examined to accurately assess symmetry, shape, and color. It is an essential skill for the pediatric health care provider, particularly when interacting with the nonverbal child, the young pediatric patient, or a child who is ill.

Palpation

Palpation is about *touching* and *feeling*, a skill used to detect temperature, vibration, position, and mobility of body organs and glands. *It* detects masses and differences in size and shape of glands, organs, muscles, and bones in all parts of the body. The fingertips are most sensitive to tactile differences, the backs of the fingers are most sensitive to temperature, and flattened fingers and palm on the chest detect vibrations. The examiner's hands should move smoothly over the body without hesitation, first using light palpation, then followed by deep, firm pressure with palpation. It is important to know the distinction between palpation and massage. Massage incorporates *rubbing*, in contrast to the technique of *palpation*, which is the movement of the fingers over an area using light to firm pressure for the purpose of identifying size, location, mobility, sensitivity, and temperature of lymph nodes, muscles, tissues, and body organs.

Percussion

Percussion is a helpful skill for mapping out the borders of the organs or sternum and for determining the presence of solid tumors. *Percussion* requires using the examiner's fingers and hands to produce sounds on the area of the body being examined. The density of the body parts is determined by the sounds emitted when the examiner's finger strikes the middle finger of the opposite hand while it is resting over the area of interest. The fingers produce sounds ranging from the least dense sound, *tympany* or *resonance*, as heard over the stomach or intestines, to the densest sound, *dullness* or *flatness*, produced by striking over bone. This technique can be useful when examining the abdomen to detect the size of an organ prior to diagnostic imaging.

Auscultation

Auscultation is listening to body sounds transmitted through the stethoscope. With infants and small children, low-pitched cardiac sounds are heard best with the bell-shaped side of the stethoscope, and high-pitched lung and bowel sounds are best heard with the diaphragm, or flat portion, of the stethoscope. The bell shape is effective in isolating cardiac sounds from stomach sounds in the young infant. For best results during the physical examination of a child, it is essential to match the size of the stethoscope head to the size of the child proportionately, or the pressure on the head of a dynamic stethoscope. In listening to the lungs and heart, it is important to develop the skill to screen out adventitious sounds that occur in infants and children. The close proximity of the organs requires the examiner to screen out stomach and abdominal sounds in listening to the heart and the respirations in the lung.

The techniques of inspection, palpation, percussion, and auscultation are among the most important tools available to the examiner for accurate diagnosis. When applied correctly, they can guide accurate diagnosis and limit unnecessary diagnostic testing and imaging for the child or adolescent and family.

REFERENCES

1. Grummer-Strawn LM, Reinold C, Krebs NF. Use of World Health Organization and CDC growth charts for children aged 0–59 months in the United States. *MMWR Recomm Rep.* 2010;59:1–15.
2. Villar J, Giuliani F, Barros F, et al. Monitoring the postnatal growth of preterm infants: a paradigm change. *Pediatrics.* 2018;141:e20172467.
3. Kliegman R, Nelson WE, Stanton B, et al. *Nelson Textbook of Pediatrics.* Elsevier; 2019.
4. Fryar CD, Carroll MD, Afful J. *Prevalence of overweight, obesity, and severe obesity among children and adolescents aged 2–19 years: United States, 1963–1965 through 2017–2018.* 2020. https://www.cdc.gov/nchs/data/hestat/obesity-child-17-18/obesity-child.htm
5. Hagan Jr JF, Shaw JS, Duncan PM. *Bright Futures: Guidelines for Health Supervision of Infants, Children and Adolescents.* 4th ed. American Academy of Pediatrics; 2017.
6. American Academy of Pediatrics. *Reference Range Values for Pediatric Care.* American Academy of Pediatrics; 2019.
7. Kumar S, Kelly AS. Review of childhood obesity: from epidemiology, etiology, and comorbidities to clinical assessment and treatment. *Mayo Clin Proc.* 2017;92:251–265.
8. Horesh A, Tsur AM, Bardugo A, Twig G. Adolescent and childhood obesity and excess morbidity and mortality in young adulthood—a systematic review. *Curr Obes Rep.* 2021;10:301–310.
9. Zhou J, Zhang F, Qin X, et al. Age at adiposity rebound and the relevance for obesity: a systematic review and meta-analysis. *Int J Obes (Lond).* 2022;46:1413–1424.
10. Moltrer M, Pala L, Cosentino C, Mannucci E, Rotella CM, Cresci B. Body mass index (BMI), waist circumference (WC), waist-to-height ratio (WHtR) e waist body mass index (wBMI): which is better? *Endocrine.* 2022;76:578–583.
11. McMorrow AM, Connaughton RM, Lithander FE, Roche HM. Adipose tissue dysregulation and metabolic consequences in childhood and adolescent obesity: potential impact of dietary fat quality. *Proc Nutr Soc.* 2015;74:67–82.
12. Pont SJ, Puhl R, Cook SR, Slusser W. Stigma experienced by children and adolescents with obesity. *Pediatrics.* 2017;140:e20173034.
13. Niven DJ, Gaudet JE, Laupland KB, Mrklas KJ, Roberts DJ, Stelfox HT. Accuracy of peripheral thermometers for estimating temperature: a systematic review and meta-analysis. *Ann Intern Med.* 2015;163:768–777.
14. Geijer H, Udumyan R, Lohse G, Nilsagård Y. Temperature measurements with a temporal scanner: systematic review and meta-analysis. *BMJ Open.* 2016;6:e009509.
15. Flynn JT, Kaelber DC, Baker-Smith CM, et al. Clinical practice guideline for screening and management of high blood pressure in children and adolescents. *Pediatrics.* 2017;140:e20171904.
16. Tsze DS, von Baeyer CL, Bulloch B, Dayan PS. Validation of self-report pain scales in children. *Pediatrics.* 2013;132:e971–979.
17. Hockenberry MJ, Wilson D, Rodgers CC. *Wong's Essentials of Pediatric Nursing.* Elsevier Health Sciences; 2021.
18. Crellin DJ, Harrison D, Santamaria N, Huque H, Babl FE. The psychometric properties of the FLACC scale used to assess procedural pain. *J Pain.* 2018;19:862–872.

Developmental, Emotional, and Behavioral Surveillance and Screening

Janis Mandac-Dy; Abbey Alkon

Children achieve developmental milestones at their own pace, yet the sequence of developmental milestones is expected to be incremental and stepwise for all children. Screening children for developmental delay and emotional and behavioral difficulties is one of the most important components of preventive health care. The goals of developmental, emotional, and behavioral surveillance and screening are to identify children with developmental delays or emotional or behavioral disorders and to improve child health outcomes. Pediatric health care providers are mandated by the Individuals with Disabilities Education Act (IDEA) and Title V of the Social Security Act to provide screening, early identification, and intervention for children with developmental delays and disabilities.[1] Early intervention to address developmental delays has been shown to improve outcomes, enhance function, and reduce the prevalence of secondary behavior problems later in life.[2]

In the United States, 17% of children 3 to 17 years of age have at least one developmental delay.[3] The most common childhood developmental and behavioral problems are speech and language delay, hearing loss, emotional and behavioral concerns, learning disabilities, and delay in other developmental milestones.[1] Pediatric primary care providers (PCPs) can identify young children with developmental and behavioral problems early in life by providing surveillance at every well-child visit and implementing standardized developmental screening tests at the 9-month, 18-month, and 24- or 30-month well-child visit.[1] Timely identification of developmental and behavioral problems and prompt referral for early intervention can resolve or lessen the impact of a delay or disability on the functioning of the child and family and promote their growth and readiness to progress toward the next developmental milestone. Effective interventions in early childhood increase a child's readiness for school entry and for optimum learning in the classroom.

Routine screening for emotional and behavioral disorders is a primary focus for health care providers caring for children and adolescents. Approximately one in four to five children have one or more mental, emotional, and/or behavioral problems, including depression, conduct disorder, and substance abuse.[4] During the COVID-19 pandemic, mental health–related emergency department visits increased by 24% for children ages 5 to 11 and 31% for children ages 12 to 17 compared with prepandemic emergency department visits.[5] Children who suffer from anxiety and depression may have difficulty forming important peer relationships, suffer from low self-esteem, and lack self-advocacy skills.[6] Children with anxiety and depression may have increased rates of school absenteeism, poor performance, and underachievement.[6]

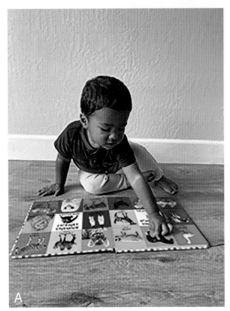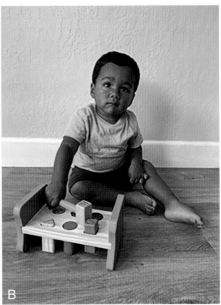

FIGURE 3.1 Toddler at play. *Courtesy Tiffany Lambright.*

DEVELOPMENTAL SURVEILLANCE

The first component of a developmental and behavioral screening program is surveillance. Developmental surveillance includes eliciting caregiver concerns, collecting and documenting a developmental history, and identifying risks and protective factors for developmental delay or emotional and behavioral problems in the child's environment. Observations of the child's development include speech and language skills, social skills, activity level, communication, and the caregiver/child relationship.

The PCP must include input from parents, other caregivers, and teachers in childcare and school settings to make informed observations of the child's developmental progress and accurately document the ongoing developmental surveillance in the health record. Guidelines for surveillance and screening during primary care visits are available at the American Academy of Pediatrics' (AAP) *Bright Futures: Guidelines for Health Supervision for Infants, Children, and Adolescents*, available at http://brightfutures.aap.org/.[7]

Developmental surveillance assists PCPs with anticipatory guidance for caregivers by identifying the developmental milestones expected and met at each age as the infant and child grows and develops. To discourage a wait-and-see approach and minimize potential delays to diagnosis, the CDC funded an AAP expert working group in 2022 to revise the CDC checklists used for developmental surveillance.[8] These checklists include evidence-informed milestones that most children (≥75%) would be expected to achieve by a certain age. Caregivers and providers are encouraged to learn and monitor the signs of healthy development and act when there is a concern. The CDC program "*Learn the Signs. Act Early.*" is a resource for caregivers, including online tools and printed materials as well as a mobile app to track developmental milestones and can be found at https://www.cdc.gov/ncbddd/actearly/milestones/index.html.

PEDIATRIC PEARLS

Caregiver concerns regarding developmental delays in fine and gross motor skills, language skills, and social/emotional development are often accurate and should always warrant further evaluation.

Surveillance for vision and hearing development includes asking caregivers about any concerns they may have about their infant or young child's developing vision or response to voices or sounds in the environment. Observable normal visual behaviors include fixing on and following near faces or objects by 3 months of age; visually tracking the caregiver at a distance of 5 feet by 4 months of age; and blinking in response to a silent sudden movement close to the face by 5 months.[9] Pediatric PCPs should also ask caregivers about their child's use of nonverbal communication and ability to hear quiet sounds and turn and locate voices. All children referred for behavioral concerns should have formal hearing and vision screening tests conducted to rule out deficits that may be contributing to delays. Reviews of vision and hearing screening practices are in Chapters 10 and 11, respectively.

Speech refers to the mechanics of oral communication, and *language* encompasses the understanding, processing, and production of communication during the early developmental years and throughout childhood. Table 3.1 presents normal developmental speech and language patterns in infancy and early childhood. Speech-language problems are the most common communication problem affecting 41% of children aged 3 to 10 years and 24%

of 11- to 17-year-olds.[10] In early childhood, children with language delay are at risk for developmental and behavioral difficulties.[11] Early referral and intervention is the key to optimizing speech and language development and outcomes for young children and their families. Pediatric PCPs need to conduct ongoing surveillance at each health encounter and screen children whose caregivers have concerns about their speech and language development. Surveillance also includes "close observation and continuity of care," where the PCP compares a child's growth and development from one point to another. A 3-year-old who has been in speech therapy may not meet all speech milestones expected of a 3-year-old, but it would be critical to note the progress they have made since the last developmental screening or assessment.

EVIDENCE-BASED PRACTICE TIP

The acquisition of language is a critical developmental skill, and pediatric PCPs can promote literacy as a component of developmental surveillance for language deficits. The *Reach Out and Read* (ROR) program, available at www.reachoutandread.org, was designed to improve the language skills of young children at risk for poor early school performance. It provides families with books and anticipatory guidance about the importance of reading to infants and young children. Several studies have shown that ROR can significantly enhance a young child's early literacy environment by increasing the frequency of caregiver-child book-sharing activities and facilitating language development.[12] With over 6000 clinics and practices utilizing the literacy program, ROR has become an important resource for PCPs to increasing the access to books for underserved families.[13,14]

Media Use

A large part of the social and emotional development of children and adolescents is now occurring while they are using mobile devices. The pediatric PCP should, therefore, include

TABLE 3.1	NORMAL RANGE OF DEVELOPMENTAL SPEECH AND LANGUAGE PATTERNS IN INFANCY AND EARLY CHILDHOOD

Age	Preverbal Communication to Developing Language and Attention to Speech Sounds
8 weeks	Emergence of social smile Grunting, crying, cooing
4 months	Squeals, yells, repeating vowel sounds or sounds in repeated patterns Turns head to look at the speaker by 4 months Laughs out loud
6 months	More complex consonant-vowel combinations ("da," "ba") Vocal play with caregiver repeating sounds Responding to own and family names by 6 months
8–10 months	Multisyllable babble, including vowel-consonant combinations Appears to listen to conversation of others by 8 months Looks at or gives common objects used at home by 8 months Word-like sounds with intonation 9 months Waves bye-bye and/or plays patty-cake by 10 months Looks for family members when asked, "Where's mama?"
10–12 months	Infant learns favorite sounds of caregiver's language and responds in a predictable manner Enjoys peek-a-boo Waves "bye-bye" back
12–13 months	Emergence of first word ranges from 8 to 18 months (mean 13 months) Consonant-vowel word 12 months Single words, other than mama/dada, with consistent meaning from 12 to 13 months Infant communicates actively by pointing
13–15 months	Follows familiar requests by 12–15 months Names one object
18–20 months	Understands about 50 words Speaks about 20 words Points to three objects when named Emergence of two-word combinations
24 months	Median speaking vocabulary 300 words 10th percentile speaking 60 words 90th percentile speaking 500 words

Adapted from Sharma A, Cockerill H. *From Birth to Five Years: Practical Developmental Examination*. Taylor & Francis; 2021; Davies D. *Child Development: A Practitioner's Guide*. 3rd ed. New York: The Guildford Press; 2011; and Scharf RJ, Scharf GJ, Stroustrup A. Developmental milestones. *Pediatr Rev*. 2016;37:25–38.

questions around screen time when conducting developmental surveillance. In the United States, 98% of children under the age of 8 live in a home with an internet-connected device and spend over 2 hours a day on screens.[15] Population-based studies have shown associations between excessive screen time and cognitive, language, and social-emotional developmental delay.[16,17] Infants with more handheld screen time are at increased risk for expressive speech delay.[18] Temperament may also influence how much media children consume. Excessive media use is often more likely in young children with self-regulation problems, and these children will present greater challenges with caregiver limit setting.[16]

Caregiver use of mobile devices is associated with fewer verbal and nonverbal interactions between caregivers and children; therefore, reducing caregiver media use and enhancing caregiver-child interactions may be an important area of family behavioral change.[16] Daily interactions between the caregiver and child will enhance the child's speech and language development. In early childhood, caregivers should ensure that media programming is of high quality and be co-viewed when possible.[16] It is also important for caregivers to monitor children's social media, gaming, web, and cell phone activities for their potential impact on the child's or adolescent's emotional health. Children's virtual lives constitute a large part of their social interactions daily. Excessive screen time in middle childhood and adolescence may involve bullying or peer-to-peer communications that pose potential risks to their privacy and safety.

The AAP has a Media and Children Communication Toolkit that provides caregivers with resources to help them manage screen time through the creation of a Media Plan, promoting thoughtful and appropriate media use to enhance daily life and achieve the purpose of its use as determined by the school and family. Further information about the toolkit and a Family Media Plan in English and Spanish are available at https://www.aap.org/en-us/advocacy-and-policy/aap-health-initiatives/Pages/Media-and-Children.aspx

PEDIATRIC PEARLS

The AAP recommends no screen exposure for children before 18 months of age other than for video chatting, limiting screen time to no more than 1 hour per day for 2 to 5 year olds, and that children 6 years of age and older receive consistent limits on the quantity and timing of recreational screen use.[19]

EVIDENCE-BASED PRACTICE TIP

Children who participate in early educational or literacy programs demonstrate increased receptive and expressive language skills and outperform children at school entry without access to these resources.[20]

Developmental, Emotional, and Behavioral Health Screening

Clinical assessment during a well-child visit or surveillance of development without using standardized screening assessments results in low detection of children with developmental delays.[1] Over 20% of children under 5 years of age are at risk for developmental, emotional, and behavioral problems, but only approximately one-third of children receive the recommended developmental screening assessment.[21] Many caregivers with children under 6 years of age are concerned about their child's development or behavior, yet caregivers often report that developmental screening was not conducted at their child's primary care visits prior to entering kindergarten.[22] The AAP's recommendations for developmental screening are based on evidence that indicates standardized screening tools capture up to 80% of children with early developmental delays.[1] Table 3.2 presents normal developmental milestones of communication, fine and gross motor, problem-solving, and social/emotional skills from 6 months to 5 years of age in accordance with a commonly used developmental screening tool, the *Ages and Stages Questionnaire, 3rd edition (ASQ-3).*[23]

Emotional health screening is recommended at every well-child visit, beginning in the newborn period with the family unit.[7] In infancy, the screening is more focused on the psychosocial assessment of the caregiver and family, such as with maternal depression screening, and gradually incorporates evaluation of the child as their socioemotional development progresses. The AAP recommends that PCPs be alert to caregiver or youth reports

TABLE 3.2	ASQ-3 DEVELOPMENTAL MILESTONES BY AGE	
Age	**Communication-Linguistic Skills**	**Gross Motor**
6 months	Makes sounds like "da," "ba"; makes high-pitched squeals; turns in direction of loud noise	Rolls from back to tummy, sits with support of own hands, bears weight with feet flat on surface
12 months	Makes 2 similar Sounds, such as "ba-ba," "da-da"; plays "peek-a-boo"; says 3 words; points to objects	Walks holding on to furniture or holding both your hands; stands alone
18 months	Points to objects and pictures in book; says 8 or more words; imitates 2-word sentence	Picks up object from the floor; walks; climbs; walks downstairs; kicks large ball
2 years	Points to correct picture in book; imitates 2-word sentence; follows directions; names objects	Walks downstairs holding rail; kicks large ball; runs; jumps with both feet;
3 years	Points to 7 body parts; speaks with 3 to 4 word sentences; follows directions; identifies action in picture book; knows own first and last name	Kicks ball by swinging leg forward; jumps forward at least 6 inches; walks upstairs; stands on one foot for 3 to 5 sec; throws ball overhand
4 years	Follows simple directions; follows 3 directions; speaks in complete sentences	Jumps forward at least 6 inches; catch a large ball with both hands; climbs a ladder
5 years	Follows 3 unrelated directions; uses 4 to 5 word sentences; used past tense and comparison words; answers questions	Throws ball at least 6 feet away; catches large ball with both hands; stands on one foot for 5 s; walks on tiptoes for 15 feet; hops on one foot 4–6 feet; skips

Fine Motor	Problem Solving	Social-Emotional
Grabs toy, picks up small toy with one hand, reaches for crumb with thumb or raking motion	Reaches or grasps toy using both hands, looks for fallen object, picks up toy and mouths it	Smiles or coos in front of mirror; grabs own foot while lying on back; tries to get toy out-of-reach
Picks up string; uses pincer grasp; throws ball with forward arm motion; turns pages of book	Claps 2 toys together; looks for hidden object (object constancy); copies scribbles on paper (Fig. 3.2)	Helps with dressing; rolls or throws a ball; hugs stuffed animal or doll
Throws small ball; stacks 2–3 blocks; marks paper; turns pages of book; uses spoon	Dumps things out of container; copies single line drawing	Gets attention by pulling on your hand or clothes; comes to you for help; drinks from a cup; copies activities
Uses spoon without spilling; turns pages of book; flips switch on and off; stack 7 blocks; string beads	Copies line drawing; pretends play; puts things away; climbs on chair to reach object	Drinks from cup without spilling; copies activities such as sweep, comb hair; pushes toys on wheels
Draws line in vertical direction and circle; strings beads; cuts paper; hold crayon between fingers and thumb	Lines up 4 objects in a row; repeats 2 numbers; makes a bridge with blocks	Pushes and steers wagon or toy on wheels; dresses self; knows gender; takes turns
Traces a circle; cuts paper with scissors; puts together 5 to 7 piece puzzle	Repeats 3 numbers; identifies small versus large circle; pretends play	Dresses self with coat and shirt; takes turns; serves self food; washes hands using soap and water
Draws picture of person with 3 or more body parts; cuts with scissors; copies shapes and letters; prints first name	Identifies colors; counts up to 15; knows opposites; names 3 numbers and 4 letters	Serves self food; washes and dries hands and face without help; knows phone number and city of residence; dresses and undresses self; uses toilet by self; takes turns and shares with others

From Squires J, Bricker D. *Ages and Stages Questionnaires*. 3rd ed. (ASQ-3). Baltimore. Brooks Publishing Company; 2009.

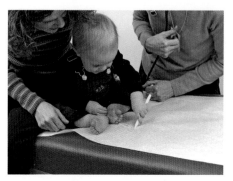

FIGURE 3.2 Toddler scribbling.

of anxiety during the psychosocial history at any age and administer a validated screening tool as appropriate.[7] The U.S. Preventive Services Task Force (USPSTF) recommends that all children 8 years and older be universally screened for anxiety. Beginning at the 12-year-old visit, annual depression and suicide screening are also universally recommended, and as clinically indicated in younger children.

The emotional health history should include eliciting a history from the caregiver and child. Adolescents should be assessed without a caregiver present, and adolescent confidentiality should be explained prior to taking an emotional health history (see Chapter 4 for information on adolescent confidentiality). The PCP should be aware that differing family and cultural perspectives regarding the stigma of developmental delay or emotional health concerns may be a barrier to reporting symptoms during screening. Providing anticipatory guidance and conducting surveillance and mental health screening at every well-child visit is an important part of normalizing the need to address developmental, emotional, and behavioral health in the pediatric population.

Children with special health care needs (CSHCN) have a high prevalence of co-occurring mental health conditions; in a recent national study of CSHCN, 34% also had anxiety, 25% had depression, and 39% had ADHD.[24] Medical or developmental complexity in CSHCN may present unique challenges for proper mental health screening and treatment,

making them more likely to have unmet mental health needs than children without special needs.[24] PCPs should recognize the limitations of using standardized screening tools for the assessment of mental health in some CSHCN. New screening methods are emerging that are tailored to identify co-occurring mental health conditions for some CSHCN,[25,26] but significant gaps in the field still exist. Obtaining a thorough history from the child's caregiver (and the child, as developmentally appropriate) and consulting with the child's interdisciplinary care coordination team can be helpful strategies for mental health evaluation in this special population.

Standardized Screening Tools

Identification of a deficit or delay on a developmental screening test does not provide a diagnosis, but it identifies children who need further evaluation, referral, and intervention services. There are numerous developmental and emotional health screening tools available. PCPs should consider a variety of validated screening tools for their practice, taking into consideration their patient population, clinical practice resources, and staff skill level. Screening tools should be directly administered by providers or trained staff or be caregiver-report questionnaires. Table 3.3 presents standardized developmental screening tools used in infancy and early childhood, and Table 3.4 presents standardized tools used to screen for emotional, behavioral, and mental health problems during early and middle childhood and adolescence.

The psychometric properties of screening tools are important considerations when deciding which screening tool to use in the pediatric health care setting.[1] Psychometric properties include test-retest reliability, validity, sensitivity, and specificity.[1] Test-retest reliability is the ability of a measure to produce consistent results. The validity of a screening test is its ability to discriminate between a child with a problem and a child without such a problem. Sensitivity is the accuracy of the test

TABLE 3.3	GENERAL DEVELOPMENTAL SCREENING TOOLS			
Tool	Age Range	Informant, Time to Administer	Description	Access
Ages and Stages Questionnaires-3 (ASQ-3)	0–5 years	Caregiver; 5 min	10–15 items for each age range available in multiple languages and using simple directions Screens communication, gross motor, fine motor, problem solving, personal-social skills Available in multiple languages Sensitivity = 70%–90%; Specificity = 76%–91%	Paul H. Brooks Publishers P.O. Box 10624 Baltimore, MD 21285 (800) 638-3775; http://age-sandstages.com/prod-ucts-services/asq3/
Parent's Evaluation of Developmental Status (PEDS)	0–8 years	Caregiver; 2 min	10 items elicit caregiver's concerns for children 0–8 years Screens for developmental and behavioral problems Available in multiple languages Sensitivity = 75%; Specificity = 74%	Ellsworth and Vandemeer Press, Ltd. P.O. Box 68164 Nashville, TN 37206 615-226-4460; http://www.pedstest.com/default.aspx
Survey of Wellbeing in Young Children (SWYC)	2–60 months	The Milestones 10 items per age; BPSC 18 items; PPSC 25 items; 10–15 min	Comprehensive tool made up of several scales: The Developmental Milestones, Baby Pediatric Symptom Checklist (BPSC), Preschool Pediatric Symptom Checklist (PPSC), Parent's Observations of Social Interactions (POSI), and Family Risk Factors. Covers cognitive, motor, language, social-emotional-behavioral functioning, autism, family factors; Available in English. Sensitivity (55%–100%) Specificity (63%–96%)	http://www.theswyc.org

in identifying a problem, and specificity is the accuracy of the test in identifying individuals who do not have a problem. Tables 3.3 and 3.4 list the sensitivity and specificity of the screening tool, developmental domains, number of items, available languages, and time to complete and score the developmental, behavioral, and emotional screening tools.

The AAP endorses the use of standardized, reliable ($\geq$80%), well-validated, and accurate

TABLE 3.4	EMOTIONAL, BEHAVIORAL, AND MENTAL HEALTH SCREENING TOOLS	
Tool	**Age Range**	**Informant, Time to Administer**
Ages and Stages Question-naires-SE-2 (ASQ-SE-2)	1–72 months	Caregiver, 10–15 min
Brief Infant/Toddler Social Emotional Assessment (BITSEA)	12–36 months	Caregiver; 5–7 min
Modified Checklist for Autism in Toddlers (M-CHAT-R/F)	18–24 months	Caregiver; <5 min stage 1; Professional and caregiver 5–10 min stage 2
Pediatric Symptom Checklist (PSC35; Y-PSC)	4–16 years of age	Caregiver (PSC) or child over 11 years (Y-PSC); 5 min
Patient Health Questionnaire Screening for Depression-9 (PHQ-9) or -Adolescent (PHQ-9A)	12 years and up	Caregiver or adolescent over 12 years; 5 min
Ask Suicide-Screening Questions (ASQ)	8 years and up	Child or adolescent self-report; less than 1 min
Children's Depression Inventory 2 (CDI 2)	7–17 years of age	Caregiver report, teacher report, self-report; 5–10 min for short form
Screen for Child Anxiety Related Disorders (SCARED),	8 years of age through adolescence	Caregiver, child, adolescent; short 5-item questionnaire
Generalized Anxiety Disorder 7-Item Scale (GAD-7).	13 years of age through late adolescence	Adolescent; self-reported 7-item questionnaire

Description	Access
30 items; Screens self-regulation, compliance, communication, adaptive behaviors, autonomy, affect, interaction with people Available in English and Spanish Test-retest reliability = 89% Sensitivity = 81% Specificity = 83%	
42-item report measure for identifying social emotional/behavioral problems with domains for externalizing, internalizing, dysregulation, and competence Available in different languages Sensitivity = 80%–85%; Specificity= 75%–80%	Pearson Assessments http://www.pearsonclinical.com
2-stage screen: (1) 20 Pass/Fail items; (2) Structured follow-up questions for children with positive screen in stage 1 Identifies children at risk of autism spectrum disorders (ASD) Sensitivity = 91%; Specificity = 96%	http://www.mchatscreen.com
35 items elicit caregiver or teen's response on short statements about problem behaviors including conduct, depression, anxiety, adjustment Available in English, Spanish, Japanese Sensitivity = 80%–95%; Specificity = 68%–100%	https://www.brightfutures.org/mentalhealth/pdf/professionals/ped_sympton_chklst.pdf
9-item survey of depression symptoms experienced over the previous 2 weeks; Modified version for adolescents includes additional suicide screening questions	https://www.aacap.org/App_Themes/AACAP/docs/member_resources/toolbox_for_clinical_practice_and_outcomes/symptoms/GLAD-PC_PHQ-9.pdf
Four brief questions to elicit suicidal ideation or behaviors; Available in 14 languages Sensitivity = 91%–99% Specificity = 84%–90%	https://www.nimh.nih.gov/research/research-conducted-at-nimh/asq-toolkit-materials
12–28 items Measures cognitive, affective, and behavioral signs of depression	http://www.mhs.com
Discriminates anxiety from other conditions including depression	https://www.pediatricbipolar.pitt.edu/resources/instruments
Assesses severity of generalized anxiety	https://adaa.org/sites/default/files/GAD-7_Anxiety-updated_0.pdf

screening tools with a sensitivity and specificity of $\geq 70\%$ for the early identification of developmental and behavioral problems.[1] Use of developmental screening tests with lower sensitivity and specificity may identify children without significant delays and may result in unnecessary referrals. Emotional and behavioral screening tests with low specificity may identify mental health symptoms that are below the level of a *Diagnostic and Statistical Manual of Mental Disorders* (DSM-5-TR) diagnosis.[27] However, these children may benefit from early interventions in the home or improved developmental learning opportunities to address developing behavioral problems. Continual tracking of a child's developmental status and follow-up on referrals is critical to optimize child health outcomes.

Developmental Screening Tools

The ASQ-3[23] and the Parents' Evaluation of Developmental Status (PEDS)[28] use caregiver report for identifying children with possible developmental delays. Caregiver-completed developmental screening tools are found to be efficient, feasible, and cost-effective compared with provider-completed screening tools.

A comprehensive caregiver-completed screening tool is the Survey of Wellbeing of Young Children (SWYC)[29] that is composed of 12 age-specific forms, linked to the pediatric periodicity schedule. The SWYC contains several brief questionnaires: Developmental Milestones, Baby Pediatric Symptom Checklist (BPSC), Preschool Pediatric Symptom Checklist (PPSC), Parent's Observations of Social Interactions (POSI), Family Questions, and Parent's Concerns, and focuses on three domains of child functioning: Development, Behavior, and Family. Together these scales cover cognitive, motor, language, social-emotional-behavioral functioning, autism, and family risk factors. The tools are available at https://www.tuftschildrenshospital.org/The-Survey-of-Wellbeing-of-Young-Children/Overview.

Mental Health, Emotional, and Behavioral Screening Tools

The Ages and Stages Questionnaire: Social-Emotional-2 (ASQ:SE-2) is a caregiver-completed questionnaire designed to monitor the social and emotional development of infants and young children and to screen for adaptive behaviors, communication, autonomy, affect, and interaction with adults.[30] The Brief Infant/Toddler Social Emotional Assessment (BITSEA) is a caregiver-report screening tool of children's social emotional and behavioral development.[31] The ASQ-SE and BITSEA both identify children with developing social and emotional disorders who may benefit from a more in-depth evaluation.

The Modified Checklist for Autism in Toddlers—Revised with Follow-Up (M-CHAT-R/F) is a two-stage screening tool to identify children at risk for autism spectrum disorder (ASD).[32] The initial stage is a caregiver-completed pass/fail survey followed by a second stage for positive screens with a 5- to 10-minute interview by a health professional. It has a high sensitivity and specificity for identifying children with possible ASD and assists PCPs in assessing the need for referral for early intervention services.

The M-CHAT caregiver-completed survey includes 20 items, such as: Does your child play pretend or make-believe? Does your child point with one finger to ask for something or to get help? Does your child like climbing on things? Does your child respond when you call his or her name? Does your child try to copy what you do? Does your child get upset by everyday noises? If a child fails three items, the follow-up questions are administered. If a child has more than seven fails, referral for a diagnostic evaluation is indicated. Children at risk for other developmental disorders or delays may be identified with the M-CHAT screening tool.

The Pediatric Symptom Checklist (PSC)[33] is a commonly used mental health screening tool for middle childhood and adolescence in pediatric primary care practices. The PSC has 35 items and screens children and adolescents from 4 years to 16 years of age. Beginning at 11 years of age, the PSC can be completed by the child or adolescent. The Patient Health Questionnaire-9 (PHQ-9)[34] and Children's Depression Inventory 2 (CDI2)[35] are used to screen children and adolescents 11 to 17 years of age and 7 to 17 years of age, respectively, for cognitive, affective, and behavioral signs of depression. The PHQ-9 and CDI2 are administered as a caregiver-report, teacher-report, and/or self-report screening tool. The Ask Suicide-Screening Questions (ASQ) tool is a set of four brief suicide screening questions that can be administered in clinical settings and includes versions for youth and adult self-report.[34] The Screen for Child Anxiety Related Disorders (SCARED) is a caregiver and child self-report instrument to assess clinical symptoms of anxiety.[36] The Generalized Anxiety Disorder 7-Item Scale (GAD-7) is a valid and efficient self-report screening tool for assessing severity of anxiety in adolescents 13 years old to late adolescence.[37]

DEVELOPMENTAL, EMOTIONAL, AND BEHAVIORAL HEALTH CONDITIONS

Developmental Risk Factors

Several genetic and environmental risk factors increase the likelihood that a child will exhibit developmental delays. Biological risk factors that influence a child's development include prenatal conditions, such as maternal substance abuse, infection, chronic health conditions, medications, and severe toxemia. Neonatal risk factors include a history of prematurity, gestational age less than 33 weeks, birth weight less than 1500 g, Apgar score less than 3 at 5 minutes, neonatal infections (sepsis or meningitis), and severe hyperbilirubinemia. Social risk factors include a family history of maternal depression, low maternal education, lack of maternal bonding, child abuse and neglect, lack of developmentally appropriate opportunities for learning, and family economic status and income stability. Environmental risk factors, such as under-resourced neighborhoods, high lead levels, exposure to environmental toxins, and limited access to health care services may also contribute to developmental delays.[38]

Children at risk require especially diligent developmental surveillance, including implementing the recommended use of developmental screening tools in the first 3 years of life and prompt referral for early intervention services, including a pediatric neurologist, pediatric developmental specialist, or genetic testing when indicated. Table 3.5 presents developmental red flags in infancy and early childhood that indicate developmental deficits and the need for referral and early intervention. Box 3.1 provides further resources for pediatric PCPs.

BOX 3.1	WEB RESOURCES

AAP Children's Mental Health: Chapter Action Kit; https://www.aap.org/en/patient-care/mental-health-initiatives/childrens-mental-health-chapter-action-kit/

Addressing Mental Health Concerns in Pediatrics: A Practical Resource Toolkit for Clinicians, 2nd edition; https://shop.aap.org/mentalhealthtoolkit/

Caring for Children with Autism Spectrum Disorder: A Practical Resource Toolkit for Clinicians, 3rd edition; https://publications.aap.org/toolkits/pages/Autism-Toolkit

Caring for Children With ADHD: A Practical Resource Toolkit for Clinicians. https://publications.aap.org/toolkits/pages/ADHD-Toolkit

CDC's Learn the Signs Act Early; Includes fact sheets on developmental screening, resource kits, growth charts; https://www.cdc.gov/ncbddd/actearly/

Developmental Red Flags: A medical reference for primary care and emergency clinicians; https://fpnotebook.com/Peds/Neuro/DvlpmntlRdFlgs.htm

| TABLE 3.5 | DEVELOPMENTAL RED FLAGS IN EARLY CHILDHOOD INDICATING NEED FOR REFERRAL |

Age	Developmental Red Flag	Developmental Deficit and Need for Referral
3 months	Rolling over prior to 3 months Persistent fisting Failure to alert to environmental stimuli Failure to alert to visual/auditory stimuli	Evaluate for hypertonia Evaluate for neuromotor dysfunction Evaluate for sensory impairment
4–6 months	Poor head control while sitting Failure to reach for objects by 5 months No social smile Lack of fixation Lack of visual tracking by 4 months Failure to turn to sound or voice at 6 months	Evaluate for hypotonia Evaluate for motor, visual, or cognitive deficits Evaluate for visual loss, attachment problems, maternal depression, consider child neglect or abuse Requires evaluation for hearing loss
6–12 months	Persistence of primitive reflexes after 6 months Inability to sit by 9 months No babbling by 6 months No reciprocal vocalizations by 9 months Inability to localize sound by 10 months Absent stranger anxiety until 7 months	Evaluate for neuromuscular disorder Evaluate for unilateral or bilateral hearing loss Evaluate for maternal attachment or may be related to multiple care providers
12–18 months	Not verbalizing consonant by 15 months Hand dominance before 18 months Lack of imitation by 16 months Simple commands not understood Lack of pointing by 18 months Advanced noncommunicative speech Inability to walk independently by 18 months	Evaluate for mild hearing loss May indicate contralateral weakness with hemiparesis Evaluate for cognitive or socialization deficit Problem in social relatedness Evaluate for autism spectrum disorder (ASD) Evaluate for neuromotor dysfunction
18–24 months	No two-word sentences by 24 months No word other than mama/dada by 18 months Unable to follow simple command by 24 months Cannot name one picture in book by 24 months; echolalia beyond 24 months Does not associate toys with function-push car to make it go Inability to walk up/down stairs by 24 months	Evaluate for hearing deficit Evaluate for cognitive or socialization deficit Evaluate for cognitive or socialization deficit May lack opportunity rather than motor deficit Evaluate for autism spectrum disorder (ASD)

Adapted from Gerber R, Wilks T, Erdie-Lalena C. Developmental milestones: motor development. *Pediatr Rev.* 2010; 31(7):267–277; Wilks T, Gerber R, Erdie-Lalena C. Developmental milestones: cognitive development, *Pediatr Rev.* 2010; 31(9):364–367; Moses S. Developmental red flags, *Family Practice Notebook*, 2015, available at http://www.fpnotebook.com/Peds/Neuro/DvlpmntlRdFlgs.htm.

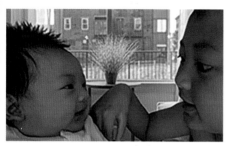

FIGURE 3.3 Infant social smile. *Courtesy Janis Mandac-Dy.*

Autism Spectrum Disorders

ASD is a complex neurodevelopmental disorder that is characterized by persistent deficits in social communication and social interaction, repetitive patterns of speech or motor behavior, delays in communication and language skills, and social and behavioral development that limit and impair family functioning and daily activities.[39] Concerning behaviors identified by 18 months of age are no social smile (Fig. 3.3) in response to the caregiver's face, not responding to their name, not using the index finger to point to objects, not taking an interest in other children, and not playing peek-a-boo or hide-and-seek. Making unusual finger movements near their face and wandering or staring without a purpose are additional early behaviors identified with ASD.

ASDs include autism; pervasive developmental disorder, not otherwise specified (PDD-NOS); and Asperger syndrome.[27] The onset of ASD symptoms is before 3 years of age, although diagnosis may occur at a later age. ASD is at least partially genetically linked, though no single gene abnormality or mode of inheritance has yet been identified. Studies have shown an increased prevalence in siblings, especially in monozygotic twins, and an elevated risk with increased relatedness, as well as an unequal sex distribution.[39] These findings further support a strong genetic contribution in the development of ASD. The complexity and variations in ASD presentation suggest a combination of interactions between multiple genes, epigenetic factors, and exposure to environmental toxins that may impact the pathogenesis of ASD.[39,40]

As of 2023, the Centers for Disease Control and Prevention (CDC) reports the prevalence of ASD is currently 1 in 36[40] children, and the ratio of ASD in children is 4:1 male to female.[40] According to the AAP, ASD screening is recommended for all children before 24 months of age, and the M-CHAT-R/F should be completed at the 18- and/or 24-month well-child visit.[1] Early identification and intervention has been shown to be highly effective in helping children with ASD gain social and emotional skills.[39]

Learning and Neurodevelopmental Disorders

Learning disorders may result from neurodevelopmental or genetic causes or co-exist with other physical or mental disabilities. *Learning disability* refers to difficulty in acquiring and using basic reading skills, reading comprehension, oral expression, listening comprehension, mathematical reasoning, and mathematical comprehension that occurs without an environmental precipitant in otherwise normally intelligent children. Learning disorders are neurologically based and persist into adulthood. The definition requires at least a 2-year discrepancy between the child's expected level of achievement and his or her performance.

Fifteen percent of all children 1 to 17 years of age receive services under a special education or early intervention plan, with twice as many males affected compared with females[41] (Fig. 3.4). Pediatric PCPs can assist with the diagnosis of learning disabilities by performing an initial thorough history and physical examination,

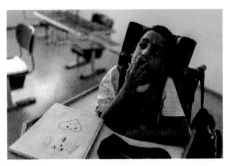

FIGURE 3.4 Boy with special needs in the classroom. *Credit: iStock/FG Trade*

including a complete neurological examination and an evaluation of school performance. The confirmation of learning disabilities includes referral for neuropsychological testing and evaluation by a licensed psychologist.

Attention Deficit Hyperactivity Disorder

Attention deficit hyperactivity disorder (ADHD) is a cluster of behaviors that appear early in a child's life and persist throughout childhood and adolescence. According to a recent National Survey of Children's Health, 9% of children 3 to 17 years of age have ever been diagnosed with ADHD, with males outnumbering females 3:1.[42] The diagnosis of ADHD is based on a characteristic clinical presentation and observable behaviors. Behavior symptoms include inattention, hyperactivity, and/or impulsivity and must be present in two or more settings. The practitioner must rule out the possibility that such behaviors merely represent variations in normal development or temperament and that they are not attributable to environmental factors such as response to a traumatic event, or a poor fit with the teacher and/or classroom. Furthermore, ADHD may coexist with other disorders or conditions that must be addressed before an appropriate diagnosis can be given. It is not uncommon for children with ADHD to also have a learning disability. Schools are federally mandated to perform a learning evaluation if a child is suspected of having a learning disability.

Pediatric PCPs should initiate an evaluation for ADHD by gathering a comprehensive history, with careful attention given to developmental milestones: performing a complete physical examination, including neurological exam; and obtaining input from teachers regarding behavior and classroom performance. Assessment of lead and hematocrit levels should be considered in preschool children, as well as vision and hearing screening at any age, to rule out other etiologies for behavior symptoms. Caregivers should be assisted in initiating an individualized education plan (IEP) coordinated with the child's school. The AAP created a resource for pediatric providers, Caring for Children With ADHD: A Practical Resource Toolkit for Clinicians, which includes the Vanderbilt Assessment Scales by the National Institute for Children's Healthcare Quality (NICHQ).[43] The Vanderbilt Assessment Scales have been validated in both community and referral settings with evidence to support its use as a diagnostic rating scale for ADHD.[44,45] Further evaluation and treatment of children with ADHD may include follow-up and referral to a developmental-behavioral specialist, mental health professional, and/or pediatric neurologist, when indicated.

Depression, Anxiety, and Suicide

The global prevalence of youth depression and anxiety symptoms has doubled since the start of the COVID-19 pandemic.[46] Combined with a critical shortage of mental health providers, the role of the pediatric PCP in identifying and managing emotional health diagnoses is essential. Depression and anxiety can be experienced by children of all ages, although it most often presents in older childhood or adolescence.[47] Youth from communities who have been marginalized due to race, gender, or sexual orientation may be at high risk for depression or anxiety related to persistent experiences of discrimination or long-standing health, social, or systemic inequities, yet they remain underdiagnosed and undertreated.[4]

The well-child visit presents an opportunity for providers to ask questions about persistent emotional distress, such as sadness, worry, or anger, as well as environmental risk factors such as isolation or bullying. Providers should also consider screening for depression or anxiety as part of the diagnostic workup for chronic symptoms without a clear organic etiology (such as headache or abdominal pain), or unexplained disruptions to activities of daily living such as sleep or appetite. A thorough family mental health history is a valuable component of assessment, as depression and anxiety are both known to have some genetic inheritability.[47] Identification of protective factors in the child's life is also important, for example asking about healthy coping strategies or having the child name a trusted adult whom they talk to about their feelings.

Suicide is the second leading cause of death in young people ages 10 to 24 years.[34] As of 2022, the AAP Bright Futures guidelines recommend universal suicide screening for all youth 12 years and older, and to screen youth ages 8 to 11 years old if clinically indicated.[7] Evidence demonstrates that screening for depression alone is not enough, and specific assessment for suicidal thinking and behavior is critical for prevention.[34] The AAP Blueprint for Youth Suicide Prevention offers several resources to support suicide screening and intervention, and can be accessed at: https://www.aap.org/en/patient-care/blueprint-for-youth-suicide-prevention/

TELEHEALTH TIPS

The widespread utilization of telehealth due to the COVID-19 pandemic, facilitated by emergency authorization from governmental agencies and insurers to allow for reimbursement of telehealth visits, has enabled pediatric clinicians to provide ongoing developmental surveillance and screening of infants and children. PCPs should continue to use validated caregiver-completed questionnaires along with caregiver concerns and clinical findings to properly assess a child's developmental status. Observation alone through video telehealth is not sufficient due to limitations in screen and sound clarity and variations in how children interact via screens in early childhood. Any caregiver concerns or concerns on review of the caregiver-completed developmental screening tools may require an in-person visit to assess the infant or child before initiating a referral. Validated caregiver-completed screening instruments can be used by the PCP either in-person or via telehealth. However, diagnostic screening tools have not yet been validated for use over telehealth and further research is needed at this time.

Telehealth services may be more feasible for mental health assessment and treatment, due to the limited need for hands-on physical examination. Several studies of youth have demonstrated similar effectiveness between face to face and telehealth delivery of mental health services.[48] Youth may be particularly receptive to tele-mental health services due to their technology literacy and access. Prior to conducting mental health assessment, the provider should confirm the location of the child or adolescent, and the contact information for an available trusted adult, which can be used in case of concerns for safety.[48] An alternate form of contact should be identified at the start of the visit so that the worry of technological malfunction does not interfere with rapport. Privacy is also essential to protect confidentiality, and the provider should ask the child or adolescent whether they are in a space where they feel comfortable discussing mental health topics. Earbuds or headsets may be encouraged to facilitate a more private conversation between patient and provider. Video calls may enhance the experience for patients who desire face-to-face interaction when discussing their emotional health; conversely, mobile applications or text-based platforms may be preferred by others who are more accustomed to these modalities for engagement.[48]

SUMMARY OF DEVELOPMENTAL, EMOTIONAL, AND BEHAVIORAL SURVEILLANCE AND SCREENING

- The most common childhood developmental problems are speech and language delay, hearing loss, emotional and behavioral concerns, learning disabilities, and other neurodevelopmental disorders.

- Developmental surveillance is an important component of all pediatric primary care visits, and developmental psychometric testing should be performed routinely at well child visits at 9 months, 15 months, 18 months, and 24 or 30 months of age. Timely identification of developmental delay and behavioral and mental health problems and prompt referral for early intervention can significantly impact a deficit or disability on the long-term development and functioning of the child and family.
- With a rise in mental health conditions in children and adolescents, pediatric providers must be vigilant in screening for self-injurious behaviors, suicidal ideation, and mood disorders and be informed about mental health resources in their communities.
- Developmental, emotional, and behavioral health assessment can be successfully completed via telehealth if clinically appropriate but may require an in-person visit for further assessment and/or before initiating a referral.

DOCUMENTATION

A Healthy 9-Month-Old Infant With Typical Development
Crawling, pulls to stand, bangs handheld toy against another toy on the table, demonstrates thumb-finger grasp, exhibits some stranger anxiety, consolable when upset, verbalizing sounds. Passed ASQ for communication, fine motor, gross motor, and social/emotional behaviors.

DOCUMENTATION

14-Year-Old Adolescent With Depression
Well-appearing adolescent in no acute distress. Engaged and focused in conversation, no evidence of disorientation or psychomotor agitation. Generally euthymic mood, occasional tearfulness congruent with discussion content. Physical exam negative for obvious signs of self-harm. PHQ-9 score: 7 (mild depression) including negative suicidal ideation.

REFERENCES

1. Lipkin PH, Macias MM. Promoting optimal development: identifying infants and young children with developmental disorders through developmental surveillance and screening. *Pediatrics*. 2020;145.
2. Scharf RJ, Scharf GJ, Stroustrup A. Developmental milestones. *Pediatr Rev*. 2016;37:25–37. quiz 38, 47.
3. Zablotsky B, Black LI, Maenner MJ, et al. Prevalence and trends of developmental disabilities among children in the United States: 2009–2017. *Pediatrics*. 2019;144:e20190811.
4. Ghandour RM, Sherman LJ, Vladutiu CJ, et al. Prevalence and treatment of depression, anxiety, and conduct problems in US children. *J Pediatr*. 2019;206(256–267):e3.
5. Leeb RT, Bitsko RH, Radhakrishnan L, Martinez P, Njai R, Holland KM. Mental health-related emergency department visits among children aged <18 years during the COVID-19 pandemic—United States, January 1-October 17, 2020. *MMWR Morb Mortal Wkly Rep*. 2020;69:1675–1680.
6. Martinsen KD, Neumer SP, Holen S, Waaktaar T, Sund AM, Kendall PC. Self-reported quality of life and self-esteem in sad and anxious school children. *BMC Psychol*. 2016;4:45.
7. Hagan Jr JF, Shaw JS, Duncan PM. *Bright Futures: Guidelines for Health Supervision of Infants, Children and Adolescents*. 4th ed. American Academy of Pediatrics; 2017.
8. Zubler JM, Wiggins LD, Macias MM, et al. Evidence-informed milestones for developmental surveillance tools. *Pediatrics*. 2022;149 e2021052138.
9. Bowman R. Assessing vision in a baby. *Community Eye Health*. 2016;29:16–17.
10. Black LI, Vahratian A, Hoffman HJ. Communication Disorders and Use of Interventions Services Among Children Aged 3-17 Years: United States, 2012. 2015. NCHS Data Brief No. 205.
11. Thurm A, Manwaring SS, Cardozo Jimenez C, et al. Socioemotional and behavioral problems in toddlers with language delay. *Infant Ment Health J*. 2018;39:569–580.
12. High PC, Klass P. Literacy promotion: an essential component of primary care pediatric practice. *Pediatrics*. 2014;134:404–409.
13. Zuckerman B, Needlman R. 30 years of reach out and read: need for a developmental perspective. *Pediatrics*. 2020;145:e20191958.
14. Erickson E, Caldwell A, Shearman N, et al. Clinician experiences with reach out and read: An exploratory qualitative analysis. *Acad Pediatr*. 2021;21:961–967.
15. Rideout V, Robb MB. The Common Sense census: Media use by kids age zero to eight. San Francisco, CA. *Common Sense Media*. 2017 https://www.commonsensemedia.

org/research/the-common-sense-census-media-use-by-kids-age-zero-to-eight-2017.

16. Council on Communications and Media Media and young minds. *Pediatrics.* 2016;138:e20162591.

17. Madigan S, Browne D, Racine N, Mori C, Tough S. Association between screen time and children's performance on a developmental screening test. *JAMA Pediatr.* 2019;173:244–250.

18. van den Heuvel M, Ma J, Borkhoff CM, et al. Mobile media device use is associated with expressive language delay in 18-month-old children. *J Dev Behav Pediatr.* 2019;40:99–104.

19. Madigan S, McArthur BA, Anhorn C, Eirich R, Christakis DA. Associations between screen use and child language skills: a systematic review and meta-analysis. *JAMA Pediatr.* 2020;174:665–675.

20. Williams PG, Lerner MA. School readiness. *Pediatrics.* 2019;144:e20191766.

21. Child and Adolescent Health Measurement Initiative. 2020-2021 National Survey of Children's Health (NSCH) data query. U.S. Department of Health and Human Services, Health Resources and Services Administration, Maternal and Child Health Bureau. www.childhealthdata.org

22. Khan L. Detecting early developmental delays in children. *Pediatr Ann.* 2019;48:e381–e384.

23. Squires J, Bricker D.*Ages and Stages Questionnaires (ASQ-3).* 3rd ed. Paul H. Brookes; 2009.

24. Parasuraman SR, Anglin TM, McLellan SE, Riley C, Mann MY. Health care utilization and unmet need among youth with special health care needs. *J Adolesc Health.* 2018;63:435–444.

25. Scahill L, Lecavalier L, Schultz RT, et al. Development of the parent-rated anxiety scale for youth with autism spectrum disorder. *J Am Acad Child Adolesc Psychiatry.* 2019;58:887–896.e2.

26. Kalb LG, Hagopian LP, Gross AL, Vasa RA. Psychometric characteristics of the mental health crisis assessment scale in youth with autism spectrum disorder. *J Child Psychol Psychiatry.* 2018;59:48–56.

27. American Psychiatric Association.. *DSM-5-TR(tm) Classification.* American Psychiatric Association Publishing; 2022.

28. Glascoe FP.*Collaborating with parents: Using parents' evaluation of developmental status to detect and address developmental and behavioral problems.* Ellsworth & Vandermeer Press; 1998:viii 157.

29. Sheldrick RC, Perrin EC. Evidence-based milestones for surveillance of cognitive, language, and motor development. *Acad Pediatr.* 2013;13:577–586.

30. Squires J, Bricker D, Twombly E. *Ages and Stages Questionnaires: Social-Emotional-2 (ASQ SE-2). A parent-completed, child-monitoring system for social-emotional behaviors.* Baltimore, MD: Paul H. Brookes Publishing Co., Inc.; 2013.

31. Briggs-Gowan MJ, Carter AS, Irwin JR, Wachtel K, Cicchetti DV. The Brief Infant-Toddler Social and Emotional Assessment: screening for social-emotional problems and delays in competence. *J Pediatr Psychol.* 2004;29:143–155.

32. Robins DL, Casagrande K, Barton M, Chen CM, Dumont-Mathieu T, Fein D. Validation of the modified checklist for Autism in toddlers, revised with follow-up (M-CHAT-R/F). *Pediatrics.* 2014;133:37–45.

33. Jellinek MS, Murphy JM, Little M, Pagano ME, Comer DM, Kelleher KJ. Use of the Pediatric Symptom Checklist to screen for psychosocial problems in pediatric primary care: a national feasibility study. *Arch Pediatr Adolesc Med.* 1999;153:254–260.

34. Kemper AR, Hostutler CA, Beck K, Fontanella CA, Bridge JA. Depression and suicide-risk screening results in pediatric primary care. *Pediatrics.* 2021;148 e2021049999.

35. Kovacs M. The Children's Depression, Inventory (CDI). *Psychopharmacol Bull.* 1985;21:995–998.

36. Runyon K, Chesnut SR, Burley H. Screening for childhood anxiety: a meta-analysis of the screen for child anxiety related emotional disorders. *J Affect Disord.* 2018;240:220–229.

37. Spitzer RL, Kroenke K, Williams JB, Löwe B. A brief measure for assessing generalized anxiety disorder: the GAD-7. *Arch Intern Med.* 2006;166:1092–1097.

38. Sharma A, Cockerill H.*From Birth to Five Years: Practical Developmental Examination* Taylor & Francis; 2021.

39. Hyman SL, Levy SE, Myers SM. Identification, evaluation, and management of children with autism spectrum disorder. *Pediatrics.* 2020;145:e20193447.

40. Maenner MJ, Warren Z, Williams AR, et al. Prevalence and characteristics of autism spectrum disorder among children aged 8 years—Autism and Developmental Disabilities Monitoring Network, 11 Sites, United States, 2020. *MMWR Surveill Summ.* 2023;72:1–14.http://dx.doi.org/10.15585/mmwr.ss7202a1 In this issue.

41. National Center for Education Statistics. Students with Disabilities. U.S. Department of Education, Institute of Education Sciences. Accessed October 19, 2022. https://nces.ed.gov/programs/coe/indicator/cgg

42. Bitsko RH, Claussen AH, Lichstein J, et al. Mental health surveillance among children—United States, 2013–2019. *MMWR Suppl.* 2022;71:1–42.

43. Zurhellen W, Lessin HR, Chan E, et al.*Toolkit Chapter. Caring for Children With ADHD: A Practical Resource Toolkit for Clinicians.* 3rd. American Academy of Pediatrics; 2019 In this issue.

44. Wolraich ML, Bard DE, Neas B, et al. The psychometric properties of the Vanderbilt attention-deficit hyperactivity disorder diagnostic teacher rating scale in a community population. *J Dev Behav Pediatr.* 2013;34(2):83–93. In this issue. https://doi.org/10.1097/DBP.0b013e31827d55c3.

45. Bard DE, Wolraich ML, Neas B, et al. The psychometric properties of the Vanderbilt attention-deficit hyperactivity disorder diagnostic parent rating scale in a community population. *J Dev Behav Pediatr.* 2013;34(2):72–82. In this issue. https://doi.org/10.1097/DBP.0b013e31827a3a22.

46. Racine N, McArthur BA, Cooke JE, Eirich R, Zhu J, Madigan S. Global prevalence of depressive and anxiety symptoms in children and adolescents during COVID-19: a meta-analysis. *JAMA Pediatr.* 2021;175:1142–1150.

47. Ogundele MO. Behavioural and emotional disorders in childhood: a brief overview for paediatricians. *World J Clin Pediatr.* 2018;7:9–26.

48. Holland M, Hawks J, Morelli LC, Khan Z. Risk assessment and crisis intervention for youth in a time of telehealth. *Contemp Sch Psychol.* 2021;25:12–26.

CHAPTER 4

COMPREHENSIVE INFORMATION GATHERING

Naomi Ann Schapiro; Adam J. Leonard

Despite the many technologic advances in health care, a comprehensive, holistic health history remains the most important diagnostic tool. Accurate diagnosis is most influenced by observing, listening, and thinking critically in a clinical setting. Recognizing patterns of health and illness in infants, children, and adolescents involves obtaining relevant data from the health history, thinking about their meaning, and explaining them logically. Taking a comprehensive history with families not only develops a profile to guide physical assessment, diagnosis, and treatment, but also contributes to the development of a trusting, collaborative relationship between the family and the pediatric health care provider. Information gathered from the family history is also key to identifying social determinants and genetic patterns of inheritance in health conditions and can help illuminate priorities for and barriers to implementing healthy behaviors in the child and adolescent. Identifying particular risks for chronic health conditions such as tooth decay, behavioral health conditions, diabetes, and cardiometabolic diseases begins with gathering a comprehensive family history.

Anticipatory guidance about growth, development, emotions and behavior, diet, exercise, and sleep are cornerstones of pediatric primary care and benefits all children.[1] However, it is rarely possible to gather all needed information and provide guidance in all of these areas in one visit. Although it is practical to deliver anticipatory guidance while taking a health history, giving advice early in the visit may affect developing a collaborative conversation, may increase family resistance to the information, and may not address the family's most urgent concerns.[2] Box 4.1 gives some resources with links to handouts for anticipatory guidance.

TRAUMA-INFORMED CARE

A trauma-informed approach to the visit begins with history taking. Trauma-informed care (TIC) involves a *realization* that traumatic events are widely prevalent in children, adolescents, and their families, *recognition* of the physical signs and behavioral and emotional symptoms of trauma, compassionate *response* to these signs and symptoms of trauma whether or not families disclose trauma histories, and changes in the behavior of pediatric health clinicians and the systems in which they work, in order to *resist re-traumatizing* children and families.[3,4] Some of these systematic changes might include less punitive policies about late or missed appointments, explaining in advance the rationale for intake and screening questionnaires, explaining importance of and limits to privacy and confidentiality of information, interviewing the child and adolescent while dressed, asking age-appropriate permission and any concerns about being touched before physical examinations, and asking permission before offering advice and anticipatory guidance.[5,6] Discussions about privacy and the limits to confidentiality are especially important when disclosures may trigger mandatory reporting of maltreatment, family information that may be released for billing purposes, or when explaining state-specific adolescent confidentiality protections.

BOX 4.1   ANTICIPATORY GUIDANCE RESOURCES

Bright Futures—Anticipatory Guidance Handouts for Well Child Visits
https://brightfutures.aap.org/families/Pages/Well-Child-Visits.aspx
Oral Health Risk Assessment Tool and Protective Factors
https://www.smilesforlifeoralhealth.org/wp-content/uploads/2020/06/Oral_Health_Assessment_Tool.pdf
The Health Care Toolbox: Pediatric Medical Traumatic Stress and Trauma-Informed Care

https://healthcaretoolbox.org
Equipment Guide to Safe Car and Booster Seats
https://www.nhtsa.gov/equipment/car-seats-and-booster-seats
State by State Guide to Car Seat Regulations
https://saferide4kids.com/car-seat-laws-by-state/
Social Media and Teens
https://www.aacap.org/AACAP/Families_and_Youth/Facts_for_Families/FFF-Guide/Social-Media-and-Teens-100.aspx

---

TIC benefits patients, providers, and clinic staff by creating a sense of safety for all in the clinic, encouraging self-care and peer support for staff and families, and paying attention to cultural, historical, and gender issues that might affect all relationships in the clinic. TIC can lay the groundwork for the family's trust in the pediatric provider and staff. Thus, TIC provides a context for family-centered care and comprehensive history taking.

CULTURAL HUMILITY AND EQUITY

Health equity, attaining optimum health for all, is linked to social, economic, structural, and environmental factors, which affect the life course of the child, adolescent, and family.[7,8] Trauma exposure or adverse childhood experiences (ACEs) including physical, sexual, or emotional abuse or neglect, intimate partner violence, parental substance abuse, parental incarceration, and parent-child separation through death, divorce, immigration, or deportation can result in toxic stress, which negatively affects the life course.[9,10] Further, inclusion of an assessment of the *social determinants of health* for all families (e.g., food insecurity, unstable housing, family or neighborhood violence, structural racism, discrimination) has become a priority in taking a comprehensive health history and an important part of the family-centered encounter, along with assessment of family strengths and protective factors.[1,11]

Cultural humility involves engaging in "self-reflection and self-critique as lifelong learners and reflective practitioners" about power imbalances between health care providers and families, in order to "develop and maintain mutually respectful and dynamic partnerships with families."[12] Rather than trying to become experts in the culture of others, cultural humility involves active listening and asking patients and families about their own lives and their multiple identities, to the extent they are willing to share, including gender, sexuality, race, ethnicity, immigration, economic stresses, and histories of discrimination.[13] Cultural humility is especially important in asking families about what they think is going on with their child, and their views on the origins of the illness. The goal is not to correct their views, but rather to develop a collaborative alliance in promoting the health of their children.[13,14] As one example, traditional Western psychiatry has framed physical and mental health as separate, in contrast to many non-Western cultures,[15] yet emerging research on the long-term health impacts of toxic stress indicates the importance of a more integrated view.[9]

FAMILY HEALTH HISTORY

The *family health history* (FHH), also known as the *genetic family history*, can be an important tool in the comprehensive health history to identify a child's and adolescent's risk for developing diabetes, hypertension, cardiac disease, and a wide range of chronic health conditions.[16] Family patterns of genetic, behavioral, and environmental factors that influence the occurrence of health conditions often emerge in the course of developing a three-generation FHH.[17,18] The FHH can use a *family pedigree* or *genogram* as a visual way to enhance recognition of patterns of inheritance. This approach leads to insights in patterns of inheritance across generations; it gives pediatric health care providers an opportunity to counsel families on prevention and offer referrals for further genetic testing.[16] Knowledge of the genetic family history can aid in the diagnosis of rare single-gene disorders such as cystic fibrosis, fragile X syndrome, Huntington disease, and familial hypercholesterolemia.

The American Academy of Pediatrics' *Bright Futures*[1] recommends taking a comprehensive FHH at the 1-month visit. Some practices take a FHH for all new patients, updated during yearly well-child checks. Challenges related to taking a thorough FHH include time constraints and some families' lack of access to biological relatives to obtain information about heritable conditions.[16] A recent systematic review of pediatric primary care history-taking practices found little consistency in frequency and depth of FHHs, and that electronic health records can either facilitate or hinder efficient collection of FHH data.[19] Beyond these logistical issues, it is important for the provider to be aware that taking a FHH can raise emotionally laden family issues and questions of trust between the family and provider. For example, families may be reluctant to discuss patterns of mental health and substance abuse or complex heritance issues such as egg or sperm donors or biological parents of adopted children.

There is evidence that genetics and medical research have played a harmful role in promoting racial and ethnic stereotypes and justifying discrimination toward *minoritized* populations.[20,21] Families who have experienced bias due to perceived race, socioeconomic, or immigrant status may be wary of disclosing their complete family medical and behavioral health histories. It is important for providers who are taking health histories to be aware of their own implicit biases and how these may impact history taking and preventive counseling about genetically related conditions.[22]

It is also important to use gender-inclusive language when gathering history about sex-related heritable conditions and household members. Using terms like "designated" or "assigned" female/male at birth, and asking whether there are any transgender or nonbinary family members, can improve communication with caregivers and children and increase the accuracy of the FHH.[23] Historically, genograms were constructed using sex-based symbols, such as for male and for female, with solid and dotted lines to represent relationships such as intimate partner or parent/child. Many practitioners continue to use them in primary care notes. With the switch to electronic records, constructing a genogram is impractical without additional software, usually available only in specialty clinics. In addition, the traditional sex-based symbols do not adequately represent intersex individuals or those incorrectly designated at birth, nor do they represent the varieties of gender identification, expression and phases of transition that are relevant to current practice. Currently, there are no standard trans-inclusive pedigree symbols.[24]

It is important to be aware of emotional and ethical issues that may arise when patterns of serious heritable conditions emerge, such as a potential hereditary link with breast cancer in female-designated relatives. Pediatric health care providers can provide support to individuals and families in making decisions about seeking genetic testing. Pediatric providers are well positioned to counsel families as they provide primary care and anticipatory guidance for children from birth to young adulthood, the period during which many genetically linked conditions emerge.

FAMILY-CENTERED HISTORY

The following key strategies are involved in developing a successful family-centered relationship with children and families in the pediatric setting:

- Listen actively to the concerns of the family throughout the visit.
- Ask families about languages spoken by adults and children in the home. Conduct the health interview in the family's preferred language, if possible, to promote family engagement. Ask families about their preferences for spoken and written language, as they may differ, and whether the use of interpreters is acceptable and beneficial.
- Ask about the family's expectations for the encounter. To successfully establish a collaborative relationship, the caregivers' agendas must be identified and addressed during the encounter.
- Ask open-ended questions and pause to give families time to answer, thereby allowing relevant data to unfold.
- Ask about the health and well-being of household and extended family members to develop a more comprehensive FHH and to assist in building a collaborate relationship with the family.
- Ask about positive childhood experiences, including shared leisure time, sports, hobbies, cultural events, and religious observances.
- Identify the caregiver's hope for the child's future, assessment of the child's strengths, and family or social support in addition to the caregiver(s).

- Show your respect for caregivers by noticing and praising their strengths in caring for their child or adolescent. This approach also facilitates an open relationship between the family and health care provider.

Family trust in their pediatric provider is based on the knowledge, understanding, respect, and care that the pediatric provider demonstrates during the encounter with their child. Electronic medical records and telehealth have transformed the ways in which pediatric providers interact with children and families. Best practices in the exam room include sitting when possible while gathering health history, maintaining eye contact with the child and family as much as possible, and using the screen to share growth charts, lab results, and other health information. If the visit is conducted over telehealth, ask about and adapt to the family's technology access, whether using their own, shared, or borrowed portable electronic device or computer. Ask about any barriers to privacy or accessibility and integrate the family's preference for language interpretation.[25]

By integrating the social context in the family-centered interview, you may identify unmet needs such as food insecurity or parental unemployment, which are important child health determinants and may warrant further discussion and referral to community services.[11] Box 4.2 provides links to questionnaires about social determinants of health (SDH) and resources for TIC.

COMPONENTS OF INFORMATION GATHERING

The information gathered during a health history reflects the child's or caregiver's opinions and experience and is therefore *subjective* information. The subjective information guides the *objective* findings of the physical examination and assists the health care provider in evaluating the family functioning, the family's approach to health and illness, and the reliability of the historian and their relationship to the

---

BOX 4.2   TRAUMA INFORMED CARE & SCREENING FOR SOCIAL DETERMINANTS OF HEALTH

Resources for Child Trauma Informed Care (SAMHSA)
https://www.samhsa.gov/childrens-aware-ness-day/past-events/2018/child-traumatic-stress-resources
Trauma Transformed Trauma Informed Tools
https://traumatransformed.org/resources/Trauma-Tools.asp
The Everyone Project (American Academy of Family Practice) guide to social needs screening

https://www.aafp.org/dam/AAFP/documents/patient_care/everyone_project/hops19-physician-guide-sdoh.pdf
Safe Environment for Every Kid (SEEK)—SDH and some ACE
https://seekwellbeing.org/seek-materials/
PEARL screener—ACE and SDH
https://www.acesaware.org/learn-about-screening/screening-tools/screening-tools-additional-languages/

---

child. Children beginning at 3 years of age can effectively participate in the health interview. Involving children at this age begins to establish the importance of the child's contribution to their own health, gives voice to the concerns of the child, and facilitates the provider's relationship with and ability to advocate for the child. It also allows the provider to observe another aspect of the caregiver/child relationship during the interview process.

The type of health history gathered during an encounter depends on whether the child and family are presenting for a *comprehensive well-child visit, acute care visit, symptom-focused visit*, a *confidential adolescent visit*, or for a *preparticipation sports physical examination* (see Chapter 18).

INFORMATION GATHERING OF SUBJECTIVE DATA

Child Profile

The demographic and biographical information for a child and family is typically gathered at registration for the visit and should be verified by the provider. In an initial visit, the child's profile should include information on the previous health care provider, date of the child's or adolescent's last health care visit, and emergency contact information, including confidential contact information for adolescent patients. Family units change, and this information should be updated at each health encounter.

The Open-Ended Question

Begin the encounter with an open-ended question such as, "What brings you here today?" This allows the family to tell their story in their own words, centers the health visit around the family concerns, and establishes the basis of the *family-centered interview*. Although the child or adolescent may have presented for a well visit or with a primary complaint, it is important to be open to other health issues that may arise during the encounter. Clarifying the expectations for the child or adolescent and family for the health visit and negotiating a time frame and plan for care are important to establishing trust in a provider/parent relationship.

Present Concern

After summarizing the family concerns gathered in the initial phase of the interview, transition to a more focused approach to gathering information on the present health history and past medical history. For a *symptom-focused* or *acute care visit*, begin gathering information in the following areas to clarify information the family has not already addressed. A mnemonic such as OLDCART (onset, location, duration, characteristics, aggravating factors, relieving factors, treatment) can help organize the questioning for many chief complaints:

- When did you first notice the symptoms? Or date/time child was last well?
- Where are the symptoms (name, point to parts of body, document whether indicating discrete location or larger area)?
- Character of symptoms (time of day, location, intensity, duration, quality)?
- Progression of symptoms (How is child doing now? Symptoms getting better or worse?)
- Associated symptoms (vomiting, fever, rash, cough etc.)? Anything else bothering child?
- Exposure to household member, classmates, or others who have been ill? Pets in home?
- Any recent travel? If travel outside the United States, staying in tourist areas or with family?
- Changes in appetite or activity level (eating regularly, school/day care attendance, sleeping pattern)?
- Medications taken (dosage, time, date)? Did the medication help or relieve the symptoms?
- Home management (What has the family tried? What has helped?) Use of alternative therapies or healing practices? Family belief about the illness?
- Pertinent family medical history?
- What changes have occurred in the family as a result of this illness (effects or secondary gain)?
- Has the family seen other health care providers for the concern?

COMPREHENSIVE HEALTH HISTORY

This section will cover content relevant for a comprehensive visit, such as a well-child or new patient visit. For a *symptom-focused* or *acute care visit*, the health care provider should include only pertinent parts of the comprehensive history presented below.

Prenatal and Birth History

The prenatal and birth history is important in relation to the first 2 years of life and may be particularly relevant at any age for infants and children with a history of preterm birth, developmental delays, atypical neurologic findings, or congenital syndromes.

Prenatal History

- Gestational parent's GTPAL (Gravidity, number of pregnancies; Term deliveries; Premature deliveries; Abortions, spontaneous or induced; Living children)
- Age of biological parents, month prenatal care initiated
- Family/community support or lack of support or conflicts related to the pregnancy
- Length of pregnancy, history of fetal movement/activity
- Gestational parent's health before and during pregnancy—weight gain; hypertension; diabetes; history of infectious diseases including tuberculosis (TB), human immunodeficiency virus (HIV), hepatitis, sexually transmitted infections (STIs), group B streptococcal (GBS) status; asthma, allergies, or other chronic health conditions; hospitalizations
- Gestational parent's alcohol and tobacco use; prescription drug use; over-the-counter (OTC) or recreational drug use
- Intimate partner violence or exposure to abuse or family violence
- Caregiver depression, anxiety, or other mental health conditions

Birth and Neonatal History

- Length of labor, caesarean or vaginal delivery, epidural/anesthesia? Vacuum-assisted vaginal birth? Breech or shoulder presentation?
- Gestational age: born on or near expected due date, preterm, or postterm? *If preterm*: Was infant in neonatal intensive care unit (NICU)? Intubated? Length of stay in NICU?
- Born at home, birthing center, hospital? Place of birth, if outside of present location/country, date of arrival to present location/country?
- Birth weight and length?

- Apgar score (see Chapter 6), if known? Breathing, cardiac, or other problems noted immediately after birth?
- Who was present at delivery, how soon after birth did parent(s) touch or hold baby?
- Difficulties in feeding or stooling? Irritability or jitteriness? Jaundice?
- Length of hospitalization at birth? Was infant discharged with biological parents or other caregivers?

Past Medical History

A comprehensive health history includes a review of the *past medical history* from birth to adolescence. For symptom-focused or acute care visits, past medical history information is often focused on system-specific symptoms, which are presented in the system chapters that follow. The following are components of the past medical history:

- **Chronic conditions**: Seasonal or household allergies, wheezing or asthma; recurrent cough; frequent ear infections or fluid in ears; hearing or vision problems; hypertension or other cardiovascular conditions; over- or underweight; diabetes; gastrointestinal, liver, or kidney conditions; bedwetting; dental decay or poor oral health? Immunosuppressed? Chronic constipation? Chronic abdominal pain? Onset of chronic condition?
- **Hospitalizations**/surgeries: Date and reason for hospitalization, length of stay, complications after hospitalization? History of surgery, trauma, or head injury?
- **Unintentional injuries**: Falls, nature of injury, age of child when injury occurred, problems after injury? Motor vehicle, bicycle, scooter/skateboard, or pedestrian-related injuries?
- **Intentional injuries**: History of family violence, physical abuse, or intimate partner violence? Child interview should include the following questions: Has anyone hurt you? Have you felt afraid someone would harm you? Is there any bullying or verbal abuse from family members, surrounding community, or during school, after-school programs, or at childcare?
- **Allergies**: Allergic to prescription medications or antibiotics; reaction to OTC medications? Any food allergies noted? What type of reaction occurred? Severity of the reaction? Was an epinephrine pen (EpiPen) recommended? Reaction to insect bites or bee stings? Pets in home? Environmental triggers (dampness, mold, household dust, dust mites)?
- **Medications**: Is child taking vitamins, fluoride, or medications regularly? Type of medication? Use of OTC medications? Use of herbs or natural or homeopathic medicines? Traditional healing practices?
- **Immunization**: Review immunization dates and current status including status of annual flu vaccine; ask parent/caregiver about reactions to vaccines; travel history and date of last tuberculin purified protein derivative (PPD) or TB symptom screening? If under-immunized, reasons for withholding vaccines or parental concerns about vaccine safety?
- **Laboratory tests**: Result of newborn hearing screening? Review of newborn screening results? Hemoglobin or hematocrit screening for anemia? Lead screening? Blood test for TB (QUANTIferon)?

Family History

As discussed above, a FHH is an essential component of a comprehensive history and may be gathered in depth or briefly, depending on the type of visit. Table 4.1 presents the SCREEN mnemonic for an initial genetic family history.[18] This mnemonic represents an initial series of questions used to quickly identify potential genetically influenced health conditions in the family that may require further intervention, counselling, referral, or screening by a geneticist. These conditions could include hypertension, heart disease, diabetes, stroke, overweight or obesity, cancer, asthma, nasal allergy, eczema, mental health problems, family history of headaches or migraine, congenital

TABLE 4.1	THE SCREEN MNEMONIC FOR FAMILY HISTORY GATHERING	
SC	Some concerns	"Do you have any (some) concerns about diseases or conditions that run in the family?"
R	Reproduction	"Have there been any problems with pregnancy, infertility, or birth defects in your family?"
E	Early disease, death, or disability	"Have any members of your family died or become sick at an early age?"
E	Ethnicity	"How would you describe your ethnicity?" or "Where were your parents born?"
N	Nongenetic	"Are there any other risk factors or nonmedical conditions that run in your family?"

From Trotter TL, Martin HM. Family history in pediatric primary care, *Pediatrics*. 2007; 120(Suppl 2):S60–S65.

anomalies or mental retardation, sickle cell trait or disease, kidney disease, learning problems, neonatal loss or death in infancy, early death from heart attack or any cause before 50 years of age, seizures, or epilepsy. (Information gathered should include age of family member if known and be incorporated into the electronic record's FHH.)

- **Relevant infectious disease history** (especially important for children who have lived or travelled abroad): History of transmissible infections in gestational parent or other family members, including hepatitis, HIV, Zika virus, syphilis, TB; history of malaria, Chagas disease; history of parasitic infections, or COVID-19 variants.[26]

Social History

- **Socioeconomic history**: Employment status, parental occupations, parental or caregiver work schedules, parental education and parental literacy level in native language and current language if different, access to health insurance, medical or health care home, uninsured or underinsured. Does family experience periods of food insecurity? Have difficulty paying bills?
- **Home and housing situation**: Who lives in the household? Currently living with spouse or partner? Parental separation or divorce? Any separation due to incarceration, immigration, deportation or death of a parent

or other family member? Has child always lived with current caregivers? Number of adults and children living in home? Type of home, apartment, or housing situation? Living with extended family members or relatives? Is housing secure or temporary? Unstable housing problems? Any habitability concerns, such as mold or pests? Is the neighborhood and community safe? Sleeping arrangements?
- **Support systems**: With whom do you talk when you have a problem? Family support or extended family living near or in home? Help with childcare? Supportive or close friends? With which ethnicity(ies), race(s), religion(s) does family identify, and are they living in a culturally congruent or supportive community?
- **Family violence or intimate partner violence**: Do you feel safe in the home? Is there a history of family violence or intimate partner violence in home? Has the child or adolescent witnessed or been involved in family violence?
- **Family substance use**: Is smoking, alcohol, e-cigarette, or drug use a concern in your family? Is your child or adolescent exposed to substance abuse or overuse or abuse of prescription drugs?
- **Caregiver history**: Any feelings of depressed mood, feeling down, or loss of interest or pleasure in activities? Feeling

TABLE 4.2	REVIEW OF SYSTEMS FOR MIDDLE CHILDHOOD AND ADOLESCENCE
General	General health/well-being, weight gain/loss, fevers, appetite, sleep, malaise, fatigue, mood
Skin	Rashes, eruptions, skin infections, nodules or lumps, easy bruising, variations in skin pigment, congenital birthmarks
Eyes	Itching, redness, dryness, mucous discharge, tearing, rubbing eyes frequently, vision screening results, vision problems, squinting, trouble reading and/or holding screen close, sitting close to TV, has glasses or wears glasses, has contact lenses
Ears	History of frequent infections, ear pain, pulling at ears, ear drainage, ear wax impaction, trouble hearing, newborn hearing screening results, history of failed audiogram
Nose	Frequent nasal congestion, runny nose or nasal allergy, frequent upper respiratory infection, nose bleeds, difficulty breathing at night, snoring
Mouth/ throat	Frequent sore throats, large tonsils, mouth breathing, speech difficulties, number of teeth, signs of teething, most recent dental visit, history of dental caries, thumb sucking
Neck/ lymphatic	Pain or stiffness in neck, swollen or tender lymph nodes or glands, any lumps or masses noted
Chest	Any breast development or breast swelling—noted at what age? For pubertal males: Any breast swelling or gynecomastia?
Respiratory	Frequent cough, nighttime cough, shortness of breath when exercising, respiratory distress, nasal flaring, retractions, rate, wheezing, cyanosis, pain on respiration, tuberculosis exposure and testing, previous chest x-rays, history of asthma, sleep apnea, snoring, smoke exposure
Cardiovascular	Shortness of breath, tire easily with exercise, history of heart murmur, any chest pain, hypertension, history of anemia
Gastrointestinal	Appetite, weight gain/loss, food intolerance, frequent abdominal pain or stomachaches, vomiting (description), constipation, history of colic, lactose intolerance, frequent loose stool or diarrhea, anal itching, blood or mucus in stool
Genitourinary	Frequency of urination, blood in urine, burning/dysuria, urgency, hesitancy, wetting during day or at night, history of urinary tract infections, testicular pain
Gynecologic	Age of puberty, age of first menses, frequency of periods and onset of last menstrual period, duration of periods, pain with menses, pelvic pain, vaginal discharge, vaginal itching
Musculoskeletal	Pain, redness, or swelling around joints; sprains or strains; history of injuries; recent change in gait; hip or feet deformities; family history of flat feet; weakness; awkwardness; or clumsiness when walking or running
Neurologic	Headaches, dizziness, fainting, tremors, tics, breath-holding spells, night terrors, sleepwalking, history of head trauma, convulsions or seizures, concussions, unconsciousness, falls
Endocrine	Polyuria, polydipsia, polyphagia, any hair/skin changes (including acne, skin pigmentations, extra body hair), parental or child concerns about rate of growth, early or late puberty, elevated blood glucose
Hematologic	History of anemia, blood transfusions, any problems with bleeding, frequent bruising, sickle cell trait or disease, hepatitis exposure
Psychosocial and behavioral	Behavioral problems, frequent mood changes, concerns about unusual behavior, difficulty focusing, learning problems, anxiety, nervousness, extreme shyness, fearful, or depressed

anxious or unable to control worrying? Stress related to current, recent or past traumatic events?

Review of Systems

The *review of systems* is often included in the comprehensive health history for children and adolescents, particularly those with chronic health conditions affecting multiple systems in the body. Table 4.2 presents a guide for the information gathered in a review of systems. Experienced providers will incorporate the *review of systems* questions into the physical examination to prompt families to remember areas of history that may have been overlooked in the initial interview. Interview questions for the *review of systems* are also found in the system-specific chapters that follow.

ACTIVITIES OF DAILY LIVING

Age-Specific Nutritional Information Gathering

Infancy

Adequate nutrition in the first 2 years of life is critical for the period of rapid growth and brain development. A thorough dietary history in the infant recognizes problems early and allows the health care provider to counsel families later in the visit for developing issues related to growth or nourishment. (See Box 4.1 for anticipatory guidance counseling resources.) Dietary history for the first year of life includes the following:

- **Breastfeeding**: Frequency and duration of infant feeds; use of supplemental formula feedings or water; difficulties with latching or feeding patterns? Concern about infant weight gain? Any vomiting after feeds? Breastfeeding parent's diet or dietary restrictions?[27] Other family participation in feeding routines? Breastfeeding parent receiving adequate rest? Experiencing nipple soreness? Plans for return to work? Plan for expression of breast milk or weaning?
- **Formula feeding**: Type of infant formula, how is formula stored? How is powdered formula prepared? Amount and frequency of feeds? Concern about infant weight gain? Bottle-feeding at night? How often? Difficulty feeding or slow feeder? Plans for bottle weaning and transition to cup?
- **Formula and breastfeeding**: Feeding both breast milk and formula? How often and quantity of formula daily? Frequency and length of breastfeeding? Number of nighttime feedings with breast or bottle?
- **Fluids**: Drinking anything besides breast milk or formula before introduction of solid foods? Drinking sugar-sweetened beverages (SSB)? Amount and type? Drinking SSB in cup or bottle? Amount of water daily (after introduction of solids)? Introduction of cup?
- **Solid foods**: Age at introduction of solid foods? Portion size/amount of baby foods? Introduction of table foods and finger foods? Regular meal pattern? Infant interested in table foods? Family members frequently feeding infant table foods?

Early Childhood (1 to 4 Years of Age)

A careful history of dietary intake in the infant, toddler, and young child can provide the basis for anticipatory guidance about nutrition needed for growth, prevention of anemia or caries, and food safety, including choking prevention. The history should include information about breastmilk, formula, water, juices, and whether delivered by breast, bottle, or cup; type and consistency of solid foods, preparation and servings of solid foods.

Dietary history for early childhood includes the following:

- Obtain a 24-hour dietary history.
- Document servings and variety of fruits and vegetables, sources of protein, iron, vitamin C, vitamin D, and calcium (Ca^{2+}).
- Food likes and dislikes? Any food struggles developing around mealtime or portion size?
- Snacking and meal pattern? Frequency of juice and soda?

- Any parental concerns about the child's appetite, age-appropriate intake? Any food insecurity, lack of resources for storing or preparing food?

Middle Childhood (5 to 10 Years of Age)

It is important to obtain a comprehensive history of the food environment, available nutritional resources, and eating habits during the health history interview with the school-age child and caregiver. Determine the role of food in the family and if there are family mealtimes, considering available resources. Dietary history for middle childhood should include the following:

- Obtain a 24-hour dietary history. Begin with the child's recall of dietary intake and then elicit dietary information from caregiver.
- Document servings and variety of fruits and vegetables, sources of protein, iron, vitamin C, vitamin D, and calcium (Ca^{2+}).
- Review daily meal pattern and snacking habits, amount of fast foods and carry-out foods weekly, daily quantity of juice and water, amount of sugar-sweetened beverages, soda and carbonated beverages daily or weekly, consumption of sports drinks or caffeinated drinks daily or weekly.
- How many meals does child eat away from home daily or weekly? Does child contribute to preparation or planning of family meals at home? Does the child have any interest in cooking?
- Any parental concerns about lack of appetite, overeating, or portion size at meals? Any family struggles around food and weight gain or weight loss?

Adolescence (11 Years of Age to Young Adulthood)

Adolescence is a time of tremendous physical development, second only to infancy, but longer in duration. As such, nutritional requirements during adolescence may be greater than any other time in life. The evolving independence during this developmental stage also impacts long-term eating behaviors that may continue into adulthood. Supporting healthy nutrition in adolescence is essential for adequate growth and maturation as well as imprinting lifelong health promoting behaviors.[28] "Disordered eating" is unfortunately the norm for many adolescents who do not necessarily otherwise meet diagnostic criteria for a clinical eating disorder. According to the 2019 National Youth Risk Behavior Surveillance System, 7.9% of adolescents reported no vegetable intake, 16.7% reported no breakfast intake in the 7 days before the survey, 44.6% reported drinking less than the recommended amount of plain water daily, and 15.1% drank one or more cans or bottles of soda daily.[29] Teens may skip breakfast, either because of lack of time, lack of available food, or the misconception that skipping breakfast will aid in weight loss. A vegetarian diet is often a healthy choice for adults or for children who have been raised as vegetarians; however, young people who adopt a vegetarian diet because of weight concerns are at increased risk of developing an eating disorder.[30] Even though eating disorders are more common among adolescents who identify as female, males are also at risk. Eating disorders may present differently among males, with an increased focus on muscularity, and certain subpopulations such as athletes as well as racial/ethnic, sexual, and gender minority males are at increased risk.[31] A 24- or 48-hour diet recall can be helpful in evaluating nutrition status. While an assessment of the context of nutrition and activity can take longer than a traditional diet recall (e.g., "Tell me how eating and activity fit into your day yesterday"), this contextual information can be very useful in client-centered counseling techniques, such as motivational interviewing, for improved nutritional and dietary habits.

In asking adolescents about body image, the provider should avoid the assumptions that an adolescent with a low BMI for age is satisfied with his or her weight or that an adolescent with a high BMI wants to lose weight. See Box 4.3 for examples of two screening tools used to evaluate adolescents for eating disorders.

Eating disorder Screen for Primary care (ESP):
- Are you satisfied with your eating patterns?
- Do you ever eat in secret?
- Does your weight affect the way you feel about yourself?
- Have any members of your family suffered with an eating disorder?
- Do you currently suffer with or have you ever suffered in the past with an eating disorder?

Sick, Control, One, Fat, and Food (SCOFF) questionnaire:
- Do you make yourself Sick because you feel uncomfortably full?
- Do you worry you have lost Control over how much you eat?
- Have you recently lost more than One stone (14 lb or 7.7 kg) in a 3-month period?
- Do you believe yourself to be Fat when others say you are thin?
- Would you say that Food dominates your life?

Data from Cotton M-A, Ball C, Robinson P: Four simple questions can help screen for eating disorders. *J Gen Intern Med.* 2003;18:53–56; and Kutz AM, Marsh AG, Gunderson CG, Maguen S, Masheb RM. Eating disorder screening: a systematic review and meta-analysis of diagnostic test characteristics of the SCOFF. *J Gen Intern Med.*2020;35:885–893.

Family Meal Patterns

- Is there a time daily when the family has a common meal? Are there usual family meal patterns? How often does the family eat a meal together? Who does the food shopping? How often are meals prepared at home? Daily or number of times per week? Number of fast food or carry-out meals per week?
- Does family have a vegetarian or vegan diet? Are there any special cultural or religious food rituals or preferences?
- Does the family participate in any supplemental food programs? WIC (Special Supplemental Nutrition Program for Women, Infants, and Children) or SNAP (Supplemental Nutrition Assistance Program)? Does the family run out of food during the month or are they worried about running out of food?

Stooling and Elimination Patterns

- **Infancy**: Stooling pattern, frequency, and consistency for breastfed or formula-fed infants? Irregular or hard stool pattern?
- **Early childhood (1 to 4 years of age)**: Stooling pattern and frequency? Signs of readiness for toilet training? Plan for initiating toilet training? Any resistance to toilet training or difficulty with bowel or bladder control? Age when bowel and bladder control was attained for daytime? Age of bladder control for nighttime?
- **Middle childhood (5 to 10 years of age)**: History of constipation, frequent stooling, or diarrhea? Daytime or nighttime wetting? Parental concern or attitude toward wetting incidents? Soiling or difficulty with bowel control? History of encopresis? History of diurnal or nocturnal enuresis?

Oral Health and Dentition

- **Infancy**: Number of teeth? Use of night bottle or frequent breastfeeding? Weaning occurred at what age? Does infant have juice in a bottle or cup? Cleaning or brushing teeth daily?
- **Early childhood to adolescents**: Number of teeth? Tooth eruption and tooth loss pattern? Brushing teeth twice daily? Flossing daily? SSB intake? Sugary snacks and snacking frequency? Has child or adolescent seen a dentist? Does the family have a dental provider? Last dental appointment? History of dental caries? Recent application of fluoride varnish or dental sealants?

Sleep

Sleep is essential for the optimal health of children and adolescents, and sleeping the recommended number of hours regularly is associated with improved attention, memory, and learning; behavior and emotional regulation;

TABLE 4.3	RECOMMENDED GUIDELINES FOR AMOUNT OF SLEEP PER AGE
4–12 months	12–16 h daily including naps
1–2 years of age	11–14 h daily including naps
3–5 years of age	10–13 h daily including naps
6–12 years of age	9–12 h daily
13–18 years of age	8–10 h daily

Data from Paruthi S, Brooks LJ, D'Ambrosio C, et al. Recommended amount of sleep for pediatric populations: a consensus statement of the American Academy of Sleep Medicine. *J Clin Sleep Med.* 2016; 12:785–786.

improved immune function and improved health outcomes.[32] Insufficient sleep has been associated with an increased risk for childhood overweight and obesity and also an increase in risk in adolescents of depression and self-harm.[33] Table 4.3 shows the recommended guidelines for the amount of sleep needed each night to promote optimal health across the pediatric age span.[32]

- **Infancy**: What are the infant's sleeping patterns and amount of sleep during the day and at night in the first year? Where does the infant sleep? Back to sleep on firm surface? Avoiding soft bedding?
- **Early childhood (1 to 4 years of age)**: Sleep pattern and amount of sleep? Bedtime routines? Regular bedtime? Hours of sleep nightly? Where does the child sleep? Co-sleeping until what age? Does the child sleep in one or more than one household? Concerns about nightmares, night terrors, night waking, somnambulism (sleepwalking)?
- **Middle childhood (5 to 10 years of age) and adolescents**: Regular bedtime? Hours of sleep nightly? Does child sleep in one or more than one household? Share bed, bedroom, or sleep in common areas of

household? Concerns about difficulty falling asleep, insomnia, nightmares, night terrors, night waking, somnambulism (sleepwalking)? Screen or cell phone time after bedtime?

Physical Activity

- **Infancy:** Opportunities for observed time on abdomen, sitting, cruising, age-appropriate active play?
- **Early childhood (1 to 4 years of age):** Opportunities for active play, indoors and out, access to and safety around playgrounds, natures? Introduction to scooters, tricycles or bicycles, playing with balls? Family active time? Organized activities such as sports, gymnastics, swimming, or dance?
- **Middle childhood (5 to 10 years of age) and adolescents**: Amount of time spent in walking, running, biking, active play? Time in nature? Organized sports, dance?

INTERESTS/HOBBIES/SPORTS

- Screen time? Number of hours daily of TV, video gaming, cell phone use, tablet, nonacademic laptop or computer use, and computer gaming?
- After-school activities? At school or in the community? Interests or focus (music, art, etc.)?
- Interested in sports? Involved in competitive or recreational sports? Participates in after-school sports programs?

School/After-School Programs/Child Care

- **Infancy (birth to 11 months)**: Who is the infant's primary caregiver? For infants in day care or childcare, is the infant in home day care or in a childcare center? Number of children in home day care and ratio of caregivers to children? Hours spent daily in childcare?
- **Early childhood (1 to 4 years of age)**: Where does the child spend the day? Who is primary caregiver? What is your child's school experience? Day care or childcare,

preschool, or prekindergarten experience? How well did your child adapt to child care or school entry? Assessment of child's performance in childcare or preschool?

- **Middle childhood (5 to 10 years of age):** School performance? Likes school? What are child's strengths? Number of missed school days? Reason for school absence? Teacher or caregiver has concerns about learning? Attends special education classes? Any history of bullying in the classroom or during school hours? Attends after-school program?
- **Adolescence (11 years to young adulthood):** See adolescent-specific content later in this chapter.

SAFETY[1]

- **Infancy:** *Car seat*: Rear-facing car seat in back seat of car? Any concern about installation of car seat? Safely installed? If preterm infant or infant with special health care needs, is infant using supports in car seat or car bed for safe transport?[34,35] Using sunscreen for outdoor activities? *Household*: Is household water temperature set at 120°F or less? Avoiding choking hazards? Installation of safety locks and gates? Avoiding screen time? Is infant in smoke-free environment? Discuss avoidance of parental vaping, tobacco or drug use and counsel on smoking cessation. Adults should avoid drinking hot liquids while holding an infant.
- **Early childhood (1 to 4 years of age):** *Car seat*: Rear-facing car seat in back seat of car until at least age 2 years, and as long as possible, given car seat weight limits?[36] See Box 4.1. Front-facing car seat until at least age 4 or until reaching weight/height limits for the particular seat? Any concern about installation of car seat? Safely installed? Transition to booster seat and belt positioning? Bicycle or scooter safety? Helmet use? *Household*: Childproofing of household? Preventing burns and falls? Are medications, recreational drugs, detergent pods, and other potential toxins locked away

out of reach? Number for poison control? Choking hazards? Tobacco or vaping use in home? Presence of gun in home, loaded/unloaded, locked, how stored? Stranger safety taught? Teaching pet safety? Drowning risks? Cleaning buckets, bathtub? Home or community pool? Sunscreen use? Monitoring screen time and content (cell phone, tablet, and TV)?

- **Middle childhood (5 to 10 years of age):** *Car safety*: Transition to booster seat at what age? For children who are above the height and weight limit for a car seat, a belt-positioning booster seat is recommended by the AAP and required in some states until the child's height reaches 4 feet 9 inches or until child is at least 8 years of age.[36] Seat belt used regularly? Riding in back seat of motor vehicle?[36] Pedestrian safety? Bicycle, skateboard, or scooter safety? Helmet use? Sports safety equipment used? Swimming safety? Sunscreen use? Stranger safety taught? Supervision with friends/peers, in person and online? *Household*: Presence of gun in home? Loaded/unloaded, locked, how stored? Fire safety? Smoke detectors? Monitoring screen time and content (cell phone, tablet, computer, and TV)? Discussion about tobacco, vaping, alcohol, and drug use risks with child?
- **Adolescence (11 years to young adulthood):** See later section on adolescent health history.

DEVELOPMENTAL HISTORY

Normal developmental progress and achieving developmental milestones on time is a critical marker of health during infancy and early childhood. Parental concerns about delayed physical growth or delayed psychomotor or cognitive development are of primary importance in the health history interview. Parental expectations of developmental markers vary widely in families, so it is important to elicit in the history not only what the infant or child is doing but also what the parent or family expects and allows.[1] Always note in the electronic health record the ages at which key developmental milestones were attained. (See Chapter 3 for developmental and behavioral screening questions to ask caregivers of infants and children up to 4 years of age.)

Middle Childhood (5 to 10 Years of Age)

Middle childhood provides an opportunity to foster positive health habits, particularly in the areas of nutrition and physical activity.[1] The health care provider should explore developing interests with the school-age child and parent and encourage participation in recreational or organized sports as well as creative hobbies. The clinician should assess what physical activities the child enjoys and the duration and frequency of activity. Exploring the quality of the child's friendships and the school performance and experience (current grades, relationship with teacher, responsibility for homework) gives a view into the child's world. Habits such as nail biting and tics should be explored.

With advancements in technology and digital communication it is important for the provider to be aware that children's peer interactions also include online formats such as social media or gaming chat rooms. Children who are bullying, being bullied, or both should be counseled and considered for possible referral. Increased use of social media can also affect mental health; particularly, heavy use is associated with depression, anxiety, and stress.[37] At the same time, social media may be used by adolescents to foster peer connection and learn about mental health resources in ways that promote wellbeing.[38] Providers should assess the amount and type of social media used and level of caregiver monitoring.

- **Gross and fine motors skills**: Physical balance and coordination appropriate for age? Participating in sports? Handwriting ability?
- **Communication**: Readiness to learn? Speech or language delays? Communication patterns with peers and adults? Problem-solving skills?
- **Social/emotional**: Increasing independence? Self-esteem? Relationships with

parents, siblings? Peer relationships and best friend? Experienced bullying in school or from family members? Mood or symptoms of depression? History of suicidal ideation, whether or not youth reports depression? See Chapter 3 for more details on psychosocial and behavioral health assessment.

- **Temperament/personality**: Congenial with peers? Positive self-image? Able to name best friend? Ability to adapt to change?
- **Discipline**: What type of discipline is used when your child misbehaves? When is it used? Is it effective? Are parenting styles consistent? Does child live at more than one home? Are there behavior issues at home or at school?
- **Sexual development**: Gender and sexual identity, congruity with sex designated at birth, child or family questions about gender expression; sex education provided in the home and/or at school? Signs of body odor, breast development or pubic hair noted?

Adolescence (11 Years to Young Adulthood)

See adolescent-specific content later in this chapter.

CHILDREN WITH SPECIAL HEALTH CARE NEEDS AND MEDICAL COMPLEXITY

Children with special health care needs (CSHCNs) are those who have a chronic physical, developmental, behavioral, or emotional condition and who also require health and related services of a type or amount beyond that required by children generally.[39] Children with medical complexity are medically fragile, have severe functional limitations often requiring assistive technology, and frequent needs for specialized health care.[40] In gathering information on health history, CSHCNs require special consideration. Assessing the level of impact on family functioning, family cohesion, sibling relationships, and care management required for a child with special health care needs is an important part of the health history. The role of the pediatric health care provider is to assist families in optimizing the daily functioning of the child in the home and school environment; focusing on the strengths of the child and family; coordinating pediatric specialty referral as indicated; and providing support and a framework for continuity of care in a medical home or health care home setting.[1] The CSHCN screener is a five-item survey-based tool completed by the parent; it is an efficient and flexible standardized method of identifying children across the range and diversity of chronic health conditions and special needs.[41] Implementing the CSHCN screener can be an effective part of the comprehensive health history and child and family assessment. Although the National Survey of Children's Health using the screener was updated for 2016, the original screener for individual children remains in use.[39] The CSHCN screener is available at https://www.childhealthdata.org/docs/cshcn/technical-summary-of-cshcn-screener.pdf.

ADOLESCENT PSYCHOSOCIAL HISTORY AND CONFIDENTIALITY

The most important caveat of the adolescent psychosocial history is that it should be conducted without the parent or guardian in the room. A review of studies on adolescent access to health care services shows that a perceived lack of confidentiality is a barrier to care and discussing sensitive topics improves the adolescent's satisfaction with care, yet only a minority of adolescents have ever discussed the importance of the confidentiality of the health visit with a health care provider.[42]

It is crucial for the provider to become familiar with the specific state laws pertaining to adolescent consent, confidentiality, privacy, child abuse reporting, and the amount of control the adolescent has over the release of medical records related to confidential services. In all 50 states, there are some limitations to confidentiality. Providers are generally required to notify parents and/or police or child protective services if an adolescent under 18 years of age reports thoughts of self-harm or of harming others. Reporting requirements would also apply to cases where an adolescent has been abused or neglected.

In addition, some states have mandatory reporting laws about consensual sexual activity, depending on the age discrepancy between an adolescent and the sexual partner; other states encourage reporting but give the provider some discretion. All 50 states have laws allowing adolescents to consent to testing for STIs and to treatment; however, confidential access to contraception, prenatal care, abortion, adoption, medical care of the minor's child, and mental health services vary from state to state, as do laws restricting or requiring disclosure of confidential care to a parent.[43]

Federal regulations under the Health Insurance Portability and Accountability Act (HIPAA), as well as the adoption of electronic health records (EHRs), affect the control and privacy of medical records for services the adolescent may have accessed confidentially.[44] The 21st Century Cures Act passed by the United States Congress in 2016 has unique privacy implications for adolescent patients in the era of EHRs. The law, which took effect in 2021, requires documented medical information in the EHR be viewable to patients and the caregivers of minor patients. There are exceptions to information sharing, including a privacy exception, which is particularly relevant to adolescent medical care. Providers need to be aware of local laws regarding adolescent confidentiality, EHR functionality, and institutional policies in order to ensure adolescent privacy is not breached in the documentation process.[45]

Adolescent Psychosocial Screen: From HEADSSS to SSHADESS

The SSHADESS psychosocial history (Box 4.4) is a key part of a comprehensive adolescent health history and assessment.[46,47] The SSHADESS psychosocial history is preferred by many adolescent providers to the more familiar HEADSSS mnemonic, which covers a similar health

| BOX 4.4 | SSHADESS—REVIEW OF ADOLESCENT HISTORY |

Strengths
- What are some of your strengths that help you cope with stress?
- How would your friends describe you?
- If you were applying for a job, how would you describe yourself to encourage someone to hire you?

School
- Are you in school? (Regular or continuation? English learner/bilingual? Special education/504 plan?) Attend regularly? Suspensions?
- Favorite/most difficult subjects?
- What are your grades/GPA?
  - Low: Recent if changes in GPA? Is work too difficult? Not doing homework?
  - High: Any stress about college goals or grades?
- Plans after high school graduation? (Realistic? Is teen taking right courses/activities? Sending college applications on time? Taking vocational training?)
  - If no specific plans, end of high school can be a difficult, vulnerable time.

Home
- Who lives with you? (One or both parents, grandparents, aunts/uncles, adult siblings, group home, foster care?) Do you live with boyfriend/girlfriend and family?
  - Immigrant teens may live with adult siblings/extended family while parents live in home country.
- Have you lived with…your whole life? Changes because of divorce or death of parent? Separation/reunification with parents resulting from immigration? Conflict with parents/guardians? Illness, incarceration, homelessness of family members?
- How do you get along with…? How are conflicts handled at home?

Activities
- How do you spend free time? What do you do for fun? Sports/other extracurricular activities? Exercise? How many hours of physical activity per day? Hobbies? Church or community activities?

- Responses reflect a measure of connection to school, extra motivation for attendance/grades
- Jobs? (Number of hours/week, schedule, location, hazards)
- Names of friends, best friend?

Drugs/Alcohol/Tobacco
Introduce the subject gently, especially with young teens; can be more direct with older teens
- Does anyone at your school… ? Do any of your friends… ? Then, have you…?
- If yes, use CRAFFT questions (see Box 4.5).
- Attempts to quit?
- Family members using drugs/alcohol/tobacco?

Emotions
- How would you describe your moods? (Elicits rich information if teen is given time to elaborate)
- Depression/anger: Changes in energy, appetite, weight? Sleep disturbances, difficulty concentrating? Irritability is hallmark of depression in teens. Difficulty with homework, school? How teen copes with anger?
- Present/past suicidal ideation, attempts? Suicide gesture versus self-cutting without suicidal intent?
  - Suicidal gestures/attempts may be impulsive acts after disagreement with parents, peers; teen may not self-identify as depressed.
- Warn parent/guardian if teen contemplating suicide, even if not at immediate risk.

Sexuality, Gender Identity, and Sexual Abuse
Warn the teen of limits of confidentiality in your setting or state.
- "Have you ever had sex or ever come close to having sex?"
  - "Come close to" covers a broad range, includes oral/anal sex, which teens often do not define as sex. For teens with the intention to initiate sexual activity, it is important to explore choice and decisions about sex in relationship. It is important to elicit history before discussing safer sex, contraception, and need for pelvic exam.

Continued

BOX 4.4   SSHADESS—REVIEW OF ADOLESCENT HISTORY—CONT'D

- "Are your partners of the same or different genders?" or "Are you attracted to people of the same or different genders than you?"
  - Ask of everyone. Be sensitive to teens engaging in same-sex activities.
- Condom/barrier (if appropriate): "At what point in the sexual encounter do you use condoms?" ("late use" problem). Condom education in school? Knowledge of other barriers (gloves, dental dams)? Difficulties in negotiating condom use with partner?
  - Teens with less formal education may lack awareness of anatomy/physiology of genitals and reproductive organs.
- Are you doing anything to prevent pregnancy (if indicated)? Are you experiencing any pressure from partners or family to not use birth control or interference with condom or birth control use?
- "Has anyone ever touched you sexually without permission or tried to force you to have sex?" *If yes,* history of childhood sexual abuse? Acquaintance or date rape? Stranger assault?
- "Have you ever gone on dates or had sex in exchange for food, money, clothing, drugs or a place to stay? Has anyone asked you to have sex with another person? Has anyone ever taken sexual pictures of you or posted such pictures on the internet? How many sexual partners have you had in your lifetime?"

- "Has anyone you were seeing ever put you down or made you feel ashamed? Pressured you to go the next step when you are not ready? Grabbed your arm, yelled at you, or pushed you when they were angry or frustrated? Treated you badly when you were alone but acted differently in front of friends and family? Pushed you to have sex or do sexual things when you didn't want to?"

Safety Issues
- Do you have to do anything special to be safe in your home, at school, or in your neighborhood (e.g., positive climates, presence of gangs, etc.)?
- Have you run away or been thrown out of your home?
- Guns or other weapons in home or school?
- Physical fighting/abuse in home (between siblings, parents, parent-child)?
- Teen involved in physical fights at home, neighborhood, school?
- Adolescent relationship abuse? (See previous questions under Sexuality.)
- Friends in gangs? Have you ever been a gang member or do you wear a color/insignia? Teen, peers, siblings/cousins involved in gangs?
  - Be sensitive to potential reluctance to disclose.

Data from Ginsburg KR, Ramirez McClain ZR. *Reaching Teens: Strength-Based Communication Strategies to Build Resilience and Support Healthy Adolescent Development. Chicago:* American Academy of Pediatrics; 2020. 2nd ed; Griswold KS, Aronoff H, Kernan JB, Kahn LS. Adolescent substance use and abuse: recognition and management. *Am Fam Physician.* 2008;77(3):331–336; Hornor G, Quinones SG, Bretl D, et al. Commercial sexual exploitation of children: an update for the forensic nurse. *J Forensic Nurs.* 2019;15:93–102; Miller E. Trauma-informed approaches to adolescent relationship abuse and sexual violence prevention. *Pediatr Ann.* 2019;48:e274–e279.

history.[48] The SSHADESS offers the advantages of a strength-based approach and a more holistic exploration of the adolescent's emotional states.[49] The order of questioning, in general, proceeds from less private and sensitive questions to more sensitive ones, giving the provider and adolescent an opportunity to establish rapport. The SSHADESS can be tailored to early, middle, or late adolescents by modifying the questions. Remember that early adolescents and occasionally middle adolescents can have concrete thinking[50] and may wonder why the provider is asking such unusual questions. It is important to explain to early adolescents that you ask all teens the same questions; it is also important that you start the health history interview by asking questions about the activities of peers before asking about the teen directly.

BOX 4.5   PARTIAL CRAFFT + N 2.1 SUBSTANCE ABUSE SCREENING INTERVIEW*

Begin: *"I'm going to ask you a few questions that I ask all my patients. Please be honest. I will keep your answers confidential."*

Part A

During the PAST 12 MONTHS, on how many days did you:	No. of Days
1. Drink more than a few sips of beer, wine, or any drink containing **alcohol**? Say "0" if none.	
2. Use any **marijuana** (cannabis, weed, oil, wax, or hash by smoking, vaping, dabbing, or in edibles) or **"synthetic marijuana"** (like "K2," "Spice")? Say "0" if none.	
3. Use **anything else to get high** (like other illegal drugs, pills, prescription or over-the-counter medications, and things that you sniff, huff, vape, or inject)? Say "0" if none.	
4. Use a vaping device* containing nicotine and/or flavors, or use any tobacco products†? Say "0" if none. *Such as e-cigs, mods, pod devices like JUUL, disposable vapes like Puff Bar, vape pens, or e-hookahs. †Cigarettes, cigars, cigarillos, hookahs, chewing tobacco, snuff, snus, dissolvables, or nicotine pouches.	

If the patient answered...

"0" for all questions in Part A	"1" or more for Q. 1, 2, or 3	"1" or more for Q. 4
↓	↓	↓
Ask 1st question only in Part B below, then STOP	Ask all 6 questions in Part B below	Ask all 10 questions in Part C on next page

Part B

	Circle One	
C Have you ever ridden in a **CAR** driven by someone (including yourself) who was "high" or had been using alcohol or drugs?	No	Yes
R Do you ever use alcohol or drugs to **RELAX**, feel better about yourself, or fit in?	No	Yes
A Do you ever use alcohol or drugs while you are by yourself, or **ALONE**?	No	Yes
F Do you ever **FORGET** things you did while using alcohol or drugs?	No	Yes
F Do your **FAMILY** or **FRIENDS** ever tell you that you should cut down on your drinking or drug use?	No	Yes
T Have you ever gotten into TROUBLE while you were using alcohol or drugs?	No	Yes

NOTICE TO CLINIC STAFF AND MEDICAL RECORDS:
The information on this page is protected by special federal confidentiality rules (42 CFR Part 2), which prohibit disclosure of this information unless authorized by specific written consent.

*Note: Content presented shows only the first page of the tool. Additional questions related to nicotine and vaping (Part C) are available on the second page of the tool, which is accessible at www.crafft.org.

Avoid medical jargon and try to use the teen's own terminology without sounding as though you are trying to talk like a teen. Remember that adolescents tend to be oriented in the here and now. A "long time ago" may refer to years or months ago or as little as a few weeks ago.

Begin the interview with an opening such as "I'm going to ask you questions that I ask all teens about sex, drugs, and feelings. What you tell me is private, unless you tell me that you have been hurt by someone else, you are thinking of hurting someone else, or you are thinking of hurting yourself." Questions are asked in as neutral and nonjudgmental manner as possible to avoid making assumptions about the family structure, kinds of sexual activity, or sexual orientation of the adolescent. Asking open-ended questions such as, "How are things at home?" sets a neutral tone.

SSHADESS Assessment for Adolescence[46]

(S) Strengths: Personal characteristics that help youth cope and succeed

(S) School: Connection to or disconnection from school

(H) Home: Family structure and living arrangement, supports, and any problems at home

TABLE 4.4	TAKING A SEXUAL HISTORY: THE FIVE "P"S
Partners	• Are you currently having sex of any kind—so, oral, vaginal, or anal— with anyone? (Are you having sex?) • If no, have you ever had sex of any kind with another person? • In recent months, how many sex partners have you had? • What is/are the gender(s) of your sex partner(s)? • Do you or your partner(s) currently have other sex partners?

Practices	• What kind of sexual contact do you have, or have you had? What parts of your body are involved when you have sex?
	  • Do you have genital sex (penis in the vagina)?
	  • Anal sex (penis in the anus)?
	  • Oral sex (mouth on penis, vagina, or anus)?
	  • Are you a top and/or bottom?
	• Do you meet your partners online or through apps?
	• Have you or any of your partners used drugs?
	• Have you exchanged sex for your needs (money, housing, drugs, etc.)?

Protection from STIs	• Do you and your partner(s) discuss STI prevention? • Have you received HPV, hepatitis A, and/or hepatitis B shots? • Are you aware of PrEP, a medicine that can prevent HIV? Have you ever used it or considered using it?
Past History of STIs	• Have you ever been tested for STIs and HIV? Would you like to be tested? • Have you been diagnosed with an STI in the past? When? Did you get treatment? • Have you had any symptoms that keep coming back? • Has your current partner or any former partners ever been diagnosed or treated for an STI? Were you tested for the same STI(s)? Do you know your partner(s) HIV status?
Pregnancy Intention	• Do you think you would like to have (more) children at some point? • When do you think that might be? • How important is it to you to prevent pregnancy (until then)? • Are you or your partner using contraception or practicing any form of birth control? Would you like to talk about ways to prevent pregnancy? Do you need any information on birth control?

Data from Reno H, et al. *A Guide to Taking a Sexual History.* Atlanta: Centers for Disease Control and Prevention; 2022. Available at: https://www.cdc.gov/std/treatment/SexualHistory.htm.

(A) Activities: Sports, physical activity, school activities (school connection), hobbies, church involvement, youth groups, jobs, social media, and hours per week for each

(D) Drugs: Drug, alcohol, tobacco experimentation and abuse (Box 4.5)

(E) Emotions/eating/depression: Positive and negative emotional states, including potential depression and suicidal ideation, healthy and unhealthy eating habits

(S) Sexuality and gender identity: Sexual attractions, sexual identity, sexual activity or intentions, and any history of coercion or sexual abuse (Table 4.4). Gender identity, congruity with sex designated at birth[51]

(S) Safety issues: Protective factors (seat belts, helmets, problem-solving skills) and risk factors (guns in home, engaging in fights, gang activity), home and neighborhood safety, social media use and online interactions

Menstrual History

- Age at menarche, last menstrual period, regularity of menses, days of menstrual flow, pain during menstruation, missed school due to painful menses, gender dysphoria with menses?

See Chapter 17 for detailed information on menstrual history.

Mental and Behavioral Health History

Assessing for behavioral and mental health symptoms in middle childhood and adolescence is a crucial component of a pediatric health history. See Chapter 3 for detailed information.

REFERENCES

1. Hagan J, Shaw J, Duncan P, eds. *Bright Futures: Guidelines for Health Supervision of Infants, Children, and Adolescents*. 4th ed. Elk Grove Village: American Academy of Pediatrics; 2017.
2. Miller WR, Rollnick S. *Motivational Interviewing: Helping People Change*. 3rd ed. New York: The Guilford Press; 2013.
3. Substance Abuse and Mental Health Services Administration.. *SAMHSA's Concept of Trauma and Guidance for a Trauma-informed Approach*. Rockville: Substance and Mental Health Services Administration; July 2014.
4. Marsac ML, Kassam-Adams N, Hildenbrand AK, et al. Implementing a trauma-informed approach in pediatric health care networks. *JAMA Pediatr*. 2016;170:70–77.
5. Fleishman J, Kamsky H, Sundborg S. Trauma-informed nursing practice. *OJIN: The Online Journal of Issues in Nursing*. 2019;24(2): N.PAG.
6. Forkey H, Szilagyi M, Kelly ET, Duffee J. Trauma-informed care. *Pediatrics*. 2021:148.
7. Henry TL, Britz JB, St, Louis J, et al. Health equity: the only path forward for primary care. *Ann Fam Med*. 2022;20:175–178.
8. Kuruvilla S, Sadana R, Montesinos EV, et al. A life-course approach to health: synergy with sustainable development goals. *Bull World Health Organ*. 2018;96:42–50.
9. Bhushan D, Kotz K, McCall J, et al. *Roadmap for Resilience: The California Surgeon General's Report on Adverse Childhood Experiences, Toxic Stress and Health*. Office of the California Surgeon General; 2020.
10. Gilgoff R, Singh L, Koita K, Gentile B, Marques SS. Adverse childhood experiences, outcomes, and interventions. *Pediatr Clin North Am*. 2020;67:259–273.
11. Garg A, Homer CJ, Dworkin PH. Addressing social determinants of health: Challenges and opportunities in a value-based model. *Pediatrics*. 2019;143 e20182355.
12. Tervalon M, Murray-García J. Cultural humility versus cultural competence: a critical distinction in defining physician training outcomes in multicultural education. *J Health Care Poor Underserved*. 1998;9:117–125.
13. Kibakaya EC, Oyeku SO. Cultural humility: a critical step in achieving health equity. *Pediatrics*. 2022;149 e2021052883.
14. Foronda C, Baptiste DL, Reinholdt MM, Ousman K. Cultural humility: a concept analysis. *J Transcult Nurs*. 2016;27:210–217.
15. Gangamma R, Shipman D. Transnational intersectionality in family therapy with resettled refugees. *J Marital Fam Ther*. 2018;44:206–219.
16. Saul RA, Trotter T, Sease K, Tarini B. Survey of family history taking and genetic testing in pediatric practice. *J Community Genet*. 2017;8:109–115.
17. Tarini BA, McInerney JD. Family history in primary care pediatrics. *Pediatrics*. 2013;132:S203–210.
18. Trotter TL, Martin HM. Family history in pediatric primary care. *Pediatrics*. 2007;120(Suppl 2):S60–65.
19. Kwong L, Bodurtha J, Busch DW. An integrative review of family health history in pediatrics. *Clin Pediatr (Phila)*. 2020;59:1282–1287.
20. Amutah C, Greenidge K, Mante A, et al. Misrepresenting race—The role of medical schools in propagating physician bias. *N Engl J Med*. 2021;384:872–878.
21. Sabatello M, Jackson Scroggins M, Goto G, et al. Structural racism in the COVID-19 pandemic: Moving forward. *Am J Bioeth*. 2021;21:56–74.

22. Lowe C, Beach MC, Roter DL. Individuation and implicit racial bias in genetic counseling communication. *Patient Educ Couns.* 2020;103:804–810.

23. Barnes H, Morris E, Austin J. Trans-inclusive genetic counseling services: Recommendations from members of the transgender and non-binary community. *J Genet Couns.* 2020;29:423–434.

24. Tuite A, Dalla Piazza M, Brandi K, Pletcher BA. Beyond circles and squares: a commentary on updating pedigree nomenclature to better represent patient diversity. *J Genet Couns.* 2020;29:435–439.

25. Curfman A, McSwain SD, Chuo J, et al. Pediatric telehealth in the COVID-19 pandemic era and beyond. *Pediatrics.* 2021;148 e2020047795.

26. Linton JM, Green A.Council on Community Pediatrics Providing care for children in immigrant families. *Pediatrics.* 2019;144 e20192077.

27. Bartick M, Stehel EK, Calhoun SL, et al. Academy of Breastfeeding Medicine Position Statement and Guideline: Infant feeding and lactation-related language and gender. *Breastfeed Med.* 2021;16:587–590.

28. Das JK, Salam RA, Thornburg KL, et al. Nutrition in adolescents: physiology, metabolism, and nutritional needs. *Ann N Y Acad Sci.* 2017;1393:21–33.

29. Merlo CL, Jones SE, Michael SL, et al. Dietary and physical activity behaviors among high school students—Youth Risk Behavior Survey, United States, 2019. *MMWR Suppl.* 2020;69:64–76.

30. Zickgraf HF, Hazzard VM, O'Connor SM, et al. Examining vegetarianism, weight motivations, and eating disorder psychopathology among college students. *Int J Eat Disord.* 2020;53:1506–1514.

31. Nagata JM, Ganson KT, Murray SB. Eating disorders in adolescent boys and young men: an update. *Curr Opin Pediatr.* 2020;32:476–481.

32. Paruthi S, Brooks L, D'Ambrosio C, et al. Recommended amount of sleep for pediatric populations: a consensus statement of the American Academy of Sleep Medicine. *J Clini Sleep Med.* 2016;12:785–786.

33. Zhang J, Paksarian D, Lamers F, Hickie IB, He J, Merikangas KR. Sleep patterns and mental health correlates in US adolescents. *J Pediatr.* 2017;182:137–143.

34. O'Neil J, Hoffman B.Council on Injury, Violence, and Poison Prevention Transporting children with special health care needs. *Pediatrics.* 2019;143:e20190724.

35. Davis NL, Shah N. Use of car beds for infant travel: a review of the literature. *J Perinatol.* 2018;38:1287–1294.

36. Durbin DR, Hoffman BD.Council on Injury, Violence, and Poison Prevention Child passenger safety. *Pediatrics.* 2018;142 e20182460.

37. Shannon H, Bush K, Villeneuve PJ, Hellemans KG, Guimond S. Problematic social media use in adolescents and young adults: systematic review and meta-analysis. *JMIR Ment Health.* 2022;9:e33450..

38. O'Reilly M, Dogra N, Hughes J, Reilly P, George R, Whiteman N. Potential of social media in promoting mental health in adolescents. *Health Promot Int.* 2019;34:981–991.

39. Ghandour RM, Hirai AH, Kenney MK. Children and youth with special health care needs: a profile. *Pediatrics.* 2022;149 e2021056150D.

40. Cohen E, Berry JG, Sanders L, Schor EL, Wise PH. Status complexicus? The emergence of pediatric complex care. *Pediatrics.* 2018;141(Supplement_3):S202–S211.

41. Bethell CD, Blumberg SJ, Stein RE, Strickland B, Robertson J, Newacheck PW. Taking stock of the CSHCN screener: a review of common questions and current reflections. *Acad Pediatr.* 2015;15:165–176.

42. Schapiro NA, Mejia J. Adolescent confidentiality and women's health: History, rationale, and current threats. *Nurs Clin North Am.* 2018;53:145–156.

43. Sharko M, Jameson R, Ancker JS, Krams L, Webber EC. *Rosenbloom ST State-by-State Variability in Adolescent Privacy Laws. Pediatrics.* 2022;149(6). https://doi.org/10.1542/peds.2021-053458.

44. Schapiro NA, Mihaly LK. The 21st century cures act and challenges to adolescent confidentiality. *J Pediatr Health Care.* 2021;35:439–442.

45. Carlson J, Goldstein R, Hoover K, Tyson N. NASPAG/SAHM statement: the 21st century cures act and adolescent confidentiality. *J Pediatr Adolesc Gynecol.* 2021;34:3–5.

46. Ginsburg KR, Ramirez McClain ZR.*Reaching Teens: Strength-Based Communication Strategies to Build Resilience and Support Healthy Adolescent Development.* 2nd ed. Chicago: American Academy of Pediatrics; 2020.

47. Klein DA, Paradise SL, Landis CA. Screening and counseling adolescents and young adults: A framework for comprehensive care. *Am Fam Physician.* 2020;101:147–158.

48. Doukrou M, Segal TY. Fifteen-minute consultation: communicating with young people—how to use HEEADSSS, a psychosocial interview for adolescents. *Arch Dis Child Educ Pract Ed.* 2017;102:226–229.

49. Svetaz MV, Miller K, Gewirtz O'Brien J, McPherson L. Adolescent health: communication with adolescent patients. *FP Essent.* 2021;507:11–18.

50. Neinstein LS, Katzman DK, Callahan T, Joffe A, Rickert VI.*Neinsteint's Adolescent and Young Adult Health Care: A Practical Guide.* 6th ed. Riverwoods: Wolters Kluwer; 2016.

51. Shteyler VM, Clarke JA, Adashi EY. Failed assignments—Rethinking sex designations on birth certificates. *N Engl J Med.* 2020;383:2399–2401.

ENVIRONMENTAL HEALTH HISTORY

Karen G. Duderstadt

Environment is a key determinant of health, and children are vulnerable to environmental risks. The developing fetus and the young child are particularly vulnerable to the neurodevelopmental effects of environmental toxins because of their rapid periods of brain growth and development in the first 2 years of life. Environmental health hazards include physical agents; chemical agents; outdoor and indoor air contaminants; water, soil, or dust contaminants; biologic irritants; allergens; toxins; infectious agents; and extreme weather events.

ENVIRONMENTAL HEALTH

Environmental health is defined broadly and includes environment as a basic determinant of human health and illness. The long-term goal of environmental health is to safeguard children's health and improve the environments where children live, learn, and play.[1] Children can encounter environmental hazards and be exposed to many different toxic substances in the home, car, school, childcare setting, play environments, and community. Young children spend 80% to 90% of their time indoors, and the home and childcare environments are their primary sources of exposure to environmental hazards.[2]

Environmental inequities and injustices in under-resourced communities contribute to the higher burden of toxic exposures in children. In the United States, disparities exist related to toxic environmental exposures in areas predominantly populated by persons of color or persons living in poverty, such as increased rates of low birth weight, preterm births, and increased incidence of asthma.[3,4] In 2021, the U.S. Environmental Protection Agency (EPA) defined *environmental justice* as "the fair treatment and meaningful involvement of all people regardless of race, color, national origin, or income, with respect to the development, implementation, and enforcement of environmental laws, regulations, and policies."[5] Children in under-resourced communities face higher exposures to environmental pollutants and hazards and in many communities have limited access to protective factors such as quality health care services.[6]

It is critically important for pediatric health care providers to understand the impact of environmental hazards and exposures on the healthy growth and development of infants and children. Health care providers have a professional responsibility to identify and understand the environmental health risks present in the communities in which they work, to access available health risk data from community surveillance programs, and to report exposures to appropriate local and state authorities. Furthermore, providers are mandated to conduct appropriate screening tests and to educate children and families about toxic environmental health risks.

PHYSIOLOGIC VULNERABILITIES

Toxic substances are chemicals in the environment capable of causing harm. *Toxicants* are environmental hazards from chemical pollutants, and *toxins* are environmental hazards from biologic sources. Children have a larger ratio of surface area to body mass and have higher metabolic rates than adults, which increases their susceptibility to pesticides and other environmental toxicants.[6] Young children also breathe more air and drink more water per pound of body weight than adults, which results in greater exposure to toxic chemicals and air pollutants for their body weight. The skin, respiratory tract, and gastrointestinal tract in a child are particularly vulnerable to toxic substances, and children *absorb* toxic substances more readily and efficiently than adults.[7] Therefore, children absorb larger amounts of environmental toxins, kilogram for kilogram, than adults.

Children may also inhale a higher concentration of toxic substances because they live and play closer to environmental hazards on the ground. The breathing zone of a child is lower than adults, and chemical pollutants such as lead or mercury, chemicals vaporizing from carpets, flooring, or nap mats affect children at a greater rate than adults.[2] Children's higher metabolic rate increases their oxygen consumption and production of carbon dioxide (CO_2). The increased CO_2 exposes infants and children to higher levels of particulate matter in the air, which impacts lung development.[2] Children's metabolic pathways are also immature, and they *metabolize* toxic chemicals differently than adults because they lack the enzymes to break down and remove toxic chemicals from the body.[1]

DEVELOPMENTAL VULNERABILITIES

Children go through critical developmental periods or *windows of vulnerability* both prenatally and during early childhood. There are sensitive periods throughout childhood when rapid growth occurs and during which exposure to toxic or other harmful substances affects growth or damages organs or body systems. Children's genetic predisposition, social milieu, exposure to environmental hazards, and nutrition play an important role in their development.[2] Newborn immature organ systems

metabolize more slowly and make it difficult for infants to detoxify and excrete harmful substances. Prenatal exposure of the fetus to maternal smoking, substance use, and chemical or biologic agents increases the risk of absorption of toxicants and toxins. Toxicants such as illicit drugs, alcohol, cotinine from environmental tobacco smoke, mercury, and lead, all of which cross the placental barrier, contribute to low birth weight, intrauterine growth retardation, cognitive and developmental delays, and congenital birth defects. In the newborn, particular attention should be given to toxicants in breast milk or infant formula, dermal contacts, and caregiver occupations (see Fig. 5.1).

Infants and toddlers have expanded mobility, giving them increased exposure to their environment. They are particularly vulnerable to oral exposures because of their hand-to-mouth activity and inhaled substances within the physical zone they occupy near the ground. Children in early and middle childhood become susceptible to toxicants in the school, childcare settings, and playground environments. Occupational hazards are of particular concern in adolescents and young adults, as are harmful exposures that occur through experimentation with illicit drugs, alcohol, and intentional inhalation of other substances. Adolescents face increased risks to toxicants and pollutants due to short-term direct exposure through employment or recreation as well as long-term exposures.[6] Box 5.1 presents common indoor and outdoor air pollutants, contaminants in water and soil, food contaminants, and hazardous substances that children may be exposed to through parental or family employment or hobbies.

SOURCES OF ENVIRONMENTAL TOXINS

Children are at risk for environmental toxins from dust in homes containing lead-contaminated soil, paint chips, or peeling paint; industrial toxicants and oil drilling in or near neighborhoods, landfill sites, or waste treatment sites; pre-1989 plumbing in schools or

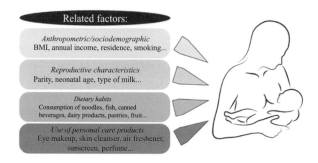

Related factors:

Anthropometric/sociodemographic
BMI, annual income, residence, smoking...

Reproductive characteristics
Parity, neonatal age, type of milk...

Dietary habits
Consumption of noodles, fish, canned
beverages, dairy products, pastries, fruit...

Use of personal care products
Eye makeup, skin cleanser, air freshener,
sunscreen, perfume...

FIGURE 5.1 Factors related to chemical exposures in breast milk. (From Iribarne-Durán L, Peinado F, Freirel C, Castillero-Rosales I, Artacho-Cordón F, Olea N. Concentrations of bisphenols, parabens, and benzophenones in human breast milk: a systematic review and meta-analysis. *Sci Total Environ.* 2022; 806:150437.)

BOX 5.1   RISK CATEGORIES OF ENVIRONMENTAL HAZARDS

Household Exposures and Indoor Air Pollutants
- Mold spores
- Animal dander
- Carbon monoxide
- Tobacco smoke
- Mercury vapors
- Radon
- Smoke from wood-burning stoves
- Lead
- Phthalates and plasticizers
- Personal care products or cosmetics

Outdoor Air Pollutants
- Pesticides
- Air particulates
- Ozone
- Insecticides
- Herbicides

School or Day Care Exposures
- Polychlorinated biphenyls
- Arsenic from pesticide-treated wood
- Pesticides
- Friable asbestos

Community and Outdoor Exposures
- Insecticides
- Herbicides

Water Pollutants
- Bacteria
- Parasites

Food Contaminants
- Mercury
- Pesticides

Unintentional Ingestions or Poisonings

Family Members' Occupations/Hobbies
- Paint contractors
- Car mechanics
- Smelters
- Agricultural workers or farm workers
- Miners
- Jewelry artists
- Stained-glass artists

Data from American Academy of Pediatrics. *Pediatric Environmental Hazards.* 4th ed. Council on Environmental Health; 2019.

---

homes with presence of lead pipes or lead solder; well water or contaminated tap water; and drinking water contaminated with lead or other toxins and toxicants. Children that play near high-traffic areas risk exposure to soil contaminated with old deposits from leaded gasoline. Children are also at increased risk for pesticide and organophosphate exposure, as they consume more fruits and vegetables per pound of body weight than adults. Children of farm workers are particularly vulnerable to pesticide and organophosphate exposure.

Children are at risk for indoor air pollutants such as environmental tobacco smoke. Over

---

BOX 5.2   PEDIATRIC HEALTH CONSEQUENCES OF CLIMATE CHANGE

The pediatric health consequences of climate change include:
- Exposure to waterborne illness
- Acute heat-related illnesses
- Adverse learning due to heat
- Negative mental health impacts including anxiety and depression

- Increased asthma and allergy exacerbations due to increases in particulate matter, pollen, and mold
- Increased risk for vector borne illnesses including those previously seen only in tropical climates such as malaria and dengue

Data from Fuller M, Duderstadt K. Environmental influences on pediatric health. In: Garzon D, Gaylord N, Driessnack M, Duderstadt K, eds. *Burn's Pediatric Primary Care*. 8th ed. Elsevier; 2023. Philipsborn RP, Chan K. Climate change and global child health. *Pediatrics*. 2018;141(6):e20173774.

40% of young children in the United States are exposed to secondhand smoke.[8] Mold, pesticide use in the home or school setting, products in the home containing lead, including pottery with lead glaze, put children at risk. Children's exposure to toxins may also occur through contact with a parent's workplace or work clothes, storage of hazardous materials, or activities of family members, such as soldering or refinishing furniture.

Children with asthma are at higher risk to exposure from outdoor air pollutants during the occurrence of extreme weather events due to climate change. Extreme weather events are associated with increased levels of pollen as well as other toxins and environmental hazards in the air and soil often as the result of hazardous smoke due to wildfires (see Box 5.2). These risks combined with increased carbon dioxide and other air pollutants lead to increased frequency and severity of pediatric asthma attacks.[9] Exposure to *particulate matter* in the air consists of extremely small particles and liquid droplets that can have adverse effects on developing lungs in infants and respiratory function in children and adolescents. Increased levels of particulate matter created by air pollution from gasoline, diesel engines, wood-burning stoves, the release of environmental toxins from industrial sources, and increased allergens can trigger and exacerbate pediatric asthma. Children living in under-resourced communities are at highest risk for exposure to outdoor air pollutants and environmental toxins due to environmental inequities and injustices.

Vaping and E-Cigarettes

Vaping and the use of electronic cigarettes (e-cigarettes) have increased significantly among the pediatric and adolescent population. Adolescents in the United States are initiating e-cigarette use at earlier ages. A recent study found that 28% of youth-initiated e-cigarette use at 14 years of age or younger, and 90% of adult smokers, begin smoking by 18 years of age.[10] E-cigarette pods are often flavored and may contain significantly more nicotine than traditional tobacco cigarettes (3% or 5% nicotine, or one pod equivalent to 1 to 2 packs of conventional cigarettes).[11] Studies have shown that the adolescent brain in particular is uniquely susceptible to nicotine addiction.[12] Most concerning is that 63% of adolescents reported that they did not know some vaping pens contained nicotine.[13] Lasting cognitive and behavioral impairments, disrupted memory, selective attention, and reduced executive function and activity of the prefrontal cortex have been associated with early uptake of traditional cigarettes and e-cigarettes.[14]

ENVIRONMENTAL HEALTH SCREENING HISTORY

All children and adolescents should have an environmental health screening history taken during routine primary care visits to establish the risk of exposures.[15] An environmental health screening history establishes known home, school, and/or community environmental health risks and a family history of parental or sibling exposure in the workplace. Environmental health screening history forms for use in establishing a risk profile for exposure to pesticides, poor indoor or outdoor air quality, contaminated drinking water, or chemical toxicants can be adapted for electronic medical record formats. A Pediatric Environmental History form for children from birth to 18 years of age with categories of environmental exposures and questions for parents and children for environmental risks is available at https://www.neefusa.org/resource/pediatric-environmental-history, and a Pediatric Asthma Environmental Health History form is available at https://www.neefusa.org/resource/asthma-environmental-history-form (see Figs. 5.2A and B).

The concept of *health risk communication* is particularly important to assessing environmental health in children and is part of a holistic approach to working with families in the clinical setting. *Health risk communication* requires active listening to identify caregiver concern and the public health risks of exposure to indoor and outdoor hazardous substances in the surrounding community. It requires determining the presence of an environmental hazard, assessment of the health risk, the severity of the exposure or dose, acceptability of the health risk, the impact on the health of the child or adolescent, and communicating the health risk effectively to the family.[8]

LEAD AND CHEMICAL EXPOSURES

No amount of lead exposure in children is safe, and children living in families with food insecurity are at risk for poor nutrition resulting in iron or calcium deficiency and at particular risk for enhanced uptake of lead and lead toxicity in the body. Immigrant and refugee children who live in under-resourced communities in the United States are also at higher risk for elevated blood lead levels

(BLLs) due to air, food, and water contaminated with heavy metals, including lead. It is important for providers to screen the pediatric immigrant population for lead toxicity from exposures in their country of origin. Fig. 5.3 illustrates the primary organs and body systems affected by exposure to environmental hazards.

Millions of homes in the United States may still contain lead paint under layers of newer paint, and children are now more likely to be exposed to lead paint by consuming paint chips or exposure to contaminated dust or soil within or around the home. Children with excess lead levels usually show no unique features on physical examination. Environmental lead exposures are often insidious and affect the internal organs and brain. Children with lead toxicity may present with one or more of the following symptoms: fatigue, malaise, abdominal pain, loss of appetite, constipation, irritability, headache, weakness, or clumsiness. Any signs of developmental delay, neurobehavioral disorders such as tics, persistent hand-to-mouth activity such as pica, unexplained seizures, anemia, chronic abdominal pain, learning difficulties, or attention deficit/hyperactivity disorder warrant an in-depth environmental health history to relate positive exposure to environmental toxins and hazards.

Pediatric health care providers should take the primary role in screening for risk of environmental exposure to lead. Lead screening in children is routinely performed in most pediatric health care settings at the 12-month and 24-month well-child visits but should not be overlooked in older children with risk factors for lead exposure. Educating individual families and monitoring the health status of children and infants with BLLs above the 97.5th percentile or greater than $2.0\,\mu g/dL$ is key in preventing long-term health effects until community and environmental investigation and mitigation have been implemented. The U.S. EPA recently updated resources to protect environmentally overburdened and under-resourced

Pediatric Environmental History (0-18 Years of Age)

The Screening Environmental History

For all of the questions below, most are often asked about the child's primary residence. Although some questions may specify certain locations, one should always consider all places where the child spends time, such as daycare centers, schools, and relative's houses.

Where does your child live and spend most of his/her time? _____

What are the age, condition, and location of your home? _____

Does anyone in the family smoke? ❑ Yes ❑ No ❑ Not sure

Do you have a carbon monoxide detector? ❑ Yes ❑ No ❑ Not sure

Do you have any indoor furry pets? ❑ Yes ❑ No ❑ Not sure

What type of heating/air system does your home have?
❑ Radiator ❑ Forced air ❑ Gas stove ❑ Wood stove ❑ Other_____

What is the source of your drinking water?
❑ Well water ❑ City water ❑ Bottled water

Is your child protected from excessive sun exposure? ❑ Yes ❑ No ❑ Not sure

Is your child exposed to any toxic chemicals of which you are aware? ❑ Yes ❑ No ❑ Not sure

What are the occupations of all adults in the household? _____

Have you tested your home for radon? ❑ Yes ❑ No ❑ Not sure

Does your child watch TV, or use a computer or video game system more than two hours a day? ❑ Yes ❑ No ❑ Not sure

How many times a week does your child have unstructured, free play outside for at least 60 minutes? _____

Do you have any other questions or concerns about your child's home environment or symptoms that may be a result of his or her environment? _____

Follow up/ Notes
_____
_____
_____

The Screening Environmental History is taken in part from the following sources:

■ American Academy of Pediatrics Committee on Environmental Health. Pediatric Environmental Health 2nd ed. Etzel RA, Balk SJ, Eds. Elk Grove Village, IL: American Academy of Pediatrics; 2003. Chapter 4: How to Take an Environmental History.

■ Balk SJ. The environmental history: asking the right questions. *Contemp Pediatr.* 1996;13:19-36.

■ Frank A, Balk S, Carter W, et al. Case Studies in Environmental Medicine. Agency for Toxic Substances and Disease Registry, Atlanta GA. 1992, rev. 2000. Taking an Exposure History.

This screening environmental history is designed to capture most of the common environmental exposures to children. The screening history can be administered regularly during well-child exams as well as to assess whether an environmental exposure plays a role in a child's symptoms. If a positive response is given to one or more of the screening questions, the primary care provider can consider asking questions on the topic provided in the Additional Categories and Questions to Supplement the Screening Environmental History, accessible at www.neefusa.org/pdf/PEHIhistory.pdf.

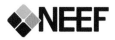

Additional resources and Spanish language materials available at www.neefusa.org/health
health@neefusa.org

A

FIGURE 5.2 **(A)** Pediatric Environmental Health History form.

Pediatric Environmental History (0-18 Years of Age)

Additional Categories and Questions to Supplement
The Screening Environmental History

For all of the questions below, most are often asked about the child's primary residence. Although some questions may specify certain locations, one should always consider all places where the child spends time, such as daycare centers, schools, and relative's houses.

General Housing Characteristics (For lead poisoning, refer to Table 3.2 in CDC Managing Elevated Blood Lead Levels Among Young Children 1.usa.gov/KAL9Yc)

Do you own or rent your home?	_____
What year was your home built? (Or: Was your home built before 1978? 1950?)	_____
Has your child been tested for lead?	❏ Yes ❏ No ❏ Not sure
Is there a family member or playmate with an elevated blood lead level?	❏ Yes ❏ No ❏ Not sure
Does your child spend significant time at another location? (e.g. baby sitters, school, daycare?)	_____

Indoor home environment (For asthma, refer to Environmental History Form for Pediatric Asthma Patient goo.gl/4JdUls)

If a family member smokes, does this person want to quit smoking?	❏ Yes ❏ No ❏ Not sure
Is your child exposed to smoke at the baby sitters, school, or daycare center?	❏ Yes ❏ No ❏ Not sure
Do regular visitors to your home smoke?	❏ Yes ❏ No ❏ Not sure
Have there been renovations or new carpet or furniture in the home during the past year?	❏ Yes ❏ No ❏ Not sure
Does your home have carpet?	❏ Yes ❏ No ❏ Not sure
Is the room where your child sleeps carpeted?	❏ Yes ❏ No ❏ Not sure
Do you use a wood stove or fire place?	❏ Yes ❏ No ❏ Not sure
Have you had water damage, leaks, or a flood in your home?	❏ Yes ❏ No ❏ Not sure
Do you see cockroaches in your home daily or weekly?	❏ Yes ❏ No ❏ Not sure
Do you see rats and/or mice in your home weekly?	❏ Yes ❏ No ❏ Not sure
Do you have smoke detectors in your home?	❏ Yes ❏ No ❏ Not sure

Air Pollution/Outdoor Environment (For asthma, refer to Environmental History Form for Pediatric Asthma Patient goo.gl/4JdUls)

Is your home near an industrial site, hazardous waste site, or landfill?	❏ Yes ❏ No ❏ Not sure
Is your home near major highways or other high traffic roads?	❏ Yes ❏ No ❏ Not sure
Are you aware of Air Quality Alerts in your community?	❏ Yes ❏ No ❏ Not sure
Do you change your child's activity when an Air Quality Alert is issued?	❏ Yes ❏ No ❏ Not sure
Do you live on or near a farm where pesticides are used frequently?	❏ Yes ❏ No ❏ Not sure

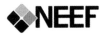

B

FIGURE 5.2—CONT'D **(B)** Pediatric Asthma Environmental Health History form.

Food and Water Contamination

If you use well water for drinking, when was the last time the water was tested?
  Coliform bacteria_____ Other microbials_____ Nitrites/nitrates_____ Arsenic_____ Pesticides_____

For all types of water sources:

Have you tested your water for lead?	❑ Yes ❑ No ❑ Not sure
Do you mix infant formula with tap water?	❑ Yes ❑ No ❑ Not sure

Which types of seafood do you normally eat?   _____

How many times per month do you eat that particular fish or shellfish?   _____

How many times a week do you eat any of the following types of fish?
  Shark_____ Swordfish_____ Tile fish_____ King mackerel_____ Albacore tuna_____ Other_____

How often do you wash fruits and vegetables before giving them to your child? _____

What type of produce do you buy? ❑ Organic ❑ Local ❑ Grocery store ❑ Other

---

Toxic Chemical Exposures (Also refer to Taking an Environmental History and Environmental and Occupational History in Recognition and Management of Pesticide Poisonings)

Consider this set of questions for patients with seizures, frequent headaches, or other unusual or chronic symptoms

How often are pesticides applied inside your home?	_____
How often are pesticides applied outside your home?	_____
Where do you store chemicals/pesticides?	_____
Do you often use solvents or other cleaning or disinfectant chemicals?	_____
Do you have a deck or play structure made from pressure treated wood?	❑ Yes ❑ No ❑ Not sure
Have you applied a sealant to the wood in the past year?	❑ Yes ❑ No ❑ Not sure
What do you use to prevent mosquito bites to your children?	_____
How often do you apply that product?	_____

Occupations and Hobbies

What type of work does your child/teenager do?	_____
Do any adults work around toxic chemicals?	❑ Yes ❑ No ❑ Not sure
If so, do they shower and change clothes before returning home from work?	❑ Yes ❑ No ❑ Not sure
Does the child or any family member have arts, crafts, ceramics, stained glass work or similar hobbies?	❑ Yes ❑ No ❑ Not sure

---

Health Related Questions

Have you ever relocated due to concerns about an environmental exposure?	❑ Yes ❑ No ❑ Not sure
Do symptoms seem to occur at the same time of day?	❑ Yes ❑ No ❑ Not sure
Do symptoms seem to occur after being at the same place every day?	❑ Yes ❑ No ❑ Not sure
Do symptoms seem to occur during a certain season?	❑ Yes ❑ No ❑ Not sure
Are family members/neighbors/co-workers experiencing similar symptoms?	❑ Yes ❑ No ❑ Not sure
Are there environmental concerns in your neighborhood, child's school, or day care?	❑ Yes ❑ No ❑ Not sure

Has any family member had a diagnosis of any of the following?
  ❑ Asthma ❑ Autism ❑ Cancer ❑ Learning disability

Does your child suffer from any of the following recurrent symptoms?
  ❑ Cough ❑ Headaches ❑ Fatigue ❑ Unexplained pain_____

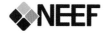

FIGURE 5.2—CONT'D

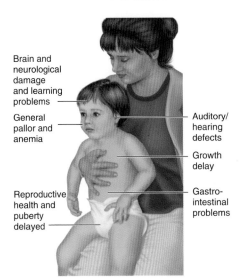

Brain and neurological damage and learning problems

General pallor and anemia

Auditory/hearing defects

Growth delay

Gastro-intestinal problems

Reproductive health and puberty delayed

FIGURE 5.3 Effects of lead exposure on a child's body.

communities from lead exposure. The culturally and linguistically appropriate resources are available at https://www.epa.gov/lead.

Lead is not the only toxic ingredient found in paint. Household paint, as well as children's craft paint, can contain volatile organic compounds (VOCs). VOCs are gasses, such as benzene, formaldehyde, toluene, and xylene, that are emitted into the air from products or processes and can be toxic by themselves but can also react with other gasses in the air to create air pollution.[16] Symptoms of acute VOC exposure are eye irritation, respiratory tract irritation, headaches, dizziness, visual disorders, and impaired memory whereas long-term exposures can cause cancer and damage the nervous system, kidneys, and liver.[17]

Per- and polyfluoroalkyl substances (PFAS) are a group of man-made chemicals that are found in a wide range of products that are used daily such as food packaging, cookware, pizza boxes, stain repellents, nonstick products, and waxes.[18] Other sources of PFAS include exposure from contaminated drinking water or eating fish caught from contaminated waters through industrial or disposal sites.[19] PFAS

exposure in childhood can accumulate and stay in the body and the environment for long periods, affecting the reproductive organs and thyroid hormone receptors. It can also cause reduced bone mineral density, a risk factor for development of osteoporosis. Prenatal exposure to PFAS chemicals has been associated with ADHD in young school-age children.[20] Counseling families about PFAS exposures and limiting risks in the home is an important component of anticipatory guidance in pediatrics.

ENDOCRINE-DISRUPTING CHEMICALS AND PESTICIDES

Endocrine-disrupting chemicals are chemically manufactured or naturally occurring substances that alter the hormonal system through environmental or developmental exposures resulting in adverse health effects.[21] They are present in the environment in food, water, soil, pesticides, plastics, personal care products, and drugs. Exposure can be through ingestion, topically, and transplacentally to the fetus. Phthalates, bisphenol A (BPA), and polychlorinated biphenyls (PCBs) are three of the high-volume chemicals present in the environment and are known endocrine disruptors. Ingestion is the primary means of exposure, though inhalation and exposure through the skin also occurs.[8] They have a high degree of stability and do not degrade rapidly once discarded, continuing to pollute the environment. As fat-soluble substances, they accumulate in the body and have a very long half-life.[22] Developing body tissues are more vulnerable to endocrine disruption than mature tissues; transplacental transfer to the developing fetus is of great concern; exposure to phthalates is associated with higher risk for preterm birth.[23]

Epoxy resins are used as coatings for liners in food and beverage cans. Phthalates are also found in personal care products, plastic toys, food packaging, car seats, floor coverings, medical tubing, and many other products. BPA is an endocrine-disrupting chemical that can cause hormonal abnormalities and adverse effects on neurodevelopment. It is found in plastic water bottles, some infant feeding bottles, water main filters, dental sealants, and paint products.[8] PCBs are synthetic organic chemicals associated with harmful effects in humans. Although PCBs are no longer manufactured in the United States, they are resistant to degradation and remain in the environment, where they are hazardous to human and animal health. Phytoestrogens, which are naturally occurring substances found in some food and soy products, also can have hormone-like activity in prepubertal children.

Endocrine-disrupting chemicals can mimic naturally occurring hormones such as estrogens and androgens (sex hormones), and thyroid hormones, producing overstimulation of the endocrine system; they affect the normal function of tissues and organs, which can result in abnormal gonadal development. Low-dose exposure over time and extremely high-dose exposures to endocrine-disrupting chemicals have significant effects on the fetus and growing and developing child, decreased sperm counts, infertility, testicular cancer, cryptorchidism, hypospadias, thyroid disorders, diabetes, and some childhood cancers.[21] Exposure to endocrine-disrupting chemicals in childhood is associated with earlier onset of puberty.[21]

EVIDENCE-BASED PRACTICE TIP

Breast milk and polycarbonate feeding bottles are the primary sources of BPA exposure among infants, and canned foods are the primary source of BPA exposure in children.[24,25] Counseling families on the use of BPA-free feeding bottles and personal care products can decrease levels of exposure.[25]

DIAGNOSTICS

Valid and reliable laboratory tests have not been developed to assess for exposure to many environmental toxins. Testing for toxins is not performed at all laboratories. There is also often a lapse between exposure and testing, and the levels may not reflect the total burden of the environmental contaminant on the developing child.

If the health care provider suspects an uncommon exposure to chemical toxins, the regional Pediatric Environmental Health Specialty Units (PEHSU) will provide expert advice on whether and how to test. Prior to ordering any tests, key questions to consider including in the health history[25]:

- Could the health problem be related to an environmental exposure? What are the possible exposures in the child's environment?
- Did the potential exposure clearly occur prior to the onset of the health problem?
- Are laboratory tests available to document the exposure? Will the laboratory measurements accurately reflect toxicity if present? What is required to perform the testing? What is the cost of testing? What is the timeline from testing to receiving results?
- Will the results change the treatment plan for the child and family? Will it inform care?

See Table 5.1 for available laboratory tests for environmental hazards. Exposure to significant levels of toxicants should be reported to local and state authorities and the regional PESHUs at https://www.pehsu.net/.

RESOURCES

Resources on environmental health and the impact on children and families are available to pediatric health care providers through governmental, public health, and environmental health agencies and are important in assisting with comprehensive screening for environmental hazards (Box 5.3). Having access to evidence-based research and resources on environmental health is key to responsible health-risk screening and health-risk communication to parents, caregivers, and families.

TABLE 5.1 LABORATORY TESTING FOR ENVIRONMENTAL TOXINS	
Environmental Hazard Exposure	Diagnostic Study
Lead	Blood lead level, free erythrocyte protoporphyrin, zinc protoporphyrin
Carbon monoxide	Carboxyhemoglobin level
Mercury	Blood mercury level, 24-hr urine sample, hair analysis with atomic absorption spectrometry
Pesticide metabolites and organophosphates	Plasma cholinesterase levels
Tobacco metabolites	Urine cotinine assays
Polychlorinated biphenyls	Gas-liquid chromatography
Heavy metals, arsenic	24-hr urine sample

Data from Fuller M, Duderstadt K. Environmental influences on pediatric health. In: Garzon D, Gaylord N, Driessnack M, Duderstadt K, eds. *Burn's Pediatric Primary Care*. 8th ed. Elsevier; 2023. Philipsborn RP, Chan K. Climate change and global child health. Pediatrics. 2018;141(6):e20173774.

BOX 5.3   ENVIRONMENTAL HEALTH RESOURCES

Air Quality Monitoring
https://www2.purpleair.com/
Children's Environmental Health Network
http://www.cehn.org
National Center for Environmental Health
http://www.cdc.gov/nceh
Center for Health, Environment and Justice
http://www.chej.org
Columbia University's Center for Children's Environmental Health
https://www.publichealth.columbia.edu/research/columbia-center-childrens-environmental-health
The National Environmental Education Foundation
http://www.neefusa.org/
Healthy Schools Network, Inc.
http://www.healthyschools.org
U.S. Environmental Protection Agency: Lead Training and Educational Outreach

https://www.epa.gov/lead/local-training-and-outreach
World Health Organization: Health Impact Assessment
https://www.who.int/health-topics/health-impact-assessment - tab=tab_1
National Institute of Environmental Health Sciences: Endocrine Disruptors
http://www.niehs.nih.gov/health/topics/agents/endocrine/index.cfm
U.S. Department of Health & Human Services: Bisphenol A (BPA) Information for Parents
https://www.niehs.nih.gov/health/topics/agents/sya-bpa/index.cfm
EPA Pediatric Environmental Health Speciality Units
https://www.pehsu.net/

SUMMARY OF ENVIRONMENTAL HEALTH SCREENING

- Children are uniquely vulnerable to environmental health hazards, including physical agents; chemical agents; outdoor and indoor air contaminants; water, soil, or dust contaminants; biologic irritants; allergens; toxins; infectious agents; and extreme weather events.
- Children have a larger ratio of surface area to body mass and have higher metabolic rates than adults, which increases their

susceptibility to pesticides and other environmental toxicants.

- The child's skin, respiratory tract, and gastrointestinal tract are particularly vulnerable to toxic substances and absorb substances more readily and efficiently than those of an adult.
- Children may inhale a higher concentration of toxic substances because they live and play closer to environmental hazards on the ground.
- Children's metabolic pathways are immature, and they metabolize toxic chemicals differently than adults due to the lack of enzymes to break down and remove toxic chemicals from the body.
- Children are at risk for indoor air pollutants such as environmental tobacco smoke, mold, contaminated dust particles, pesticides in the home or school, and products containing lead.
- Children living in under-resourced communities face higher exposures to environmental pollutants and hazards, particularly outdoor air pollutants and environmental toxins due to environmental inequities and injustices.

- An environmental health history establishes known home, school, and/or community environmental health risks and a family history of caregiver exposure in the workplace.

DOCUMENTATION

Environmental Exposure History of a 2½-Year-Old
Lives in housing built before 1978; mother reports mold on the bedroom and bathroom walls; unrepaired water damage on external walls of building for 2 years; residence overlooks a large gas station and a high-traffic area

DOCUMENTATION

Environmental Exposure History of a 5-Year-Old
Lives on a farm, pesticides used seasonally on crops; father works part-time as a crop duster; house built before 1950, current renovations to living area; house is partially heated with a wood stove; parents refinish old furniture in garage adjacent to house; primary source of drinking water for family is well water

REFERENCES

1. Landrigan PJ, Fuller R, Fisher S, et al. Pollution and children's health. *Sci Total Environ*. 2019;650:2389–2394.
2. AAP Council on Environmental Health. Children's unique vulnerability to environmental hazards. In: Etzel R, ed. *Pediatric Environmental Health*. 4th ed. American Academy of Pediatrics; 2019.
3. Bailey Z, Feldman J, Bassett M. How structural racism work-Racist policies as a root cause of U.S. racial health inequities. *N Engl J Med*. 2021;384:768–773.
4. Nardone A, Rudolph K, Morello-Frosch R, Casey J. Redlines and greenspace: The relationship between historical redlining and 2010 greenspace across the United States. *Environ Health Perspect*. 2021;129:17006.
5. Agency E.P. Environmental Justice. https://www.epa.gov/environmentaljustice
6. Mastorci F, Linzalone N, Ait-Ali L, Pingitore A. Environment in children's health: a new challenge for risk assessment. *Int J Environ Res Public Health*. 2021; 18:10445.
7. Etzel RA. The special vulnerability of children. *Int J Hyg Environ Health*. 2020;227:113516.
8. American Academy of Pediatrics *Pediatric Environmental Hazards*. 4th ed. Council on Environmental Health; 2019.
9. Poole JA, Barnes CS, Demain JG, et al. Impact of weather and climate change with indoor and outdoor air quality in asthma: a work group report of the AAAAI Environmental Exposure and Respiratory Health Committee. *J Allergy Clin Immunol*. 2019;143:1702–1710.
10. Evans-Polce R, Veliz P, Boyd C, McCabe V, McCabe S. Trends in c-cigarette, cigarette, cigar, and smokeless tobacco use among US adolescent cohorts, 2014–2018. *Am J Public Health*. 2020;110:163–165.
11. Willett J, Bennett M, Hair E, et al. Recognition, use and perceptions of JUUL among youth and young adults. *Tobacco Control*. 2019;28:115–116.
12. Smith R, McDonald C, Bergstrom H, Ehlinger D, Brielmaier J. Adolescent nicotine induces persisting changes in

development of neural connectivity. *Neurosci Biobehav Rev.* 2015;55:432–443.

13. Fadus M, Smith T, LM S. The rise of e-cigarettes, pod mod devices, and JUUL among youth: factors influencing use, health implications, and downstream effects. *Drug Alcohol Depend.* 2019;201:85–93.

14. England L, Bunnell R, Pechacek T, Tong V, MacAfee T. Nicotine and the developing brain: a neglected element in the electronic cigarette debate. *Am J Prev Med.* 2015;49:286–293.

15. National Environmental Education Foundation. Pediatric Environmental History. Accessed November 2022. https://www.neefusa.org/resource/pediatric-environmental-history

16. American Lung Association. Volatile Organic Compounds. November 2022. https://www.lung.org/cleanair/at-home/indoor-air-pollutants/volatile-organic-compounds

17. Huffling k, McLaughlin J. Pediatric chemical exposures: opportunities for prevention. *J Pediatr Health Care.* 2022;36(1):27–33. https://doi.org/10.1016/j.pedhc.2021.09.009

18. U.S. Environmental Protection Agency. Basic Information on PFAS. Accessed November 2022. https://www.epa.gov/pfas/basic-information-pfas

19. Agency for Toxic Substances and Disease Registry. Per- and polyfluoroalkyl substances (PFAS) and your health. Accessed November 2022. https://www.atsdr.cdc.gov/pfas/health-effects/overview.html

20. Vuonga A, Websterb G, Yolton K, et al. Prenatal exposure to per- and polyfluoroalkyl substances (PFAS) and neurobehavior in US children through 8 years of age: The HOME study. *Envrion Res.* 2021;195:110825.

21. Lopez-Rodriguez D, Franssen D, Heger S, Parent A. Endocrine-disrupting chemicals and their effects on puberty. *Best Pract Res Clin Endocrinol Metab.* 2021;35(5):101579.

22. Yilmaz B, Terekeci H, Sandal S, Kelestimur F. Endocrine disrupting chemicals: exposure, effects on human health, mechanism of action, models for testing and strategies for prevention. *Rev Endocr Metab Disord.* 2020;21:127–147.

23. Welch BM KA, Buckley JP, et al. Associations between prenatal urinary biomarkers of phthalate exposure and preterm birth: a pooled study of 16 US cohorts. *JAMA Pediatr.* 2022;176:895–905.

24. Iribarne-Durán L, Peinado F, FreireI C, Castillero-Rosales I, Artacho-Cordón F, Olea N. Concentrations of bisphenols, parabens, and benzophenones in human breast milk: a systematic review and meta-analysis.. *Sci Total Environ.* 2022;806:150437.

25. Fuller M, Duderstadt K. Environmental influences on pediatric health. In: Garzon D, Gaylord N, Driessnack M, Duderstadt K, eds. *Burn's Pediatric Primary Care.* 8th ed. Elsevier; 2023.

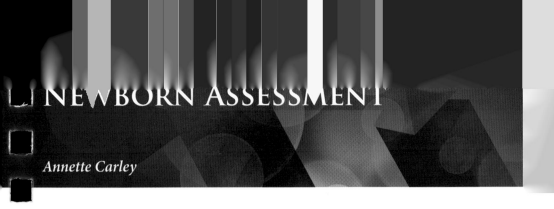

NEWBORN ASSESSMENT

Annette Carley

FETAL TRANSITION

The transition to extrauterine life for the newborn requires readily adapting from a dependent state to a newly expected independent state. Important physiologic adjustments occur in pulmonary, cardiovascular, thermoregulatory, and immunologic adaptation to the external environment.[1] During fetal life, with development of the respiratory system, pulmonary fluid occupies the evolving alveoli due to secretions from pulmonary epithelial cells necessary to ensure alveolar growth. Although production of this fluid normally decreases close to the time of delivery, residual fluid must be cleared to allow the lungs to expand with gas postnatally. Chemical stimuli such as decreased oxygen concentration and pH prompt the respiratory center receptors to initiate respirations. Paralleling these pulmonary changes are adaptations in circulatory patterns to redirect blood flow postnatally to the lungs. In utero, pulmonary blood vessels are constricted to facilitate flow away from unventilated lungs not yet participating in oxygenation. A series of circulatory shunts, the *ductus arteriosus*, *ductus venosus*, and *foramen ovale*, facilitate optimizing delivery of highly oxygenated blood from the placenta to the systemic circulation while bypassing the fetal lung (Fig. 6.1).[1,2]

Postnatally, the newborn must transition to sustained pulmonary ventilation by establishing adequate respirations for the exchange of gases. Postnatal changes in pulmonary and systemic pressure dynamics include closure of the fetal circulatory shunts to allow establishment of an adult circulatory pattern and may result in transient murmurs in some newborns.[2] The *Apgar score* reflects the transition of the newborn postnatally and is performed at 1 minute and 5 minutes of life. The score provides a summative assessment of reliable indicators of successful transition, including heart rate, respiratory effort, muscle tone, reflex irritability, and color (Tables 6.1 and 6.2). Although not predictive of long-term perinatal or neurologic outcome, it remains the standard for assessing the newborn immediately after birth.[3]

Most often postnatally, the intricate transition to extrauterine life occurs rapidly and effectively. However, infants with system immaturity or other prenatal/birth complications or anomalies may not achieve adequate or complete transition. Approximately 10% of newborns will need some assistance to achieve successful pulmonary transition, although only 1% will require extensive respiratory support measures.[1] Although tachypnea may be present during the first postnatal hours from efforts to reabsorb alveolar fluid, persistence of this symptom may indicate poor transition. Clinical findings such as nasal flaring, expiratory grunting, or chest wall retractions may indicate respiratory distress needing intervention.[1,4]

Although most systems are anatomically complete by approximately 24 weeks gestation, many systems including the pulmonary system are functionally immature until closer to term. The pediatric health care provider must

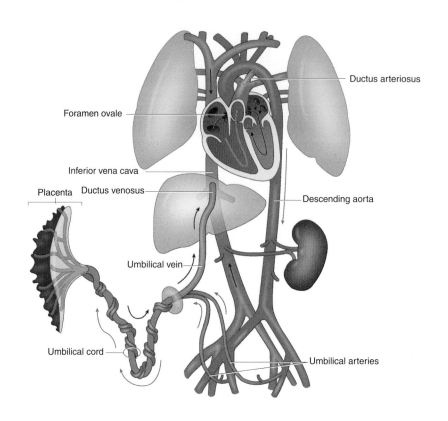

FIGURE 6.1 Fetal circulation.

TABLE 6.1	APGAR SCORING SYSTEM		
Sign	0	1	2
Heart rate	Absent	<100 beats per minute	>100 beats per minute
Respiratory rate	Absent	Irregular, slow, weak cry	Good, strong cry
Muscle tone	Limp	Some flexion of extremities	Well flexed
Reflex irritability	No response	Grimace	Cry, sneeze, active withdrawal
Color	Blue, pale	Acrocyanotic	Completely pink

Data from Apgar V. Evaluation of the newborn infant, second report. *JAMA*. 1958;168(15):1985–1988; American Academy of Pediatrics Committee on Fetus & Newborn; American College of Obstetricians & Gynecologists Committee on Obstetric Practice. The Apgar score. *Pediatrics*. 2015;136(4):819–822.

acknowledge the influences of gestational age, as well as circumstances of the ongoing fetal environment, labor and/or delivery risks, and early postnatal life in assessing the newborn to determine the need for intervention to support adequate transition.

TABLE 6.2	INTERPRETATION OF APGAR SCORES
Total Score	**Assessment**
0–2	Severe asphyxia
3–4	Moderate asphyxia
5–7	Mild asphyxia
8–10	No asphyxia

INFORMATION GATHERING OF PRENATAL AND BIRTH HISTORY

The Information Gathering table presents pertinent questions to ask about the maternal and prenatal history, neonatal history, and birth history. In addition, see prenatal and birth history in Information Gathering in Chapter 4.

INFORMATION GATHERING FOR PRENATAL AND BIRTH HISTORY

	Questions to Ask
Maternal and Prenatal History	History of prenatal care access? Maternal weight gain during pregnancy? General health during pregnancy? Any maternal infections or chronic health conditions (including diabetes, hypertension, asthma)? History of gestational diabetes or thyroid disease? Any use of drugs or alcohol during pregnancy? Maternal smoking during pregnancy? Any trauma or partner violence? History of maternal depression or anxiety disorder? Immunization status? Term birth? GTPAL (Gravidity, number of pregnancies; Term deliveries; Premature deliveries; Abortions, spontaneous or induced; Living children); medications taken during pregnancy. Results of prenatal testing, including maternal and fetal assessments. Complications in prior pregnancies.
Birth History	Vaginal or Cesarean birth? Prolonged labor with prolonged third stage? Precipitous delivery? Vacuum-assisted delivery? Breech or shoulder presentation? History of premature membrane rupture or maternal intrapartum fever? Maternal group B streptococcal (GBS) screen? Respiratory distress at birth? Apgar score and subsequent interventions? Amniotic fluid character?
Neonatal History	Risk factors for sepsis? Preterm birth? Group B streptococcal infection? Newborn screening results? Difficulties in feeding or stooling? Irritability or jitteriness? Jaundice? Length of hospitalization? Discharged with parent/co-partner?
Family and social History	Social: marital/partner status, living situation, financial, social supports. Substance use, including smoking, alcohol, and other drugs? Family: inherited diseases? Congenital anomalies? Consider a genogram if infant has a congenital disorder or disease that might have a genetic etiology.

ASSESSMENT OF GESTATIONAL AGE

An important component of newborn assessment is establishing gestational age. Obtaining an accurate assessment of gestational age begins with the prenatal and birth history and can assist the provider in anticipating conditions associated with preterm birth. Infants can be classified by gestational age as *term infant*, *preterm infant*, or *postterm infant* depending on the number of completed postmenstrual weeks. *Term infants* are born between the start of the 38th and completion of the 41st gestational week, whereas *preterm infants* are born prior to completing the 37th week and postterm infants are born following completion of the 41st week[5] (Fig. 6.2). Infants born preterm and postterm are at increased risk for postnatal complications. Preterm infants are at risk for system immaturity, notably the pulmonary, gastrointestinal, and neurologic

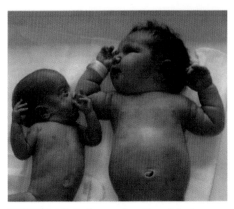

FIGURE 6.2 Preterm and postterm infant.

systems. Especially at lower gestational ages, preterm infants may develop complications such as respiratory distress syndrome, necrotizing enterocolitis, and intraventricular hemorrhage that can substantially impact survival. Postterm infants are at risk for birth complications, such as shoulder dystocia. If they are also *macrosomic* (greater than 4000 to 4500 grams), they are at added risk for poor tolerance of labor, pulmonary complications such

as meconium aspiration, and hypoglycemia. Gestational growth can be affected by maternal, placental, and fetal factors.[6] Accuracy in assessment of gestational age is thus essential for developing effective management plans.[5,6]

Gestational age can be estimated based on prenatal assessments with calculated dates based on last menstrual period, or postnatally using a standardized assessment tool that considers neuromuscular and physical criteria. The New Ballard Score (NBS) is the tool most used to evaluate gestational age postnatally (Fig. 6.3 and Box 6.1).[5,6] The NBS, consisting of six neuromuscular and six physical criteria, is validated to accurately estimate gestational age within 2 weeks for infants born between the 26th and 42nd gestational weeks if completed within 96 hours of birth (and accurate within 2 weeks for those born less than 26 weeks if completed within 12 hours of birth).[7] There is an increasing population of late preterm infants, defined as the infant whose postmenstrual age is 34 weeks 0/7 days to 36 weeks 6/7 days. These infants are not expected to be as physiologically competent as term infants and

---

BOX 6.1   TESTS FOR ASSESSING NEUROMUSCULAR MATURITY IN THE NEWBORN

Posture. With infant quiet and in supine position, observe degree of flexion in arms, legs. Muscle tone and degree of flexion increase with maturity. Full flexion of the arms, legs = 4.

Square window. With thumb supporting back of arm below wrist, apply gentle pressure with index and third fingers on dorsum of hand without rotating infant's wrist. Measure angle between base of thumb and forearm. Full flexion (hand lies flat on ventral surface of forearm) = 4.

Arm recoil. With infant supine, fully flex forearms on upper arms, hold for 5 s; pull down on hands to fully extend and rapidly release arms. Observe rapidity and intensity of recoil to state of flexion. A brisk return to full flexion = 4.

Popliteal angle. With infant supine and pelvis flat on firm surface, flex lower leg on thigh, then

flex thigh on abdomen. While holding knee with thumb and index finger, extend lower leg with index finger of other hand. Measure degree of angle behind knee (popliteal angle). Angle of <90 degrees = 5.

Scarf sign. With infant supine, support head in midline with one hand; use other hand to pull infant's arm across shoulder so that infant's hand touches shoulder. Determine location of elbow in relation to midline. Elbow does not reach midline = 4.

Heel to ear. With infant supine and pelvis flat on firm surface, pull foot as far as possible toward ear on same side. Measure distance of foot from ear and degree of knee flexion (same as popliteal angle). Knees flexed with popliteal angle of <90 degrees = 4.

Data from Hockenberry MJ, Rogers CC, Wilson D. *Wong's Essentials of Pediatric Nursing.* 11th ed, St. Louis: Mosby; 2022; Figures from Brozanski BS, et al. Neonatology. In: Zitelli BJ, McIntire SC, Nowalk AJ, Garrison J, eds. *Zitelli and Davis' Atlas of Pediatric Physical Diagnosis.* 8th ed. St. Louis: Mosby; 2023.

ESTIMATION OF GESTATIONAL AGE BY MATURITY RATING

Neuromuscular Maturity

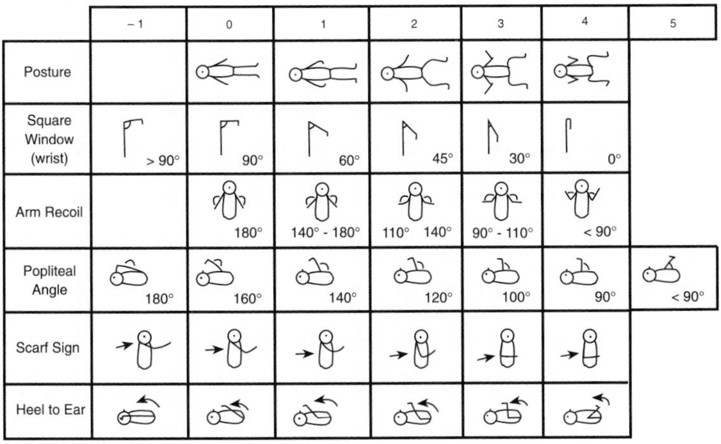

	− 1	0	1	2	3	4	5
Posture							
Square Window (wrist)	> 90°	90°	60°	45°	30°	0°	
Arm Recoil		180°	140° - 180°	110° 140°	90° - 110°	< 90°	
Popliteal Angle	180°	160°	140°	120°	100°	90°	< 90°
Scarf Sign							
Heel to Ear							

Physical Maturity

Skin	sticky friable transparent	gelatinous red, translucent	smooth pink, visible veins	superficial peeling &/or rash, few veins	cracking pale areas rare veins	parchment deep cracking no vessels	leathery cracked wrinkled
Lanugo	none	sparse	abundant	thinning	bald areas	mostly bald	
Plantar Surface	heel-toe 40-50 mm: -1 <40 mm: -2	>50 mm no crease	faint red marks	anterior transverse crease only	creases ant. 2/3	creases over entire sole	
Breast	imperceptible	barely perceptible	flat areola no bud	stippled areola 1-2 mm bud	raised areola 3-4 mm bud	full areola 5-10 mm bud	
Eye/Ear	lids fused loosely: -1 tightly: -2	lids open pinna flat stays folded	sl. curved pinna; soft; slow recoil	well-curved pinna; soft but ready recoil	formed & firm instant recoil	thick cartilage, ear stiff	
Genitals (male)	scrotum flat, smooth	scrotum empty faint rugae	testes in upper canal rare rugae	testes descending few rugae	testes down good rugae	testes pendulous, deep rugae	
Genitals (female)	clitoris prominent labia flat	prominent clitoris, small labia minora	prominent clitoris enlarging minora	majora & minora equally prominent	majora large minora small	majora cover clitoris & minora	

Maturity Rating

score	weeks
-10	20
-5	22
0	24
5	26
10	28
15	30
20	32
25	34
30	36
35	38
40	40
45	42
50	44

FIGURE 6.3 **New Ballard Score.** (From Ballard JL, Khoury JC, Wedig K et al. New Ballard Score, expanded to include extremely premature infants. *J Pediatr.* 1991; 119(3):418.)

may have issues that prolong hospitalization, including jaundice, poor feeding, hypoglycemia, apnea, and thermal instability.[1,5,6]

Congruence between growth measures and maturity is an important consideration in newborn assessment. When a newborn demonstrates expected growth at a given gestational age (if within 2 standard deviations [SDs] from the mean), the infant is classified as *appropriate for gestational age* (AGA). Infants whose growth exceeds standards for a given gestational age are considered *large for gestational age* (LGA), and conversely those whose growth is less than the standard for a given gestational age are classified as *small for gestational age* (SGA).[5,6]

Newborns are also classified by birth weight, and the terms *normal birth weight,*

TABLE 6.3	CLASSIFICATIONS OF NEWBORN BY WEIGHT
Gestational Age	Expected Growth Parameters
Appropriate for gestational age (AGA)	Growth parameters for gestational age between 10th and 90th percentile
Small for gestational age (SGA)	Weight below 10th percentile for gestational age
Large for gestational age (LGA)	Weight above 90th percentile for gestational age
Normal term birth weight	Weight between 10th and 90th percentile
Low birth weight (LBW)	Weight below 2.5 kg
Very low birth weight (VLBW)	Weight below 1.5 kg
Extremely low birth weight (ELBW)	Weight below 1 kg

Data from Chiocca EM. Assessment of the neonate. In: Chiocca EM, ed. *Advanced Pediatric Assessment*. 3rd ed. New York: Springer Publishing Company; 2019; Lopez L, Graziano PD. The neonatal physical exam. In: Koehn AR, ed. *Neonatal Nurse Practitioner Certification Intensive Review*. 1st ed. New York: Springer Publishing Company; 2019, pp. 27–57.

TABLE 6.4	CLASSIFICATION OF NEWBORNS BY GESTATIONAL AGE	
Gestational Age	**Completed Postmenstrual Weeks**	
Postterm	≥42 weeks	
Term	Completed >37 weeks	
Preterm	Born prior to 37 completed weeks	
Late preterm	Born between 34 weeks 0/7 days and 36 weeks 6/7 days	

Data from Rohan A. Common neonatal complications. In: Simpson KR, Creehan PA, eds. *Perinatal Nursing*, 5th ed. Philadelphia Wolters Kluwer-Lippincott Williams & Wilkins; 2019, pp 662–698; Trotter CW. Gestational age assessment. In Tappero EP, Honeyfield ME, eds. *Physical Assessment of the Newborn*. 6th ed. Petaluma: NICU INC, pp 23–43.

macrosomic, low birth weight (LBW), *very low birth weight* (VLBW), and *extremely low birth weight* (ELBW) are applied. Tables 6.3 and 6.4 present newborn weight and gestational age classifications. The etiologies of gestational age at birth and birth weight vary and may include maternal, placental, or fetal influences that can impact successful transition. Each of the gestational age and birth weight subgroups,

especially at extremes, carries potential for neonatal complications.[5]

Low Birth Weight Infants

LBW infants are those infants born weighing less than 2500 g. VLBW infants are those infants born weighing less than 1500 g at birth, and infants weighing ≤1000 g are considered ELBW.[5,6] Factors that contribute to the risk for LBW include maternal age, maternal health and nutrition, substance abuse during pregnancy, and access to prenatal care and health inequity.[7] Box 6.2 presents maternal risk factors for LBW and VLBW infants.

Small for Gestational Age

Infants with birth weight below the 10th percentile for age are considered SGA.[6] The head may be *microcephalic*, or small in proportion to the body, and *head circumference* may be below the fifth percentile for age. Fetal growth restriction may be symmetrical with all growth parameters smaller than expected, or asymmetrical with head sparing. The etiology of fetal growth abnormalities varies. Symmetric growth restriction may be due to intrinsic fetal conditions such as chromosomal abnormalities, whereas asymmetric growth restriction is often due to impaired placental perfusion

---

BOX 6.2   MATERNAL RISK
          FACTORS FOR LOW
          BIRTH WEIGHT AND
          VERY LOW BIRTH
          WEIGHT INFANTS

Maternal Risks
- Maternal age less than 16 or greater than 35 years of age
- Race and ethnicity
- Maternal chronic health conditions
- Maternal medications
- Nutritional status
- Environmental toxins or occupational chemical toxins
- Access to prenatal care and health inequity

Maternal Substance Abuse
- Alcoholism
- Tobacco use
- Illicit drug use
- Over-the-counter drug use

Data from LaBronte KH. Recording and evaluating the neonatal history. In Tappero EP, Honeyfield ME, eds. *Physical Assessment of the Newborn: A Comprehensive Approach to the Art of Physical Examination.* 6th ed. New York: Springer Publishing Company; 2019, pp 9–21.

BOX 6.3   MATERNAL RISK
          FACTORS FOR
          INTRAUTERINE
          GROWTH
          RETARDATION

Maternal Factors
- Maternal hypertension
- Maternal diabetes—poorly controlled
- Autoimmune disease
- Cardiac or respiratory disease
- Maternal infection
- Maternal chronic health conditions

Placental Factors
- Abnormal cord insertion or cord abnormalities
- Abnormal placentation
- Placental abruption

Fetal Factors
- Multiple gestations
- Chromosomal abnormalities
- Fetal infection

Data from Baschat, AA, Galan, HL. Fetal growth restriction. In Gabbe S, ed. *Obstetrics: Normal and Problem Pregnancies.* 8th ed. Philadelphia: Saunders.

---

or nutrient deprivation during fetal development.[6] With adequate nutrition, SGA infants experience overall catch-up growth. *Head circumference* is normally the first growth parameter to show catch-up growth, followed by weight and then length.

Newborns with intrauterine growth restriction (IUGR) have less than normal fetal weight, length, or head circumference (*occipitofrontal head circumference* [OFC]) expected for gestational age at birth due to a pathophysiologic process in utero (Box 6.3).[6] Infants with IUGR are not necessarily SGA because an IUGR infant may be below expected weight but not below the 10th percentile based on age at the time of measurement.

Large for Gestational Age

LGA is defined as birth weight greater than the 90th percentile for age.[6] The increased weight may result from fetal factors, which include genetic and chromosomal disorders, or from maternal factors, such as obesity or diabetes. *Maternal hyperglycemia* exposes the fetus to increased levels of glucose, which increases fetal insulin secretion. Increased insulin levels increase fat deposits in the fetus and often result in *macrosomia*, birth weight greater than 4000 g.[6] Diabetic mothers who are insulin dependent and in poor control during the early trimesters of pregnancy have characteristically large infants (Fig. 6.4). LGA infants are at risk for birth trauma, neonatal asphyxia, hypoglycemia, polycythemia, and hyperbilirubinemia.

Assessment of Growth Parameters

The assessment of the newborn begins with an evaluation of the stage of maturity and growth parameters. Measurements normally included in the newborn assessment are weight, length, and the OFC. Table 6.5 shows the reference values for common growth measures in term infants. The abdominal and chest circumference are not typically included in the regular

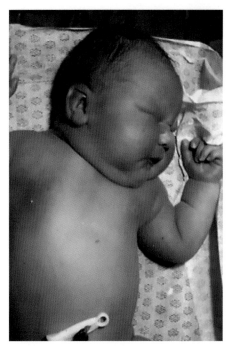

FIGURE 6.4 Macrosomic infant of diabetic mother. (From Meur S. Infant outcomes following diabetic pregnancies. *Paediatr Child Health (Oxford)*. 2007; 17(6):217–222.)

TABLE 6.5	TERM NEWBORN GROWTH PARAMETERS	
Measurement	**Normal Range**
OFC	33–36 cm Head approaches half the total body length
Length	44–55 cm
Weight	2500–3900 g
Chest circumference	30–36 cm (~1–3 cm < OFC) Average 1–2 cm less than OFC
Abdominal circumference	32–36 weeks gestation equal to OFC After 36 weeks gestation, greater than OFC

OFC, Occipitofrontal head circumference.
From Chiocca EM, ed. Assessment of the neonate. In: Chiocca EM *Advanced Pediatric Assessment*. 3rd ed. New York: Springer Publishing Company; 2019, pp 207–237; Fraser D. Chest and lungs assessment. In: Tappero EP, Honeyfield ME, eds. *Physical Assessment of the Newborn: A Comprehensive Approach to the Art of Physical Examination*. 6th ed. New York: Springer Publishing Company; 2019, pp 79–91; Goodwin M. Abdomen assessment. In: Tappero EP, Honeyfield ME, eds. *Physical Assessment of the Newborn: A Comprehensive Approach to the Art of Physical Examination*. 6th ed. New York: Springer Publishing Company; 2019, pp 111–120.

newborn examination in the absence of suspected clinical concerns.

For most accurate assessment of these measurements and subsequent plotting on a reference growth chart, the following is recommended:

- Length: measured as heel to crown with infant lying on flat surface and fully extended[8]
- Head circumference: measured with tape just above the brow line at the frontal prominence and on the occipital prominence. Note that transient head molding or overlapping of the cranial bones may affect this measurement.[9]
- Weight: obtained using a standardized scale; with infant unclothed or standardized measurement of diaper. Note that the newborn can lose up to 10% of birth weight during the first 72 hours following birth, due to contraction of the extracellular space.

The current recommendation in the United States is to use the WHO growth record for infants up to 2 years of age.[10]

PHYSICAL ASSESSMENT

Preparation for the Examination

Preparation and examination of the infant should ideally be in a well-lit room, while the infant is calm, ensuring that you are applying warm hands and warmed equipment. The infant should be weighed on an appropriately calibrated weight scale, height measurement should be obtained on a firm surface, and flexible tape measure used for head circumference. See Chapter 2 for further discussion on accurate measurement. It is best to use a pediatric or neonatal stethoscope for auscultation. An otoscope and ophthalmoscope is needed for the inspection of the ears and eyes.

The newborn assessment uses multiple examination techniques, most commonly inspection, auscultation, and palpation. Percussion and transillumination may be helpful in assessing certain organ systems (e.g., percussion with liver assessment) or to better evaluate some findings (e.g., transillumination for suspected hydrocele).[11]

Approach to Physical Examination

The best approach to physical examination of the newborn occurs with the least disruption and considers the infant's behavioral state to obtain the best results. Newborn behavioral states include: two sleep states, deep/quiet sleep, light/active sleep, as well as four awake states: drowsy, quiet alert, active alert, and crying. The examination should be conducted in a systematic manner because a consistent approach ensures that all aspects are evaluated. The provider also acknowledges that components of the exam itself (e.g., eye or kidney exam) may disturb the infant, and the unclothed infant can easily become cold stressed. Prior to touching the infant, much can be learned by observing the appearance of the undressed infant in the resting, nonstimulated state. General inspection should include assessment of external genitalia, identification of any deformities, determination of fetal nutrition, assessment of color, and newborn position and movement.[11]

The sequence of the physical assessment begins with the quiet parts of the examination—the cardiac and respiratory systems. Prior to handling, gather observational data to complement other assessment findings, such as color, perfusion, respiratory effort, level of alertness, symmetry, tone, movements, and state of arousal.[8] The overall sequence of the exam may vary with the infant's behavioral state but may then proceed systematically from head to toe and may integrate inspection of multiple systems to best take advantage of infant's behavior and tolerance of the examination. Each body system has relevant embryologic, developmental, anatomic, and physiologic variations, and the neonatal/pediatric health care provider is directed to the relevant system chapters throughout the text.

Skin

The skin of the newborn infant is composed of the same three layers as the adult; however, it is thinner and more easily disrupted than that of the adult. Additionally, the more immature the infant, the more immature and permeable the skin. The skin is assessed with the techniques of inspection and palpation. Although most skin findings are evident with inspection, palpation may enhance findings such as skin thickness and turgor. It is important to assess skin folds and scalp for additional findings. The newborn's skin is typically covered with vernix, a cheesy-white odorless protective sebaceous secretion, that may collect in the skin folds. Skin pigmentation is highly variable.[12]

Skin color is an essential element in determining perfusion of the newborn. The most reliable indicator of perfusion in the newborn is the color of the mucous membranes and tongue. Newborn infants commonly exhibit *acrocyanosis*, cool and cyanotic hands and feet due to vasomotor instability of peripheral circulation; this is a normal finding in the otherwise healthy infant. Persistence of this finding beyond the first 24 to 48 hours may indicate poor perfusion due to cold stress, hypovolemia, or polycythemia.[12] *Central cyanosis* is always considered abnormal and is evident when less than 5 g percent of desaturated hemoglobin is present. There may be associated etiologies such as cardiac or pulmonary disease, infection, metabolic and neurologic conditions, and hematologic issues such as anemia or polycythemia.[13] *Pallor*, a pale or ashen appearance, can be due to poor perfusion, acidosis, or anemia. *Plethora*, a ruddy appearance, may indicate polycythemia, with hematocrit (HCT) above the upper limits of normal for gestational or postnatal age (>2 standard deviations). Both anemia and polycythemia may be associated with hypoxemia (low oxygen saturation), although the appearance of cyanosis may be misleading. Cyanosis becomes evident when there is at least 3 to 5 g of desaturated hemoglobin, and cyanosis may readily present in polythemic infants with otherwise normal oxygenation. In newborns with anemia, cyanosis requires substantial hypoxemia and low oxygen content of the blood.

Jaundice, a yellow discoloration of the skin, may occur from deposition of bilirubin. Clinical jaundice is a common newborn finding, occurring in up to 60% of healthy-term infants during the first week of life.[1] Jaundice typically follows a cephalocaudal distribution and is initially seen in the face and upper trunk.[12] However, exaggerated clinical jaundice with associated hyperbilirubinemia in the newborn may also result from hemolysis. Jaundice occurring in the first 24 hours of life is considered pathologic and warrants investigation.[1,12]

The newborn skin assessment may reveal lesions or rashes, mostly benign in nature and requiring no intervention (Table 6.6). *Ecchymoses* may be evident over presenting parts,

TABLE 6.6   COMMON CONDITIONS IN NEWBORN AND INFANT SKIN

Condition	Photo	Description	Significance/ Treatment
Acrocyanosis		Bluish coloration of hands and feet present at birth; may persist up to 24 hr	Benign color variation in newborn; no treatment needed if gone after 24 hr
Blue-black spots		Formerly called Mongolian spots; represent infiltration of melanocytes into dermis; commonly seen over sacrum and buttocks	Benign; will fade over the first few years of life
Cavernous hemangiomas		A raised, soft, lobulated bluish-red tumor with irregular borders and involves the dermis and subcutaneous dermis layers of skin	Increases in size from 6–12 months and then involutes spontaneously
Cutis marmorata		Reddish-blue mottling or marbling of skin in response to changes in temperature; caused by dilation of capillaries and venules	Benign color variation; no treatment needed unless it does not disappear with skin warming

			Significance/
TABLE 6.6	**COMMON CONDITIONS IN NEWBORN AND INFANT SKIN—CONT'D**		
Condition	**Photo**	**Description**	**Treatment**
Erythema toxicum		Small white to yellow papules, vesicles with erythematous base; starts as early as 24 h of life, may continue until 2 weeks old	Common benign skin lesion in newborn; eosinophils in smear from papule confirms diagnosis
Jaundice		Yellow discoloration of the skin, due to bilirubin deposition; typically, cephalo-caudal presentation; initially seen in the face and upper trunk	Common finding in 60% newborns within first postnatal week; earlier or exaggerated presentation may suggest hemolysis and warrants investigation
Milia		Yellow or white 1 mm papules; represent epidermal cysts from accumulated sebaceous secretions	Benign lesions; need no treatment
Miliaria rubra, m. crystallina, m. pustulosa		Clear, thin vesicles or discrete erythematous papules seen primarily over forehead, neck, or groin or in skin folds; occurs as a result of obstructed sweat glands in humid environment	Benign skin lesion in newborn; can be treated by eliminating precipitating factors such as heat, humidity, too many clothes
Nevus simplex, Nevus flammeus		Red to purple macule with irregular borders often over the upper eyelids, bridge of nose and upper lip, increases with crying; when occurs over nape of neck called stork bite	Increases until 6 months of age and then involutes spontaneously

Continued

TABLE 6.6		COMMON CONDITIONS IN NEWBORN AND INFANT SKIN—CONT'D	
Condition	Photo	Description	Significance/ Treatment
Petechiae		Pinpoint hemorrhages; may occur over presenting part at delivery; multiple may also suggest thrombocytopenia	
Sturge-Weber, Port Wine nevi		Purplish-red lesion with clearly defined borders under the epidermis generally on face; usually unilateral; may be located over trigeminal nerve	Does not resolve spontaneously and size remains stable; may be associated with Sturge-Weber syndrome
Transient neonatal pustular melanosis		Vesicles that rupture leaving collaret of scale and pigmented macule; macules may remain for up to 3 months after birth	Benign skin lesion requiring no treatment

UNN Fig. 6.2 Blue-black spots. From Reginatto FP. Prevalence and characterization of neonatal skin disorders in the first 72 h of life. *J Pediatr (Rio J)*. 2017; 93(3):238–245. UNN Fig. 6.3 Cavernous hemangiomas. From Reginatto FP. Prevalence and characterization of neonatal skin disorders in the first 72 h of life. *J Pediatr (Rio J)*. 2017;93(3):238–245. UNN Fig. 6.6 Jaundice. From https://dftbskindeep.com/all-diagnoses/jaundice/ UNN Fig. 6.7 Milia. From Reginatto FP. Prevalence and characterization of neonatal skin disorders in the first 72 h of life. *J Pediatr (Rio J)*. 2017; 93(3):238–245. UNN Fig 6.9 Nevus simplex, Nevus flammeus. Bolognia JL, et al. *Dermatology*. 4th ed. Elsevier; 2018. Fig 104.3 UNN Fig 6.10 Petechiae. Temple R, Bull K. Petechiae in a newborn. *Am Fam Physician*. 2015; 92(11):1017–1018. UNN Fig 6.12 Transient neonatal pustular melanosis. Kliegman RM, et al. *Nelson Pediatric Symptom-Based Diagnosis*. 2nd ed. Elsevier; 2023, Fig 60.2.

such as the head or buttocks, or occur related to use of assistive devices such as forceps for delivery. *Milia* are pearly white or yellow papules typically found on the nose, brows, and cheeks. These epidermal cystic lesions are the result of accumulated sebaceous gland secretions and resolve spontaneously. *Erythema toxicum* occurs in nearly three-quarters of newborns and presents at approximately 24 to 48 hours as small yellowish-white papular lesions with erythematous bases on the face and trunk. The papules may persist or occur intermittently until 2 weeks of age. Neither of these transient skin lesions requires intervention.[8,12]

Nevi and other hyperpigmented macular lesions may be common findings on the newborn skin. *Blue-black spots or hyperpigmented macules* are seen mostly in infants with darker-pigmented skin and less often in infants with lighter-pigmented skin. These large lesions are found most often over the buttocks but may extend to the back and shoulders. These lesions represent infiltration of the dermis with melanocytes, generally fade in early childhood, but may persist into adulthood.[12] *Nevus simplex* is a common vascular lesion seen in up to 40% of newborns. It is commonly referred to as stork bite or salmon patch, is an irregularly edged macular lesion caused by dilated capillaries, and is most often found at the nape of the neck (stork bite), eyelid, bridge of nose, or lip. Due to the distended underlying capillaries, these lesions blanch with pressure and may increase in size over the first 1 to 2 years of life. *Nevus flammeus*, also known as port-wine nevus, is a flat pink to purple lesion of dilated capillaries with a regular edge. This lesion does not typically increase in size but also does not regress in size spontaneously and may require treatment with laser for elimination or reduction. Most of these lesions are isolated; however, an important variant is the lesion that follows the branches of the trigeminal nerve in the forehead and upper eyelid. This lesion may be associated with Sturge-Weber syndrome, a condition that may result in seizures and other system complications.[12]

In addition to hyperpigmented macules, the skin assessment may reveal strawberry or *cavernous hemangiomas* that consist of dilated capillaries and associated endothelial proliferation of dermis and subdermal skin layers. These lesions grow rapidly for the first 6 months and then typically begin to regress spontaneously. Important complications due to their dense capillary network are bleeding, ulceration, and infection. Depending on the location, hemangiomas may also grow in size to the point of obstructing the airway, necessitating treatment. As with *port-wine nevi*, there is an association of cavernous hemangiomas with congenital syndromes.[12]

Head

Using the techniques of inspection and palpation, the infant's head is initially assessed for size, shape, presence of abnormal hair patterns,
scalp defects, unusual lesions or protuberances, lacerations, and abrasions or contusions. Measurement of head circumference is performed and contrasted with anticipated norms (see Chapter 2, Fig. 2.2). The head size is considered normal (10th percentile to 90th percentile), *microcephalic* (<2 SD or less than the 10th percentile), or *macrocephalic* (>2 SD or greater than the 90th percentile) compared with established norms. Note that macrocephaly or microcephaly can be associated with other pediatric chromosomal and developmental conditions.[9] The scalp is examined for bruising or other disruptions, such as lacerations, that might have occurred during delivery. Due to the influences of the birth process, there may be transient deformation in head shape and size. Table 6.7 and Fig. 6.5 present some transient deformations of the head in newborns. (See Chapter 19 for further assessment of the head.)

Superficial swelling may be evident. *Caput succedaneum* is common and refers to fetal scalp edema as a consequence of labor and delivery. *Cephalohematoma* is a collection of blood between the periosteum and skill that may slowly increase in size and resolve over months. The distinguishing characteristic of caput is that it crosses suture lines with poorly defined edges, while cephalohematoma is confined by the bones and does not cross suture lines.[8] One important cause of external cranial swelling is a *subgaleal hemorrhage*.[9,14] This uncommon complication represents venous bleeding between the aponeurosis and the periosteum and can increase considerably in size over the first hours to days of life (Fig. 6.6). Exact incidence is unknown, but it occurs less commonly than caput succedaneum. Subgaleal hemorrhage has an association with mechanically assisted deliveries, due to external compressive and shearing forces, and may be exacerbated by coagulation disorders.[14] The clinical presentation of subgaleal hemorrhage is a large boggy, shifting collection of fluid over the cranial surface unrestricted by the suture lines. The swelling may extend to the neck

TABLE 6.7   HEAD ASSESSMENT—COMMON FINDINGS

Condition	Description
Caput Succedaneum	Diffuse, soft swelling superior to cranial bones; common finding due to head compression during delivery that will resolve without intervention; not confined by suture lines and is maximally evident at birth. Does not require intervention[8,9,14]
cephalohematoma	Subperiosteal collection of fluid or blood primarily associated with assisted deliveries; occurs in approximately 2% of deliveries; distinguished on exam as a soft swelling that can increase in size over the first 24–72 h but remains confined by the suture lines. Does not typically require intervention (but may be associated with skull fracture in up to 5% of cases)[8,9,14]
Cranial Molding	Temporary skull asymmetry due to overlapping of parietal bones over frontal bones, from compression during delivery; common with prolonged labor; rarely associated with other anomalies; resolved without intervention;[8] may also occur following operative delivery if the head has been descended
Subgaleal Hemorrhage	Subaponeurotic blood collection; exact incidence unknown but occurs less commonly than caput succedaneum; associated with mechanically assisted deliveries or coagulopathy; distinguished on exam as boggy, shifting mass that extends over cranial surface to neck and behind ears; may increase substantially in size; need for intervention varies with degree of blood loss into potential space[8,9,14]

Data from Chiocca EM. Assessment of the neonate. In: Chiocca EM, ed. *Advanced Pediatric Assessment*. 3rd ed. New York: Springer Publishing Company; 2019, pp 207–237. Johnson PJ. Head, eyes, ears, nose, mouth, and neck assessment. In: Tappero EP, Honeyfield ME, eds. *Physical Assessment of the Newborn: A Comprehensive Approach to the Art of Physical Examination*. 6th ed. New York: Springer Publishing Company; 2019, pp 61–77; Volpe JJ. Injuries of extracranial, cranial, intracranial, spinal cord, and peripheral nervous system structures. In: Volpe JJ, Inder TE, Darras BT, deVries LS, dePlessis AJ, Neil JJ, Perlman JM, eds. *Volpe's Neurology of the Newborn*. 6th ed. St. Louis: Elsevierr; 2018, pp 1093–1123.

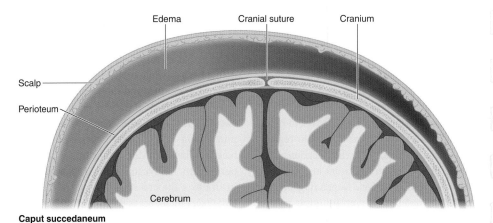

Caput succedaneum

FIGURE 6.5 Caput succedaneum.

and behind the ears, lifting the ears forward. Because this subaponeurotic space is large, infants may quickly develop hypovolemia (decreased fluid volume and dehydration) as a complication and must be vigilantly observed, as well as for the development of hyperbilirubinemia after red blood cell breakdown occurs.[14] However, infants may remain asymptomatic, and the stable infant with a subgaleal hemorrhage may be observed clinically for 24

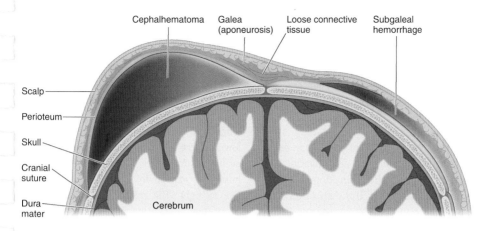

FIGURE 6.6 Subgaleal hemorrhage and cephalohematoma.

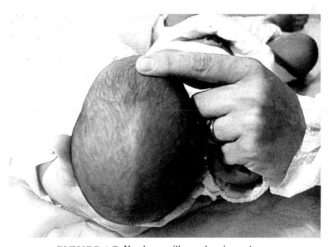

FIGURE 6.7 Newborn with overlapping sutures.

to 48 hours. Outcomes for infants who remain hemodynamically stable are good.[14]

The cranial bones are typically approximated but not fully fused until adolescence. This allows for some overlapping to occur during vaginal delivery or expansion to occur in the case of elevated intracranial pressure. There should be some slight movement appreciated at the level of the suture lines, and they may be split up to 1 cm. *Overlapping sutures* can occur during vaginal birth in the term infant (Fig. 6.7). *Craniotabes*, a softening of the cranial bones, may be evident as a ping-pong ball sensation when pressure is exerted along the parietal or occipital margins. This is often a finding in preterm infants related to incomplete ossification and, also, in breech deliveries in term infants due to pressure during delivery. In term infants, it generally disappears within a few weeks.[8,9]

The fontanels are evaluated for size, shape, and fullness; examine the fontanels while the infant is quiet as crying will increase tension. The diamond-shaped *anterior fontanelle*, at the juncture of the frontal and parietal bone, varies in size from 1 to 4 to 5 cm and typically closes by 12 to 18 months of age. The triangular-shaped *posterior fontanelle*, at the juncture of the single occipital and parietal bones, may be dimple sized at birth, typically closes by 2 to 3 months, and is no longer appreciable by 1 year of age[8] (see Chapter 19, Fig. 19.2). The hair is assessed for distribution, texture, amount, and presence of whorls or white hair tuft.[9]

Face

The facies are inspected for symmetry, gross presence of anomalies or deformation, and movement during the transition between infant behavioral states. Transient distortions can occur due to compression during delivery, prolonged delivery, and the use of forceps; these will typically resolve in a few days without intervention. Asymmetry of facies during crying or inability to close the eye may be an indication of a nerve injury occurring during delivery or from absence of musculature controlling facial movements. Typically, the infant will have decreased movement on the ipsilateral side.[8,9]

Eyes

Assessment of the eyes in the newborn is achieved by inspection, palpation, and selected use of the ophthalmoscope. Determine eye spacing and the intracanthal distance between the eyes. A narrower than normal distance between the eyes is known as *hypotelorism*; and *hypertelorism*, known as wide-set eyes, may be associated with other facial and systemic congenital anomalies. The eyes are also assessed for symmetrical placement in orbital cavity, determined by the relationship of the outer canthus with the helix of the ear. Upward or downward tilting of the eyes may be associated with congenital anomalies or syndromes.[9]

The color of the newborn's iris varies, from gray to brown to dark blue; actual eye color becomes permanent at approximately 6 months of age. The sclera is blue-white at birth and the infant may have *subconjunctival hemorrhages*, resulting from ruptured capillaries during delivery, which resolve spontaneously. Yellow sclera suggests hyperbilirubinemia and should be evaluated further.

Tears are typically absent before 2 to 3 months of age due to incomplete lacrimal duct patency for the first few months of life.[9]

The initial examination of the newborn's eyes may be difficult to perform because the eyelids often are edematous after delivery. Most infants will open their eyes spontaneously when held vertically in an environment with low ambient light. Pupillary reactivity can be evaluated in a dark room using a penlight; pupils are expectedly equal in size and reactive to light. The *retinal light reflex* should be present, indicating an intact cornea and lens. Note that in the infant, the retinal light reflex may vary from pale to slightly yellow to red depending on skin pigmentation of the infant. Unequal or a white retinal light reflex is abnormal and may indicate cataracts or other opacity.[9] Chapter 10 provides additional detail about the eye examination in the infant.

Ears

The newborn ear exam applies the techniques of inspection and palpation. The term newborn demonstrates ready recoil when the pinna is folded inward. The ears are assessed for normal positioning, presence of deformities, swelling, bruising, pits, dimples, and tags. Malformed ears may be associated with other abnormalities, including chromosomal anomalies and congenital syndromes. Uncommonly, preauricular or postauricular pits and tags may be associated with deafness or renal defects, although more often are inconsequential unless another anomaly is detected. The external auditory canals are grossly inspected for patency. The pinna is typically situated at or above an imaginary line from the inner to outer canthus of the eye; those ears situated below this line are considered low set (see Chapter 11, Fig. 11.2). The tympanic membranes are not typically visualized in the newborn due to difficulty examining the short, collapsible canals and canals obscured with vernix. However, patency of the external canal should be determined during the newborn assessment.[8] Currently, universal hearing screening of all newborns is recommended to support early intervention when hearing loss is detected[9] (Table 6.8).

Nose

The nares are inspected grossly for patency and symmetry.[8] Patency can be assessed noninvasively by listening with a stethoscope at the level of the nares or suspending a thin cotton wisp under the nare and looking for rhythmic movement of the wisp. Attention is paid to not allowing the stethoscope or wisp to touch the nare directly, and the other nare should be occluded at the time of assessment. If the results of either of these tests are inconclusive, but discontinuity of the passage is suspected, a small catheter can be introduced into the nares to the nasopharynx.[9] Assess for any nasal discharge or flaring.[8]

Mouth

The mouth, lips, gums, and palate are inspected and palpated. Assessment of the interior of the mouth includes examination of the gingiva, tongue, palate, and uvula. *Cleft lip* may be observed unilaterally or bilaterally; a unilateral cleft lip primarily occurs on the left side of the face. A bilateral cleft lip is most commonly associated with cleft palate as well.[9] Natal teeth that erupt prior to the first month of life may be present, typically as central incisors. These are similar to normal teeth but typically lack a developed root system and may fall out. Unless there is concern for aspiration or interference with feeding, there is no indication for removal. The sublingual frenulum should be inspected when the infant cries to determine position of attachment. If the sublingual frenulum is attached to the anterior portion or tip of the tongue, *ankyloglossia* or tongue-tied, this may interfere with infant feeding and require treatment.[9]

Neck

The techniques of inspection and palpation are used to determine suppleness, symmetry, and range of motion and to detect any extraneous tissue or masses. The examiner assesses for the presence of cysts, clefts, dimples, masses, and redundant skin that may suggest a syndrome. The neck is manipulated side to side;

TABLE 6.8	COMMON NEWBORN DIAGNOSTIC SCREENING TESTS
Screening	**Diagnostic Test**
Hearing screening	Universal screening recommended (but not mandated) prior to hospital discharge; testing done by either automated auditory brainstem response (ABR) or otoacoustic emission (OAE); ABR tests cochlear response to sound and auditory pathways; OAE tests cochlear transmission of sound
Screening for critical congenital heart disease	Universal screening recommended prior to discharge; testing done by pulse oximetry determination of oxygen saturation simultaneously in upper and lower extremity. Positive result warranting additional evaluations: saturation <90%; saturation 90%–95% on repeat measurements, saturation >3% difference between upper and lower sites on repeat measurements
Newborn screening	All states require newborn screening tests; however, the panel of tests vary by state; most states follow the federal *Recommended Uniform Screening Panel (RUSP)* that currently includes 35 core and 26 secondary conditions such as amino acid metabolism disorders, organic acid metabolism disorders, fatty acid oxidation disorders, endocrine disorders, hemoglobinopathies and select others. Currently, the panel of tests vary by state from 67 in CA to 33 in LA; Tests typically performed prior to discharge

Data from: American Academy of Pediatrics (AAP). Newborn pulse oximetry screening to detect critical congenital heart disease. 2021; Centers for Disease Control & Prevention (CDC). Newborn screening portal. 2020; Centers for Disease Control & Prevention (CDC). Screening and diagnosis of hearing loss. 2020.

limitations of full range of motion or head tilt may indicate *congenital torticollis*.[8,9]

Chest

The chest is inspected and palpated for size, shape, symmetry, and contour. If measured, the chest circumference at the nipple line at term is approximately 30 to 36 cm or 2 to 3 cm less than the head circumference.[4] Assess nipples and breast tissue; at term the areolae are raised and stippled and there is approximately 1 cm of evident breast tissue. Note any redness or tenderness or nipple drainage; some infants exhibit transient neonatal *galactorrhea* (breast nodules) due to the effects of maternal estrogen.[4,8] There should be symmetric movement of the chest with respiratory effort. Due to the compliant newborn chest (an advantage during delivery), the sternum is drawn inward during inspiration.[4] The clavicles are inspected and palpated to detect any swelling, tenderness, or crepitus. Any decreased movement or asymmetry of the Moro reflex on the affected side may suggest injury. Clavicular fractures, for example, are a common birth injury. These bony disruptions are evident as crepitus palpable in the clavicular region and may be confirmed by radiographic imaging. No treatment is indicated.[9]

The xiphoid process may be evident protruding at the distal end of the sternum. The measured spacing between the nipples is typically one-half of the anteroposterior diameter of the chest. The chest is inspected for presence of *supernumerary nipples*. Use of accessory muscles, evident as retractions, may indicate inability to sustain adequate inflation and may be a finding of pulmonary disease that needs further evaluation. The soft nature of the newborn's bony structures increases risks for disruptions.[4] Chest deviations may include *pectus excavatum*, an inverted sternum that is usually not medically significant, and *pectus carinatum*, a protruding sternum that occurs predominantly in males 4:1 and can be associated with other abnormalities, including scoliosis, Marfan syndrome, and congenital heart disease.[4]

Lungs

The lungs are auscultated for presence of equal, bilateral breath sounds. During the first postnatal hours, due to residual presence of alveolar fluid, the breath sounds may be moist. Respirations are typically "regularly irregular," with short periods of rapid rate followed by short pauses. However, pauses longer than 20 seconds are abnormal and warrant additional evaluation to rule out pulmonary disease or other disorders of transition.[4] Normal respiratory rate is presented in Table 6.9.

Heart

The cardiac examination commences with an inspection of the chest and palpation to determine the point of maximum impulse (PMI) of the heart. The PMI will shift in the first hours after birth once pulmonary ventilation is established and right-sided fetal heart forces diminish. Heart sounds are then auscultated, and determination of S1 and S2 and any adventitious sounds. Murmurs are common in the

TABLE 6.9	NORMAL RANGE OF NEWBORN RESPIRATORY AND CARDIAC RATES		
Heart Rate		**Respiratory Rate**	**Blood Pressure**
80–180 beats/min (70–80 during sleep; 120–160 awake)[4]		30–60 breaths/min3	57–69 systolic 44–52 diastolic[4]

Data from: Fraser D. Chest and lungs assessment. In: Tappero EP, Honeyfield ME, eds. *Physical Assessment of the Newborn: A Comprehensive Approach to the Art of Physical Examination.* 6th ed. New York: Springer Publishing Company; 2019, pp 79–91; Vargo L. Cardiovascular assessment. In Tappero EP, Honeyfield ME, eds. *Physical Assessment of the Newborn: A Comprehensive Approach to the Art of Physical Examination.* 6th ed. New York: Springer Publishing Company; 2019, pp 93–110.

early newborn period due to changing cardio-pulmonary dynamics postnatally. For example, a *patent ductus arteriosus* may be evident as a murmur best heard along the left lower sternal border. This sound typically decreases by 48 hours of age and is not associated with any other evidence of cardiac instability.[13] Normal heart rates are presented in Table 6.10. Chapter 8 reviews innocent or physiologic murmurs that may be present during infancy.

The cardiac exam also includes an assessment of pulses, including brachial and radial in the upper extremities and femoral and pedal in the lower extremities. Perfusion is determined by blanching the skin over the abdomen or chest and allowing for return of color; a capillary filling time less than 3 seconds is considered within normal limits.[8,13] Although norms exist for newborn blood pressure, it is not a typical component of the routine newborn exam unless there is suspected cardiovascular or renal disease.[13]

Abdomen

The abdomen is inspected for contour and palpated for normal presence of internal organs and any abnormal presence of masses. The abdominal circumference is measured just superior to the umbilicus at the largest diameter; it is approximately equal to head circumference by term.[15] The newborn abdomen is rounded and soft. Use light and deep palpation in a circular area examining the four regions in sequence. Bowel sounds are evident within several hours postnatally, as swallowed air progresses distally. *Diastasis recti*, a separation of the abdominal musculature, may be evident as a midline bulge extending from the xiphoid process to the umbilicus. This is due to failed fusion of the muscle and will resolve without intervention. The umbilicus is inspected for color and state of healing, as well as the presence of vessels. Typically, the cord remnant is opaque, blue-white, and odorless with evidence of two thick-walled arteries and one thin-walled vein. The presence of swelling or masses is noted because this may represent a herniation of abdominal contents.[15]

The liver is palpated as an upper right to midline region organ; the newborn liver may extend down 1 to 3 cm below the right costal margin.[15] An alternative technique to direct palpation is to use the "scratch" technique and listen indirectly with a stethoscope to detect a change in percussion note. The spleen is also palpated, although typically not appreciated on the normal exam. Kidneys in the newborn are palpated; they are expectedly smooth, round, and approximately 4 to 5 cm in size. A bimanual technique is the easiest method for assessing the kidneys, approached with deep palpation at a 45-degree angle just below and lateral to the umbilicus.[15]

Genital and Rectal

The perianal area is assessed for the presence of a patent anus. Most newborns will spontaneously pass stool within the first 48 hours of life and void within the first 24 hours of life. Failure to stool beyond this time may indicate obstruction and is an indication for further assessment.[15] The femoral area is inspected

TABLE 6.10	COMMON NEWBORN SYMPTOMS AND CONDITIONS
Presentation	**Signs and Symptoms**
Transient tachypnea of newborn	Excessively rapid respirations usually due to retained fetal lung fluid; tachypnea subsides with absorption of fluid
Acrocyanosis and circumoral cyanosis	Bluish discoloration of the surrounding the lips and of the hands and feet due to changes in newborn temperature
Transient jitteriness	Rapid movements of newborn's arms and legs often with vigorous crying generally in response to stimuli; does not persist after early neonatal period and does not involve eye movements

for bulges and palpated. An *inguinal hernia* that represents incomplete obliteration of the *processus vaginalis* may be evident as a compressible mass or swelling and may contain abdominal viscera.[15]

Bruising and swelling of the genitalia may be a common finding following delivery. When examining the genitalia, note the clitoris and labia minora are normally covered by the labia majora at term, and the urinary meatus is situated just below the clitoris. *Hymenal tags* are common, and pseudomenses may occur transiently due to the residual effects of maternal hormones.[16] For the male, the average penile length measures 2.5 to 3.5 cm at term, and the urinary meatus is situated just ventral to the tip. Deviations of placement of the meatus include *hypospadias*, a ventral urethral opening, and *epispadias*, a dorsal urethral opening that occurs less commonly, are indications for referral. The scrotum is inspected, and rugae as well as color and symmetry of the scrotal sac are assessed. The testes are palpated bilaterally for size, firmness, and tenderness. A *hydrocele* may be evident as a fluid-filled scrotal mass that transilluminates; this will resolve spontaneously (see Chapter 15 for review of male genitourinary conditions).[8,16]

Ambiguous genitalia may be suspected when phallic structures do not appear to be discretely male or female or with the inability to palpate gonads. Due to the possible association of this diagnosis with serious endocrine disorders, it is imperative to evaluate these newborns carefully with a team that typically includes an endocrinologist, genetic specialist, urologist, and psychologist/social worker.[16]

Musculoskeletal, Extremities, and Spine

Normal resting position of the term newborn is inward flexion of upper and lower extremities, although postnatal positioning is affected by the position in utero. The extremities should be assessed for size, shape, range of motion, alignment and symmetry of movement, and presence/number of digits. Note any webbing, conjoined digits, or hypoplasia.[17] The skin overlying the spine is inspected for lesions, pits, tags, and hair tufts; the dermis should be continuous without breaks. Abnormal curvature of the spine should be noted. The hips are assessed for stability and an evaluation for *developmental dysplasia* of the hips. The *Barlow maneuver* provokes an unstable hip to dislocate by adducting the hip and applying pressure laterally to force the femoral head over the lateral rim of the acetabulum. Conversely, the *Ortolani maneuver* reduces the dislocated hip by abducting the hip and allowing the femoral head to slip back toward the acetabulum, creating an audible click and palpable sensation to the examiner (see Chapter 18, Fig. 18.17).[17]

Neurologic

The neurologic assessment can be integrated throughout the physical assessment and takes notes of changes in posture, activity, state, or muscle tone during handling. Infants should exhibit changes, especially in response to stimuli. The infant who does not increase alertness when handled or exhibits tremors, clonus, or poorly coordinated activity, such as suck/swallow, deserves careful observation. Observing an infant successfully feeding, at breast or bottle, provides information about intactness of the cranial nerves. In addition to obtaining behavioral data, observe for evidence of birth trauma such as cephalohematoma, forceps marks, bruising, or localized swelling.[18] See Chapter 19, Table 19.2 for cranial nerve testing in newborn. Assessment of primitive reflexes is included in the newborn exam. Most primitive reflexes generate symmetric responses, and this provides important information about brainstem function. Common reflexes include the Moro (startle) reflex, stepping and placing, rooting and sucking, and plantar and palmar grasping (see Chapter 19, Table 19.4). These reflexes generally disappear by 3 to 6 months postnatally.[18]

SUMMARY OF EXAMINATION

A comprehensive neonatal assessment helps the pediatric provider to anticipate potential problems, detect subtle findings in the newborn that may be meaningful, and intervene readily to prevent or minimize further problems. The neonatal assessment should generally be performed within the first 24 hours of life to identify any abnormality that would alter the normal newborn course or identify any abnormal findings in the physical examination that should be investigated further.

Consistency in technique and organizational skill, as well as integration of infant behavioral state into the physical exam can help to ensure completeness in the comprehensive assessment. The comprehensive assessment of the newborn integrates components of the prenatal, perinatal, birth, and early neonatal history with a thorough physical examination.

SUMMARY OF NEWBORN PHYSICAL EXAMINATION

Vital signs	Temperature, apical pulse or PMI, respirations
Measurements:	Birth weight and discharge weight, length, head circumference, chest circumference if indicated
General	Gestational age
	New Ballard Score and Apgar score
	Inspection and observation: posture, state of arousal/alertness, activity level, tone, symmetry, self-soothing measures
Skin	Color: presence of jaundice, cyanosis, acrocyanosis, lanugo, vernix caseosa
	Skin turgor, amount of subcutaneous tissue
	Presence of birthmarks or lesions, rashes, bruises, pustules, petechiae
Head	Shape, symmetry, scalp hair
	Anterior and posterior fontanelles, sutures
	Evidence of trauma: molding, caput succedaneum, cephalohematoma
	Face: symmetry, unusual or dysmorphic features
Eyes	Shape, edema, drainage
	Sclera, conjunctiva: color, scleral hemorrhages
	Retinal light reflex, corneal light reflex, eye movement
Ears	Shape and position of pinna, skin tags, patency of external canal, visualization of tympanic membrane
Nose	Patency, discharge, nasal flaring
Mouth and Throat	Symmetry of movement, cyanosis, intact hard and soft palate
	Presence of teeth, cysts, Epstein pearls, thrush
	Size of chin and tongue, position of tongue in mouth
	Moistness of mucus membranes
Neck	Presence of webbing, masses, range of motion
	Evidence of fractured clavicle
	Presence of lymph nodes

Continued

SUMMARY OF NEWBORN PHYSICAL EXAMINATION—CONT'D

Chest	Respiratory rate, rhythm, retractions
	Shape, size, symmetry of movement
	Breath sounds
	Breast: amount of tissue, engorgement, nipples; size, symmetry, discharge
Cardiovascular	Apical pulse or PMI location and quality
	Heart rate, rhythm, identify S1 S2
	Presence of murmurs, extra heart sounds
	Radial, femoral, pedal pulses symmetry, quality
Abdomen	Shape, size, symmetry, presence of bowel sounds
	Palpate for liver, spleen, kidneys, evidence of diastasis recti
	Umbilical cord: number of vessels, color, drainage, odor, presence of hernia
Extremities	Symmetry, shape, strength, range of motion, number of digits
	Nails: texture, color of nail beds
	Creases: palms, soles
	Abduct hips for dislocation, perform Barlow and Ortolani
Back	Spinal contour
	Presence of cysts, sinuses, dimples, tufts of hair
	Uneven skin folds (check without diaper)
	Presence of nevi
Rectum	Patency, presence of any fissures, check innervation with anal wink
	Passage of meconium
Genitalia	Position of urethral meatus, passage of urine
	Prepuce covering glans, scrotum
	Testes–descended or undescended,
	Size of labia majora, labia minora, vaginal discharge, skin tags
	Labial masses, passage of urine
	Note: Consult for any concern with gender ambiguity
Neurologic	Posture, muscle tone, movement, seizure activity
	Head control, quality of cry
	Response to light and sound
	Ankle clonus
	Primitive reflexes
Screening Tests and Labs	Passage of meconium and urine
	Newborn screening tests, newborn hearing screening results,
	point-of-care glucose testing, complete blood count or hematocrit, blood type, Coombs, bilirubin

NEWBORN HEALTH HISTORY DOCUMENTATION

Newborn 8 Hours of Age
38 weeks 2 days infant, BW 3500 gm, AGA, mother 32 y/o $G_3P_{2-3}A_0L_3$, O pos. Rh neg, Rubella,

HepBsAg RPR, GBS, GC/CT—neg., breastfeeding initiated, good suck, intermittent transient tachypnea noted.

BW, birth weight; *AGA*, appropriate gestational age; *GPAL*, gravidity, parity, abortion, live births; *HepBsAg*, hepatitis B surface antigen; *RPR*, rapid plasma regain; *GBS*, Group B Streptococcus; *GC/CT*, Neisseria gonorrhea and Chlamydia trachomatis

REFERENCES

1. Rohan A. Common neonatal complications. In: Simpson KR, Creehan PA, eds. *AWHONN's Perinatal Nursing*. 5th ed. Philadelphia, PA: Wolters Kluwer-Lippincott Williams & Wilkins; 2019:650–687.

2. Fraser D. Newborn adaptation to extrauterine life. In: Simpson KR, Creehan PA, eds. *AWHONN's Perinatal Nursing*. 5th ed. Philadelphia, PA: Wolters Kluwer-Lippincott Williams & Wilkins; 2019:563–577.

3. Simpson KR, O'Brien-Abel N. Labor and birth. In: Simpson KR, Creehan PA, eds. *AWHONN's Perinatal Nursing*. 5th ed. Philadelphia, PA: Wolters Kluwer-Lippincott Williams & Wilkins; 2019:325–411.

4. Fraser D. Chest and lungs assessment. In: Tappero EP, Honeyfield ME, eds. *Physical Assessment of the Newborn: A Comprehensive Approach to the Art of Physical Examination*. 6th ed. New York, NY: Springer Publishing Company; 2019:79–91.

5. Lopez V, Graziano PD. The neonatal physical exam. In: Koehn AR, ed. *Neonatal Nurse Practitioner Certification Intensive Review*. New York, NY: Springer Publishing Company; 2019:27–57.

6. Trotter CW. Gestational age assessment. In: Tappero EP, Honeyfield ME, eds. *Physical Assessment of the Newborn*. 6th ed. New York, NY: Springer Publishing Company; 2019:23–43.

7. LaBronte KH. Recording and evaluating the neonatal history. In: Tappero EP, Honeyfield ME, eds. *Physical Assessment of the Newborn: A Comprehensive Approach to the Art of Physical Examination*. 6th ed. New York, NY: Springer Publishing Company; 2019:9–22.

8. Chiocca EM. Assessment of the neonate. In: Chiocca EM, ed. *Advanced Pediatric Assessment*. 3rd ed. New York, NY: Springer Publishing Company; 2019:207–237.

9. Johnson PJ. Head, eyes, ears, nose, mouth, and neck assessment. In: Tappero EP, Honeyfield ME, eds. *Physical Assessment of the Newborn: A Comprehensive Approach to the Art of Physical Examination*. 6th ed. New York, NY: Springer Publishing Company; 2019:61–77.

10. Centers for Disease Control & Prevention (CDC). Clinical growth charts. 2010. https://www.cdc.gov/growthcharts/

11. Honeyfield ME. Principles of physical assessment. In: Tappero EP, Honeyfield ME, eds. *Physical Assessment of the Newborn: A Comprehensive Approach to the Art of Physical Examination*. 6th ed. New York, NY: Springer Publishing Company; 2019:1–8.

12. Witt C. Skin Assessment. In: Tappero EP, Honeyfield ME, eds. *Physical Assessment of the Newborn: A Comprehensive Approach to the Art of Physical Examination*. 6th ed. New York, NY: Springer Publishing Company; 2019:45–59.

13. Vargo L. Cardiovascular assessment. In: Tappero EP, Honeyfield ME, eds. *Physical Assessment of the Newborn: A Comprehensive Approach to the Art of Physical Examination*. 6th ed. New York, NY: Springer Publishing Company; 2019:93–110.

14. Volpe JJ. Injuries of extracranial, cranial, intracranial, spinal cord, and peripheral nervous system structures. In: Volpe JJ, Inder TE, Darras BT, deVries LS, dePlessis AJ, Neil JJ, Perlman JM, eds. *Volpe's Neurology of the Newborn*. 6th ed. St. Louis, MO: Elsevier; 2018:1093–1123.

15. Goodwin M. Abdomen Assessment. In: Tappero EP, Honeyfield ME, eds. *Physical Assessment of the Newborn: A Comprehensive Approach to the Art of Physical Examination*. 6th ed. New York, NY: Springer Publishing Company; 2019:111–120.

16. Cavaliere TA. Genitourinary assessment. In: Tappero EP, Honeyfield ME, eds. *Physical Assessment of the Newborn: A Comprehensive Approach to the Art of Physical Examination*. 6th ed. New York, NY: Springer Publishing Company; 2019:121–137.

17. Tappero EP. Musculoskeletal system assessment. In: Tappero EP, Honeyfield ME, eds. *Physical Assessment of the Newborn: A Comprehensive Approach to the Art of Physical Examination*. 6th ed. New York, NY: Springer Publishing Company; 2019:139–166.

18. Heaberlin PD. Neurologic assessment. In: Tappero EP, Honeyfield ME, eds. *Physical Assessment of the Newborn: A Comprehensive Approach to the Art of Physical Examination*. 6th ed. New York, NY: Springer Publishing Company; 2019:167–192.

CHAPTER 7

SKIN ASSESSMENT

Renee P. McLeod

Careful inspection of the skin gives the pediatric health care provider clear insight into the overall health of the child. Along with inspection and a thorough health history, examination of the skin, hair, and nails provides clues to oxygenation, tissue perfusion, nutritional and hydration status of the child, and any underlying disease pathology or injury.[1] The skin of infants and children share similarities in structure and function with adults, but a child's skin reacts differently to environmental demands because of the unique skin properties of each age group. All skin, regardless of age, is affected by seasonal factors such as the heat and humidity of summer or the dryness and low humidity of winter, but the differences in an infant's skin and ability to sweat, when compared with an adult, can cause more risks and problems associated with these seasonal changes. Therefore, the manifestations of a skin disorder observed in an infant or child may vary widely from what may be seen in an adult.[1]

The skin is the largest organ in the body and has five distinct functions. The skin controls fluids, regulates temperature, protects against invasion from pathogens and foreign bodies, and protects against damage from the ultraviolet (UV) rays of the sun. Finally, the skin is an organ of communication. Touch and skin-to-skin contact is one of the ways we bond with our caregivers and families at birth and later bond with our sexual partners. Research conducted over the past 50 years has proven that touch is more important to humans than food in regard to optimal development.[2-4] Having a disease of the skin, hair, or nails that prevents or decreases human touch can be devastating to a child's self-esteem.

THE MICROBIOME AND GUT-SKIN AXIS

The human body is inhabited by large ecological communities of bacteria, fungi, and viruses that form what is called the "human microbiome." This complex system differs from person to person and is unique to each body site (e.g., skin, gut, respiratory tract). The microbiome at each of these sites is dynamic and constantly changing in composition and function and is impacted by different ages, stages of development, conditions, and internal or external influences. How it explains or predicts human health and disease states is currently being studied.[5,6]

The microbiome of the skin contains hundreds of bacterial species of which the most common are *Firmicutes, Bacteroidetes,*

Actinobacteria, and *Proteobacteria*.[5] Initial colonization of the skin may occur even before birth via hematogenous spread of the microbes *Firmicutes, Proteobacteria, Enterococcus, and Streptococcus* from the mother's oral cavity and gastrointestinal tract into the uterine cavity.[7] It is well established that the route of birth has major implications for the newborn's gut and skin microbiome and future disease risk.[7-9] Infants born by Caesarean section have been found to have higher rates of *Staphylococcus, Corynebacterium,* and *Propionibacterium ssp.* on their skin, which has been found to increase infections and may contribute to the development of atopic dermatitis.[10] The use of antibiotics during delivery and breastfeeding decreases the presence of immunoprotective *Lactobacillus* and *Bifidobacterium* species in breast milk and can lead to a decrease of these protective bacteria and bacterial diversity in the infant's gut.[7] The development of inflammatory skin diseases like acne and atopic dermatitis have been linked to gut integrity and the diversity of the gut microbiome in children and adolescents.[10]

ANATOMY AND PHYSIOLOGY

The skin consists of three layers: the *epidermis,* the *dermis,* and the *subcutaneous layer* (Fig. 7.1). The *epidermis* is the outermost layer of the skin and consists of two main layers: the *stratum corneum* and the *cellular stratum*. The *stratum corneum* is the very top layer of the skin and is composed of stacked, overlapping nonnucleated keratinized cells called *corneocytes*. The thickness of this layer depends on the region of the body. The skin is thinnest on the face and thickest over the soles of the feet.[10] The *stratum corneum* layer forms the protective barrier of the skin and contains the waterproofing protein *keratin,* that restricts water loss and the penetration of a variety of substances through the skin. The innermost layer of the epidermis consists of a single row of columnar cells called *basal cells* that reside in the *stratum basale*. These cells divide to form the *keratinocytes* that move to the surface through the *stratum spinosum, stratum granulosum,* and *stratum lucidum* to replace the cells that are sloughed off every day in the

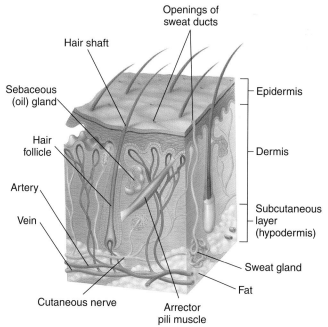

FIGURE 7.1 Anatomy of the skin. (From Thibodeau GA, Patton KT. *Anatomy and Physiology.* 9th ed. St. Louis: Mosby; 2016.)

stratum corneum.[1] The stratum basale also contains *melanocytes*, which synthesize melanin to provide color and protect the skin from damage by the UV rays of the sun. The dermal-epidermal junction lies beneath the stratum basale and is an important site of attachment in the skin. This junction allows nutrients to pass through the dermis to the avascular epidermis. *Langerhans cells* lie in the suprabasal layer of the dermis and are the immunologic cells responsible for recognizing harmful antigens to the body. They process the antigen and enter the blood stream residing in the regional lymph nodes and stimulate the production of T lymphocytes.[1,11]

The *dermis* is a richly vascular layer consisting largely of fibroblasts and collagen. The collagen matrix of the dermis supports and separates the epidermis from the subcutaneous fat layer. Papillae project up into the epidermis to provide nourishment to the living epidermal cells. In addition, the dermis contains a large network of sensory nerve fibers. These fibers provide sensations of pain, itch, and temperature. *Meissner corpuscles* are encapsulated end organs of touch found in the dermal papillae close to the epidermis. They are most numerous in hairless portions of the skin such as the volar surfaces of the hands, fingers, feet, toes, lips, eyelids, nipples, and tip of the tongue. The dermis also contains autonomic nerve fibers that innervate blood vessels, the *arrectores pilorum* muscles, the sweat glands, sebaceous glands, hair, and nails.

The *sweat glands* in the dermis control thermoregulation by releasing water through the skin. The *eccrine sweat glands* are distributed throughout the body except for the lip margins, eardrums, nail beds, inner surface of the prepuce, and the glans penis.[12] They are most abundant on the palms and soles of the feet. The *apocrine sweat glands* are larger and deeper than the eccrine glands and secrete an odorless white fluid (sweat) in response to emotional or physical stimuli. They are located in the axillae, around the nipples or areolae, anogenital area, eyelids, and external ears. Body odor in adolescence comes from the bacterial decomposition of the sweat produced by these glands; activation of these glands earlier than adolescence should be investigated. Neonates have the ability to respond to thermal stress by sweating, though it requires a greater thermal stimulus. This response is less developed in premature infants and increases with postnatal age.[8] Full-term infants are also able to respond to emotional stress by sweating, though this is not developed in the premature infant. This has clinical implications related to increased insensible water loss, dehydration, and thermoregulation in infants at risk.[13]

The *sebaceous glands* arise from the hair follicles deep within the dermis. The oil produced by these glands is called *sebum*, a lipid-rich substance that helps lubricate the skin and hair. Sebaceous glands depend on hormonal stimulation and are activated by androgens at puberty. The level of oil produced varies throughout the life span. In newborns, the production of sebum is accelerated while still under the influence of maternal hormones and the glands themselves become hyperplastic until maternal hormones wane in the infant's body. This stimulated activity results in skin conditions in the newborn such as *neonatal acne*. Overactive sebaceous glands appear again in adolescence and contribute to the common skin conditions *acne vulgaris* and *tinea versicolor*.[1]

The nail bed starts to keratinize to form a hard, protective plate around 8 to 10 weeks of gestation. It sits on a highly vascular bed that gives each nail its color. The *cuticle*, or *eponychium*, the white crescent-shaped area at the end of the nail matrix, is the root and site of nail growth (Fig. 7.2A and B). It is covered by a layer of stratum corneum that pushes up and over the lower part of the nail body. The *perionychium* is the soft tissue that surrounds the nail border on each digit. Nail health can be affected by several factors including nutrition, hydration, local infection/irritation, trauma, and systemic disease.

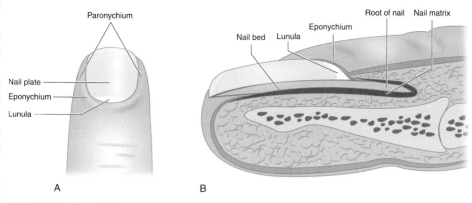

FIGURE 7.2 **A** and **B**, Anatomy of nail.

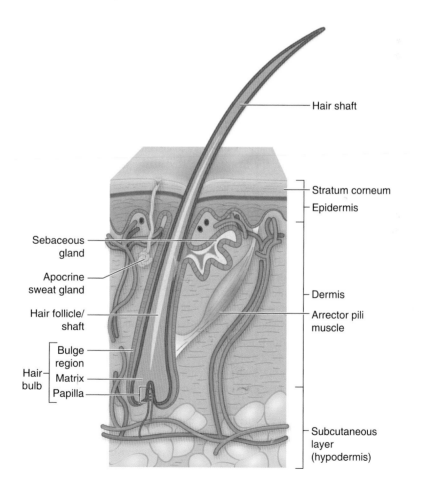

FIGURE 7.3 Anatomy of hair follicle.

The *subcutaneous* layer of the skin is composed of adipose tissue. This layer connects the dermis to underlying organs, provides insulation and shock absorption, and generates heat for the body. It also provides a reserve of calories for use by the body.[13] Premature and small for gestational age infants often lack this critical layer of insulation, which causes difficulty with thermoregulation.

Hair and eyebrows are part of the anatomical structure of the skin. Hair is formed by epidermal cells that go deep into the dermal layer of the skin and consists of a *root*, a *shaft*, and a *follicle* (Fig. 7.3). The *papilla* is the structure at the base of the hair follicle and is made of connective tissue and a loop of capillaries, which supply and nourish the hair to promote growth. *Melanocytes*, which lie in the hair shaft, supply color to the hair.

DEVELOPMENTAL VARIATIONS

In the newborn, all the hair on the body consists of fine *lanugo* hair—all of the hair is in the same phase of growth. Within the first 4 months after birth, infants undergo a period of physiologic hair shedding to convert actively growing hairs to the resting phase and start the process of nonsynchronized growth. This normal process may already be complete at birth for some infants with light hair who often appear completely bald. This process may be delayed for up to 4 months in some dark-haired infants.[13] As the lanugo is shed, it is replaced by hair that is increased in diameter and coarseness; the first to form are *vellus* hairs, which are short, fine, soft, and nonpigmented hairs on the body. Then adult-type *terminal* hairs, which are coarse, thick, longer, pigmented, and grow on the scalp and eyebrows. During adolescence, vellus hairs located in androgen-sensitive areas, pubic area, axillae, and the face in males undergo a similar transition to terminal hairs.

Hair follicles grow in a nonsynchronized fashion, with 85% to 95% in the growth phase lasting 2 to 6 years, 10% to 15% in the resting phase lasting 2 to 3 months, and less than 1%

in the involution phase that lasts 2 to 3 weeks. There are approximately 100,000 to 150,000 hairs on the scalp. Daily hair loss varies between shampoo days and nonshampoo days, with adults losing 50 to 100 hairs on a nonshampoo day and 200 to 300 hairs on a shampoo day. Hair density has to decrease by half before there is noticeable hair thinning.[14–16]

PHYSIOLOGICAL VARIATIONS

The stratum corneum does not develop until between 23 and 25 weeks of gestation. Extremely premature infants are born without this critical top layer of skin and therefore have no protective barrier and are not able to control water loss. Preterm infants need protection from the environment and can tolerate only the least amount of touching. The term newborn has a fully functional stratum corneum, but it is only about 60% of the thickness of adult skin depending on the location. A thin stratum corneum with the larger body surface area/weight ratio of the newborn may allow substances placed on the skin to pass more easily through to the bloodstream.[13] The blood vessels continue to mature into a more adult pattern of perfusion until 3 months of age. The nerves in the skin are small and poorly myelinated at birth. The growth and myelination of the nerve fibers continue on into puberty (Table 7.1).

Skin Pigmentation

Recent research has shown skin *pigmentation* or *melanin* should be considered as a factor for understanding some underlying skin properties and characteristics that are influenced by differences in genetic background. Understanding how underlying skin color and pigmentation may affect the examination and diagnosis of skin conditions allows the clinician to adjust assessment techniques and interventions using the child or adolescent's physiological characteristics rather than racial or ethnic categorization to guide care.[17,18]

Assessing skin pigmentation allows the health care provider to make clinical decisions based on tissue perfusion, jaundice, pallor, cyanosis, and blanch response. The *blanch test* differs widely based on underlying skin color. The blanch test differentiates healthy skin from erythematous skin that is nonblanchable. When gentle pressure from fingertips

TABLE 7.1	STRUCTURAL AND FUNCTIONAL DIFFERENCES OF SKIN			
Structure	**Term Newborn Infant**	**Child**	**Adolescent**	**Significance/ Implications**
Epidermis	Stratum corneum appears as adherent cell layer Greater absorption because of higher skin surface/body weight ratio	Stratum is getting thicker, starts to appear as separate sheet of cells	Stratum corneum appears as separate sheet of cells Adult-like pattern	Thin skin of infant and child allows for easy absorption of products placed on skin Apply thin layer of topical medications
Dermis	Fewer immature elastin fibers Thinner than adult	Elastin fibers are maturing	Full complement of elastin fibers	Decreased elasticity Increased tendency to blister
Melanosomes	Melanin production low Final overall skin tone is shown in genitalia where the scrotum, labia have darker pigment	Melanin production after 6 months of age like adult	Adult pattern of melanin production	Infants, young children need sunscreen/complete sun block because can sunburn easily
Eccrine sweat glands	Equivalent in structure to adult Dense distribution due to body surface area	Distribution starts becoming less dense as child grows, but has decreased neurological control until 2–3 years old	Distribution is less dense than in infant, child	Reduced sweating capability, especially first 13–24 days of life Decreased response to thermal stress
Apocrine sweat glands	Small, nonfunctional Devoid of secretory granules	Start to appear but generally nonfunctional in childhood	Apocrine sweating in response to mechanical, pharmacological stimuli	Secrete oily substance in adolescent
Sebaceous glands	Large and active but diminish rapidly in size and activity several weeks after birth	Decreased activity throughout childhood	Large, active, produce sebum in large amounts	Young infants get acne and tinea versicolor as do teens due to hormonal activity and large active sebaceous glands

Continued

TABLE 7.1	Structural and Functional Differences of Skin—cont'd			
Structure	Term Newborn Infant	Child	Adolescent	Significance/ Implications
Nervous and vascular systems	Vascular system fully organized after 3 months Most nerves are small in diameter Sensory autonomic nerves are unmyelinated Cutaneous nerve network not fully developed Meissner touch receptors[a] not fully formed	Cutaneous network continuing to develop	Cutaneous network of nerves may continue to develop into adolescence Rest of nervous, vascular systems are in adult pattern	
Hair	Lanugo covering body often shed within 10–14 days Vellus and terminal hairs appear quickly after birth Hair growth is synchronous	Vellus and terminal hairs present Hair growth is asynchronous	Vellus and terminal hairs present Hair growth is asynchronous	Dry, dull, and brittle hair may indicate protein-calorie malnutrition

[a]Meissner touch receptors are encapsulated end organs of touch found in dermal papillae close to epidermis.

is exerted on the skin, blood is temporarily forced out of the region, causing the skin to appear lighter than its typical skin color. Skin color returns swiftly as the blood refills the dermal capillaries. It may be difficult to determine this response in an individual with greater pigmentation in comparison to individuals with less pigmentation because increased melanin may obscure the view of re-perfusion. Erythema in individuals with greater skin pigmentation may appear to have a purplish tinge and often has a more follicular pattern.

Postinflammatory hypopigmentation, absence of normal melanin, and hyperpigmentation, increased melanin, occur more frequently in individuals with greater skin pigmentation, and conditions such as acne or eczema can produce significant skin color changes from postinflammatory hyperpigmentation.[19] Children with African, Asian, and Hispanic ancestry are also at higher risk of *keloid* scarring, possibly due to different genetic mutations found in these ancestral groups.[20] A keloid is a type of scar at the site of a healed skin injury resulting from an overgrowth of granular tissue composed of collagen. Individuals with less skin pigmentation may have more recognizable signs of skin breakdown, sun exposure, and tissue perfusion than individuals with greater skin pigmentation. Looking at the sclerae, conjunctivae, buccal mucosa, lips, tongue, and nail beds will assist the health care provider in assessing children and adolescents with significant clinical variations in pigmentation and skin color. Variations of skin pigmentation in individuals with greater skin pigmentation normally occur on the palms, soles of feet, nail beds, and the genital area. Freckling of the buccal cavity, gums, and tongue is also common. Areas that get regular exposure to the sun may have much greater pigmentation.

Other variations related to skin pigmentation or melanin may exist in the barrier properties of the skin and in the distribution of hair follicles.[20] Variations in barrier properties and hair follicle distribution are significant because they can impact the absorption of topically applied medications and cosmetics. The barrier function may also prevent the penetration of some toxins.[12,13,21] The variation in barrier properties of the skin contributes to individuals with greater skin pigmentation having an increased incidence of *xerosis*, abnormal dryness and increased dullness in appearance of the skin that presents as a whitish visual presence in skin with greater pigmentation.[18,22]

Hair Characteristics

Hair follicle distribution and hair quality differ greatly with racial and ethnic ancestry. For example, individuals with African ancestry typically have hair that presents with coiling of the hair shaft.[22] Children and adolescents with African ancestry have a higher incidence of *tinea capitis*, which may be due to the increased coiling of the hair shaft.

Hair, skin, and nail care practices vary widely between and within cultures. Health care providers should be sensitive and attentive to the diversity of presentations of skin quality and integrity and provide individualized care that is appropriate for each child's anatomy and physiology. Providers should also encourage and support familial cultural practices that support healthy skin care and approach all anticipatory guidance with cultural sensitivity and humility.

SYSTEM-SPECIFIC HISTORY

A careful age-appropriate history is critical to making an accurate assessment of the skin (see Information Gathering table). The health care provider needs to gather information related to current skin conditions, any significant past medical history, and family history of chronic skin conditions. Skincare routines and any recent changes in skin, hair, or nail care habits should be assessed. Sun exposure habits and application of sunscreen are also important considerations in the assessment of the skin. Box 7.1 presents symptom-focused information gathering for skin conditions in children.

BOX 7.1 SYMPTOM-FOCUSED INFORMATION GATHERING OF SKIN CONDITIONS

- Any recent changes in skin, hair, or nails? Any dryness, pruritus, sores, rashes, lumps, color changes, or changes in texture or odor noted?
- What signs or symptoms are present (rash, single or multiple skin lesions, itching, pain, exudates, bleeding, color changes)? Other symptoms of fever, malaise, loss of appetite? Upper respiratory symptoms?
- Where is the skin problem located?
- When did it start, sequence of occurrence, rapidity of onset? Is this a recurrence? Any known allergies? Any history of recent illness like strep throat?
- Any recent exposure to drugs, new skin products including insect repellent, detergent products, new foods, other environmental or occupational toxins, or family member or contact with similar condition? Family history of diseases like psoriasis? History of recent travel?
- What has been done to treat the problem, including medications (over-the-counter [OTC] or prescription) and/or lotions or other emollients applied? Did the problem get better or worse?

INFORMATION GATHERING AT KEY DEVELOPMENTAL STAGES

Age Group	Questions to Ask
Newborn	*At birth:* Vaginal or C-section birth? Were antibiotics taken during pregnancy, labor, or while breastfeeding? Breastfed or formula fed? Were probiotics taken during pregnancy or breastfeeding or was newborn given probiotics? History of skin trauma at birth or significant bruises to face/body? Presence of skin tags, dimples, cysts? Any extra digits? Moles or nevus? Hair or nail variations present at birth? Received any phototherapy?
Infant to 6 months of age	*Diaper history:* Type of disposable wipes used? Type of diapers used? *Skin care history:* Types of soap, moisturizing/cleansing lotion, other lotions, emollients, creams, oils? *Dressing habits:* Amounts/types of clothing in relation to environmental temperature, how clothing is washed, use of detergents, fabric softeners, dryer sheets? *Home environment:* Temperature, humidity, type of home heating? Air conditioning? *Feeding history:* Breast or bottle, type of formula, what foods introduced and when? *Disease history:* Constipation, diarrhea, atopic dermatitis, very dry skin, or antibiotic use?
6 months to 2 years of age	History of eating large amounts of yellow fruits, vegetables? History of prolonged crawling on hands, knees without protective clothing? History of rubbing head against furniture/walls?
Early childhood	Eating habits/types of food? History of exposure to communicable diseases? Pets/animal exposure? History of dry skin, eczema, urticaria, pruritus, nasal allergy, asthma, antibiotic use? History of nail biting, hair twisting? Excessive sweating?
Middle childhood	History of skin injuries: Cuts, falls, fractures, need for sutures? Any unexplained scarring or bruises? Outdoor exposure to plants during hiking, camping, picnics? Bee stings or contact with plants resulting in allergic reactions? Undiagnosed rashes or bites?
Adolescence	History of skin/hair changes, acne? Acne treatments used? Sports-related injuries? Body tattooing, ritual scarring, piercing? Were they done professionally using sterile techniques/supplies? History of hair removal? Problems/infections related to these practices?
Environmental risks	Exposure to tobacco smoke? Contact with chemical cleaning agents/other chemicals at home, school, work? Exposure to chemicals, toxins from caregiver's work? Living conditions, including exposures to mold, pests, or infestations? Access to resources needed for personal hygiene/cleaning, such as bathtub or shower, laundry, etc.?

PHYSICAL ASSESSMENT

The skin is one of the most accessible and easily examined organs of the body and is often the organ of most concern to children, adolescents, and parents. A complete examination of the skin using a consistent, systematic approach will increase the likelihood that important findings will not be missed. Always avoid making a quick diagnosis after only a brief inspection of an area of exposed skin or examining only the lesion of concern. A deliberate and methodical assessment of the skin will lead to a correct diagnosis and prevent missing important clues. During inspection, any changes in the skin should be palpated, inspected, and classified by morphology, size, color, texture, firmness, configuration, location, and distribution. Sterile gloves should be used for skin inspection if indicated. The color, turgor, texture, temperature, and moisture of the skin and the growth and texture of the hair and nails should also be noted.

It is important to conduct a complete skin examination before making a diagnosis. It is usually very easy to do a complete skin assessment on a newborn, but there may be a great deal of resistance from many adolescents to the idea of a complete skin exam. When the child or adolescent is uncomfortable being completely undressed because of developmental stage or cultural belief, then the assessment of the skin must be conducted using a systematic approach that divides the skin into areas that are sequentially uncovered, examined, and then re-covered before going on to the next area. In infants and young children, this may also prevent unnecessary cooling of the skin.

Inspection

Inspection of the skin is best conducted using natural light, or a well-lit room with fluorescent or incandescent lighting may be satisfactory. A magnifying glass and a measuring tool such as paper tape measure will be helpful for examining small skin lesions and moles. It may be necessary to follow the progress of lesions over time to determine an accurate diagnosis. A light for transillumination of lesions or for closer inspection may also be helpful. A photo inserted in the electronic medical record may be useful when following a skin condition or to consult with dermatology. In addition, a photo showing the tape measurement of the skin lesion can assist in evaluating changes in lesions over time.

Hair should be examined carefully by sitting the child in a chair rather than on the examination table so the hair can be viewed from above. Use a magnified light source whenever possible as overhead lighting or natural light is often not sufficient for examination of the scalp and hair.

Be sure to assess terminal and vellus hairs for changes. Note distribution, color, and quantity. Check for any lesions, dryness, oiliness, scaling, or infestation on the scalp. To assess hair density, part the hair starting at the frontal hairline and repeat the parts at 1-inch intervals, noting the spacing between the hairs. While noting color, scale, papules, pustules, and crusting on the scalp, note hair density from front to back of the scalp.

It is important for providers to assess new hair growth, temporal recession, hair loss from pulling, traction, or tension on the hair shaft, and the dimensions of hair loss in both dark hair and light hair (Fig. 7.4). Some hair loss is common in older infants and children. In infants, hair loss after the neonatal period may be due to birthmarks, birth trauma, inflammation such as seborrheic dermatitis, or infections such as *tinea capitis*. The majority of hair loss in infants and children is nonscarring, and the hair grows back once the underlying condition is corrected.[14-16] Excessive hair shedding can be measured by the *hair pull* test. Grasp 30 to 40 closely grouped hairs at the scalp using the thumb and index finger and gently but firmly pulling the hair away from the scalp. For the *hair tug* test, gather a cluster of hair at the scalp and use the other hand to tug the distal ends of the hair. This assesses hair fragility, and fragile hair will break off in small clusters.[14,15] Excessive hair loss or excessively fragile hair requires further diagnostics and referral as indicated.

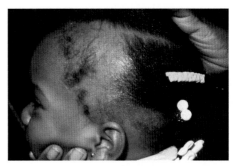

FIGURE 7.4 Traction Alopecia. (From Kliegman RM, et al. *Nelson Textbook of Pediatrics*. 21st ed. Philadelphia: Elsevier Inc.; 2020)

Nails should be examined for shape, color, and texture; artificial nails or nail polish can interfere with the assessment. Nail changes may be an early sign of systemic disease (Table 7.2). Inspect the curvature of the nail for *clubbing* (see Chapter 8, Fig. 8.5) or spooning and feel the surface for ridges. Changes in coloration or splinter hemorrhages in the nail should be noted. Finally, check the periungual tissue of the nail and note any redness, edema,

TABLE 7.2   NAIL LESIONS

Nail Symptoms	Photo	Diagnosis
Periungual blister that has coalescent tapioca-like vesicles Vesicles become turbid and opaque colored with time Usually at distal phalanx of finger Often painful, edema and erythema may be present	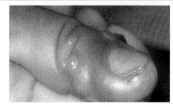	**Herpetic Whitlow**[a] **Cause:** HSV type 1 or 2 **Patient education:** Spread by touch
Dry, cauliflower-like thickened skin The absence of skin lines crossing the surface is a diagnostic sign of all warts, as are pinpoint black marks, which represent subkeratotic capillary thrombosis Usually located around the cuticle but can originate in the longitudinal grooves of the proximal or lateral nail folds Can cause fissures in the nail, pain, and embarrassment Can cause nail elevation and thickening of the nail		**Periungual warts**[b] **Cause:** HPV 1, 2, or 4 **Patient education:** Don't bite nails or bite or pick at cuticles
Thick yellow appearance to nail most often affects toenails, but check fingernails that have had acrylic or gel nails Nails are often brittle and break off or separate from the nail plate	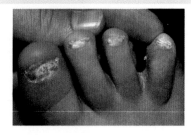	**Onchomycosis**[c] **Cause:** Fungal infection **Patient education:** Treatment is difficult and may take up to a year for a full clinical cure due to slow nail growth Prevent by keeping nails dry, change wet socks, and avoid walking with bare feet

TABLE 7.2	NAIL LESIONS—CONT'D	
Nail Symptoms	**Photo**	**Diagnosis**
Transverse grooves or furrows that originate under the proximal nail fold. Lines first appear at the cuticle and grow out with the nail Onychomadesis is proximal separation of the nail resulting from full but temporary arrest of the growth matrix	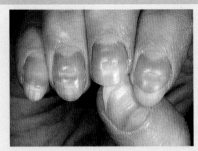	**Beau's lines and onychomadesis**[d] **Cause:** Due to any temporary disruption to the nail formation and appears several weeks or months after onset of the disease that caused the condition (hand, foot, and mouth is one such cause) **Patient education:** This is a temporary disorder and the nail will grow out normally
Punctate depressions resulting from alterations in the proximal matrix. May vary from small to large and dip pits to clusters of pits. One or more nails may be affected	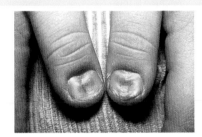	**Nail pitting**[a] **Cause:** Usually atopic dermatitis or psoriasis but can also be from trauma **Patient education:** When underlying disorder is treated this will usually allow the nail to grow out normally
Lateral edge of the nail is curved inward and penetrates the underlying tissue Erythema, edema, pain, and in chronic conditions granulation tissue are present Most commonly seen on the great toes but may occur on other nails Pseudo-ingrown nails present in newborns are self-correcting by 12 months of age	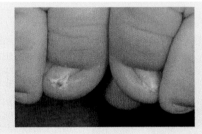	**Ingrown nails** **Cause:** Ill-fitting footwear and improper cutting of the nail (in a half-circle) **Patient education:** Provide shoes that fit correctly and cut nails straight across

Data adapted from Luckenberg EL, Silverman RA. Nail disorders in children. *Dermatol Nurs.* 2011; 22(1). Available at http://www.medscape.com/viewarticle/718695_1; Richert B, Andre J. Nail disorders in children diagnosis and management. *Am J Clin Dermatol.* 2011; 12(2):101–112; Figures:
[a]Cohen, BA. *Pediatric Dermatology.* 5th ed. Philadelphia: Elsevier Inc.; 2022
[b]Figure A from Martin JM. Spontaneous remission of recalcitrant warts in girls after human papillomavirus vaccination. *Dermatology* (Actas Dermo-Sifiliograficas, English Edition) 2016;107(6);533–535: Figure B from Paller A, Manicini A. *Hurwitz Clinical Pediatric Dermatology: A Textbook of Skin Disorders of Childhood and Adolescence.* 6th ed. St. Louis: Elsevier Inc.; 2022.
[c]Kliegman, RM, et al. *Nelson Textbook of Pediatrics.* 21st ed. Philadelphia: Elsevier Inc.; 2020.
[d]Habif T. *Clinical Dermatology.* 7th ed. Philadelphia: Elsevier, Inc.; 2021.

induration, or tenderness. Absence or atrophy of the nails in the newborn period may indicate a congenital syndrome and requires consultation and referral for further diagnostics.[23-26]

Palpation

Palpation of the skin should be done with warm hands, using gloves if you think the child or adolescent may have an infectious lesion. Palpate skin temperature using the back of your hand and compare the temperature of one area of skin to another area of skin using both hands. Temperature cannot be assessed accurately through gloves, and the presence of a fever should always be checked using a thermometer. Check for *skin turgor*, resiliency, or elasticity of the skin, by gently pinching a fold of the child's skin over the abdomen between your thumb and forefinger and then releasing it. *Skin turgor* can give important clues to the hydration and nutritional status of a child. How long the skin remains tented after it is released will provide clues to the degree of dehydration (Table 7.3).

TABLE 7.3	ESTIMATING DEHYDRATION IN AN INFANT OR YOUNG CHILD
Return to Normal After the Pinch	**Degree of Dehydration**
<2 s	<5% loss of body weight
2–3 s	5%–8% loss of body weight
3–4 s	9%–10% loss of body weight
>4 s	>10% loss of body weight

Data from Ball JW, Dains JE, Solomon BS, et al. *Seidel's Guide to Physical Examination*. 10th ed. St. Louis: Elsevier Inc.; 2023

SKIN CONDITIONS

If inspection and palpation of the skin reveals a lesion, more examination is necessary. A *skin lesion* refers to any variations or changes in the skin. Skin lesions may be *primary* or *secondary* (Tables 7.4 and 7.5). A *primary lesion*

TABLE 7.4	PRIMARY LESIONS		
Name	**Photo**	**Description**	**Examples of Conditions**
Macule/patch[a]		Flat, circumscribed lesion of any size, <1 cm is macule; >1 cm is patch; lesions usually rounded but may be oval, can be vascular, hyperpigmented, or hypopigmented	Freckle, café au lait spots, vitiligo, flat mole (nevus), blue-gray macules of the neonate (congenital melanocytosis), port-wine stain
Papule[b]		Palpable, circumscribed elevated lesions <1 cm	Dermatitis, molluscum contagiosum, papular urticaria, elevated moles, wart

TABLE 7.4 PRIMARY LESIONS—CONT'D

Name	Photo	Description	Examples of Conditions
Plaque		Circumscribed, elevated, disc-shaped lesion >1 cm; commonly formed by confluence of papules	Atopic dermatitis, lichen simplex chronicus (neurodermatitis), tinea corporis
Nodule[c]		Circumscribed, elevated, usually solid lesion that measures 0.5–2 cm; may be in epidermis or extend deeper	Fibromas, neurofibromas, intradermal nevi, erythema nodosum, hemangioma, pyogenic granuloma
Cyst[d]		Elevated, circumscribed, encapsulated lesion in dermis or subcutaneous layer filled with liquid/semisolid material	Sebaceous cyst, cystic acne
Vesicle[b]		Sharply circumscribed, elevated, fluid-containing lesion that measures ≤0.5 cm	Herpes simplex, varicella, insect bite, herpes zoster
Bullae[c]		Sharply circumscribed, elevated, fluid-containing lesion that measures ≥1 cm	Contact dermatitis, epidermolysis bullosa, pemphigus vulgaris, burn, bullous impetigo

Continued

| TABLE 7.4 | PRIMARY LESIONS—CONT'D | | |

Name	Photo	Description	Examples of Conditions
Wheal[c]		Distinctive type of solid elevation formed by local, superficial, transient edema; white to pink–pale red in color; blanches with pressure, varies in size, shape	Urticaria, insect bite, dermographia, erythema multiforme
Comedones[e]		Plugged secretions of horny material retained within pilosebaceous follicle; may be flesh-colored, closed (whiteheads); brown/black, open (blackheads)	Acne
Burrows[b]		Linear lesion produced by tunneling of animal parasite in stratum corneum	Scabies, cutaneous larva migrans (creeping eruption)
Telangiectasia[f]		Fine, irregular, red lines produced by capillary dilation	Rosacea

[a]Anderson S. Café au lait macules and associated genetic syndromes. *J Pediatr Health Care.* 2020;34(1):71–81.
[b]Cohen, BA. *Pediatric Dermatology.* 5th ed. Philadelphia: Elsevier Inc.; 2022.
[c]Eichenfeld LF, Frieden IJ, Mathes EF, Zaenglein AL. *Neonatal and Infant Dermatology.* 3rd ed. Philadelphia: Elsevier Inc.; 2015.
[d]Habif T. *Clinical Dermatology.* 7th ed. Philadelphia: Elsevier, Inc.; 2021.
[e]Brinster NK, Liu V, Diwan AH, et al. *Dermatopathology: High-Yield Pathology.* Philadelphia: Saunders; 2011.
[f]Paller A, Manicini A. *Hurwitz Clinical Pediatric Dermatology: A Textbook of Skin Disorders of Childhood and Adolescence.* 6th ed. St. Louis: Elsevier Inc.; 2022.

TABLE 7.5	SECONDARY LESIONS		
Name	**Photo**	**Description**	**Example of Diseases**
Scale[a]		Formed by accumulation of compact desquamation of stratum corneum layers; may be greasy, yellowish; silvery, fine, barely visible or large, adherent, and lamellar	Seborrheic dermatitis, psoriasis, pityriasis alba, tinea pedis, dyshidrosis, ichthyosis
Fissure[a]		Dry, moist, linear, often painful, cleavage from epidermis to dermis that results from marked drying; long-standing inflammation, thickening, loss of elasticity of integument	Chronic dermatoses, intertrigo, atopic dermatitis, lihthyosis
Lichenification[b]		Rough, thickened epidermis secondary to persistent rubbing, itching, or skin irritation; often involves flexor surface of extremity	Atopic dermatitis, chronic dermatitis
Scar[c]		Permanent fibrotic skin changes that develop following damage to dermis; initially pink/violet, fading to white, shiny, sclerotic area *Keloid:* pink, smooth, rubbery; often traversed by telangiectatic vessels; increases in size long after healing of lesion; differentiated from hypertrophic scars because surface of keloid scar tends to be beyond original wound area	Healed wound, stretch marks, keloid, burn

Continued

TABLE 7.5	SECONDARY LESIONS—CONT'D			
Name	**Photo**		**Description**	**Example of Diseases**
Crust[c]			Dried exudate on epidermis composed of serum, blood, or pus overlying a ruptured bulla or vesicle; caused by staphylococcal or streptococcal bacteria	Impetigo, epidermolysis bullosa
Erosions			Moist, slightly depressed vesicular lesion in which all or part of epidermis has been lost; may have surrounding erythema or edema; heals without scarring	Impetigo, eczematous diseases, intertrigo, candidiasis, methicillin-resistant *Staphylococcus aureus* (MRSA)
Purpura[d]			Flat lesion but may be palpable; petechiae if pinpoint; does not blanch to pressure; larger areas of bruising may be present	Henoch-Schönlein-purpura fulminans, idiopathic thrombocytopenia

Data from Eichenfield L, Frieden I, Zaenglein A, et al. *Neonatal and Infant Dermatology*. 3rd ed. Philadelphia: Elsevier Inc.; 2015; Ball JW, Dains JE, Benedict GW. *Seidel's Guide to Physical Examination*. 10th ed. St. Louis: Mosby; 2023 and Infoderm.com, Galderma Laboratories, LP, 2012.

[a]Eichenfield L, Frieden I, Zaenglein A, et al. *Neonatal and Infant Dermatology*. 3rd ed. Philadelphia: Elsevier Inc.; 2015.

[b]Chatrath S, Bradley L, Kentosh J. Dermatologic conditions in skin of color compared to white patients: similarities, differences, and special considerations. *Arch Dermatol Res*. 2022. doi:10.1007/s00403-022-02493-2.

[c]Ball JW, Dains JE, Solomon BS, et al. *Seidel' Guide to Physical Examination*. 10th ed. St. Louis: Elsevier Inc.; 2023.

[d]Paller A, Manicini A. *Hurwitz Clinical Pediatric Dermatology: A Textbook of Skin Disorders of Childhood and Adolescence*. 6th ed. St. Louis: Elsevier Inc.; 2022.

is the initial lesion of a skin condition. Identifying the *primary lesion* is the most important step in assessing skin conditions in children and assists clinicians in diagnosis. A *secondary lesion* often develops as a skin condition progresses such as infection or trauma.

Skin Lesions

Using the correct terminology facilitates accurate description of skin lesions. The *morphology* or characteristic form and structure of skin lesions should be identified when any condition is noted during the assessment of the skin. Attention should be made to the distribution and pattern of lesions. Becoming familiar with four or five distinct morphologic patterns such as acneiform, annular, or linear eruptions and the associated findings will assist in making a diagnosis. The *distribution* refers to the location of skin findings, whereas *pattern* refers to the specific anatomical or physiological arrangement of the lesions. Note the shape of skin lesions and whether they are clustered together or scattered. The border or margin, any associated findings such as central clearing, and the pigmentation of the lesion also should be identified. Find and study the primary lesion, assess for secondary lesions, and examine the distribution of any other skin lesions or skin variations. Table 7.6 illustrates the color, borders, configuration, and distribution of lesions. Table 7.7 presents a few common dermatologic conditions with differing presentations in skin with varied pigmentation. Common newborn and infant skin conditions are presented in Chapter 6, Table 6.6.

TABLE 7.6	BORDERS, CONFIGURATION, AND DISTRIBUTION OF LESIONS

Border

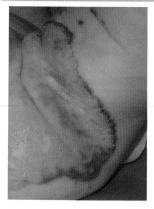

Borders of lesion may be raised or indurated, as in granuloma annulare and neonatal lupus, or indistinct, as in cellulitis or atopic dermatitis

Acrodermatitis enteropathica

Configuration
Blaschko (Linear)

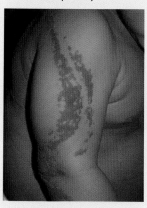

Linear lesions do not follow any known vascular, nervous, or lymphatic pattern. V- and S-shaped lines may represent patterns of neuroectodermal migration, and distribution indicates a cutaneous mosaicism

Linear epidermal nevus

Continued

TABLE 7.6	BORDERS, CONFIGURATION, AND DISTRIBUTION OF LESIONS—CONT'D

Border

Dermatomal/Zosteriform (Linear)

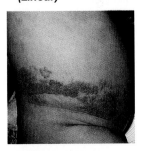

Lines demarcating a dermatome supplied by one dorsal root ganglia

Herpes zoster

Segmental Patterns

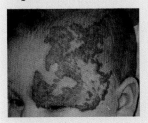

The configuration of segmental lesions is thought to be determined by the location of embryonic placodes or other embryonic territories, as can be seen in PHACE syndrome

Infantile hemangioma

Annular

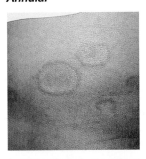

A round, ring-shaped lesion, where the periphery is distinct from the center, as in tinea corporis or neonatal lupus

Annular lesions of neonatal lupus

Nummular

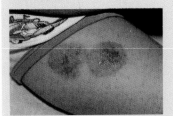

A coin-shaped lesion, with homogeneous character throughout, as in nummular eczema

Nummular eczema

TABLE 7.6	BORDERS, CONFIGURATION, AND DISTRIBUTION OF LESIONS—CONT'D

Border

Targetoid

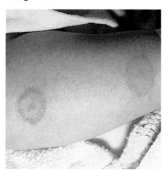

Concentric ringed lesions, often with a dusky or bullous center characteristic of erythema multiforme

Early lesions of erythema multiforme

Herpetiform

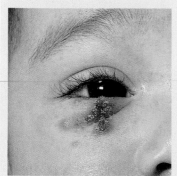

Clusters of erythematous occasionally scabbed lesions, as in herpes simplex

Herpes simplex infection

Corymbiform

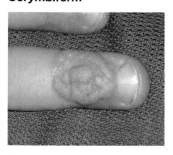

Defined as a central cluster of lesions surrounded by scattered individual lesions, as in verrucae

Verrucae

Modified from Eichenfield L, Frieden I, Zaenglein A, et al. *Neonatal and Infant Dermatology*. 3rd, Philadelphia: Elsevier Inc.; 2015; Nummular eczema image is from Weston W, Lane A, Morelli J. *Color Textbook of Pediatric Dermatology*. 4th ed. St. Louis; Mosby; 2007.

TABLE 7.7	PRESENTATIONS VARIED BY SKIN PIGMENTATION	
Diagnosis	Photo 1	Photo 2
Perioral dermatitis[a]		
Acne vulgaris[b]		
Insect bite		

TABLE 7.7	PRESENTATIONS VARIED BY SKIN PIGMENTATION—CONT'D	
Diagnosis	Photo 1	Photo 2
Urticaria[c]		
Seborrheic dermatitis of the scalp[d]		

[a]Figure A from James WD, et al. *Andrews' Diseases of the Skin.* 13th ed. Philadelphia: Elsevier, Inc.; 2020; B from Paller A, Mancini A. *Hurwitz Clinical Pediatric Dermatology: A Textbook of Skin Disorders of Childhood and Adolescence.* 6th ed. St. Louis: Elsevier Inc.; 2022.

[b]Acne Vulgaris from Chatrath S, Bradley L, Kentosh J. Dermatologic conditions in skin of color compared to white patients: similarities, differences, and special considerations. *Arch Dermatol Res.* 2022. doi:10.1007/s00403-022-02493-2.

[c]Urticaria from Chatrath S, Bradley L, Kentosh J. Dermatologic conditions in skin of color compared to white patients: similarities, differences, and special considerations. Arch Dermatol Res. 2022. doi:10.1007/s00403-022-02493-2.

[d]Seborrheic dermatitis of the scalp from Chatrath S, Bradley L, Kentosh J. Dermatologic conditions in skin of color compared to white patients: similarities, differences, and special considerations. *Arch Dermatol Res.* 2022. doi:10.1007/s00403-022-02493-2.

DOCUMENTATION

Avoid the use of a specific diagnosis when describing a lesion in the objective physical findings, such as diaper rash or *candidiasis*, a common fungal infection in infants. Accurate charting using the correct terminology and photos allows other health care providers to visualize the skin lesions and provide the necessary follow-up to evaluate a change or improvement in the skin lesions. The wide use of smartphones with high-resolution digital cameras by individuals and families makes the tracking of skin lesions and skin conditions at home a possibility for health care providers. The ability to digitally visualize lesions over time may prevent the child and family from returning to the clinical setting for frequent follow-up visits. In electronic medical record (EMR) systems, customizing a charting template for assessment of the skin with dermatological terms and adding a glossary of dermatological definitions provides accurate, consistent descriptions of skin lesions by different providers, and saves time when charting. Many EMR systems allow photos to be inserted into the medical record. These photos may be taken by the provider or by the family and submitted by text message or e-mailed to the provider to enhance accurate diagnosis, treatment, and follow-up.

TELEHEALTH TIPS

A rash cannot be diagnosed by listening to a description over the phone, and pediatric health care providers should avoid this type of assessment. Telemedicine, as a method to deliver health care, may allow a complete assessment of the skin using a computer and peripheral devices. Patients that are not able to physically come to the clinic or office may now have an option that allows both initial assessment, diagnosis, and follow-up of skin conditions and diseases. Children and adolescents are often more comfortable showing their skin, hair, and nails in the home setting using a computer. The high-resolution cameras that are available today on personal computers and tablets and the magnifier peripheral devices (dermascopes) available provide excellent visualization of the skin with proper instructions to the family or adolescent for lighting and technique. The "store and forward" feature of most telemedicine software allows the practitioner to easily forward pictures for consultation with a pediatric dermatologist when a diagnosis is uncertain.

SUMMARY OF EXAMINATION

- Skin disorders may vary widely when observed in an infant or child, as compared with the same skin disorder when seen in an adult.
- Extremely premature infants are born without the *stratum corneum*, have limited ability to control water loss, and can tolerate a limited amount of touch.
- Term newborns have a fully functional stratum corneum, which is about 60% the thickness of adult skin.

- Skin pigmentation or melanin should be considered as a factor for understanding and diagnosing some underlying skin properties and characteristics.
- A careful age-appropriate history is critical to making an accurate assessment of the skin (see Chapter 4, Information Gathering, and Box 7.1).
- A skin lesion refers to any variations or skin changes. On inspection, note distribution or location of skin findings and pattern of skin lesions.
- Identify primary lesions, the initial lesion of a skin condition, and secondary lesions, which develop over time as a skin condition progresses.
- Palpation of the skin should be done with warm hands or with gloves when infection is suspected.
- Assessment of the skin must be conducted using a systematic approach that divides the skin into areas that are sequentially uncovered, examined, and then re-covered.
- Avoid making a quick diagnosis after only a brief inspection of partially exposed skin.
- A rash in children cannot be diagnosed by listening to a description over the phone.
- Accurate charting using the correct terminology and photos allows other health care providers to visualize the skin lesions and provide the necessary follow-up to evaluate change or improvement in skin lesions.
- When charting, avoid use of a specific diagnosis when describing a lesion in the objective physical findings.
- Telemedicine, as a method to deliver healthcare, may allow a complete assessment of the skin using a computer and peripheral devices.

DOCUMENTATION

14-Month-Old With Candidiasis
Skin: Discrete, red papules and pustules over the perineum with satellite lesions over the legs and abdomen; otherwise, skin lightly pigmented and clear.

DOCUMENTATION

15-Year-Old With Moderate Acne Vulgaris
Skin: Moderate amount of open and closed comedones over nose and cheeks, discrete pustular lesions on forehead, no nodules or cyst noted. Skin oily with moderate papular, erythematous lesions over upper back.

REFERENCES

1. Paller AS, Mancini AJ. *Hurwitz Clinical Pediatric Dermatology: A Textbook of Skin Disorders of Childhood and Adolescence.* 6th ed. Philadelphia: Elsevier; 2021.
2. Bowlby J. *Attachment and loss.* New York: Basic Books; 1969.
3. Klaus MH, Kennell JH. *Maternal-Infant Bonding: The Impact of Early Separation or Loss on Family Development.* St. Louis: Mosby; 1976.
4. Spitz RA. *The First Year of Life: A Psychoanalytic Study of Normal and Deviant Development of Object Relations.* New York: International Universities Press; 1965.
5. Pintas S, Lio P. Manipulating the microbiome: What is known, what is unknown. J Integr Dermatol. Published online February 25, 2022.
6. Marchesi JR. The vocabulary of microbiome research: a proposal. *Microbiome.* 2015;3:31.
7. Dunn AB, Jordan S, Baker BJ, Carlson NS. The maternal infant microbiome. *MCN Am J Matern Child Nurs.* 2017;42:318–325.
8. Gronlund MM, Lehtonen OP, Eerola E, Kero P. Fecal micro flora in healthy infants born by different methods of delivery: permanent changes in intestinal flora after cesarean delivery. *J Pediatr Gasteroenterol Nutr.* 1999;28:19–25.
9. Pandey PK, Verma P, Kumar H, Bavdekar A, Patole MS, Shouche YS. Comparative analysis of fecal microflora of healthy full-term Indian infants born with different methods of delivery (vaginal vs cesarean): Acinetobacter sp. prevalence in vaginally born infants. *J Biosci.* 2012;37:989–998.
10. Meylan P, Lang C, Mermoud S, et al. Skin colonization by Staphylococcus aureus precedes the clinical diagnosis of atopic dermatitis in infancy. *J Invest Dermatol.* 2017;137:2497–2504.
11. Dinulos JGH. *Habif's Clinical Dermatology: A Color Guide to Diagnosis and Treatment.* 7th ed. Philadelphia: Mosby; 2020.
12. Ball JW, Dains JE, Flynn JA, Solomon BS, Stewart RW. *Seidel's Guide to Physical Examination: An Interprofessional Approach.* St. Louis: Mosby; 2022.
13. Eichenfield LF, Frieden IJ, Mathes EF, Zaenglein A. *Neonatal and Infant Dermatology.* 3rd ed. Saunders; 2015.
14. Jackson AJ, Price VH. How to diagnose hair loss. *Dermatol Clin.* 2013;31:21–28.
15. Xu L, Liu KX, Senna MM. A practical approach to the diagnosis and management of hair loss in children and adolescents. *Front Med (Lausanne).* 2017;4:112.
16. Castelo-Soccio L. Diagnosis and management of hair loss in children. *Curr Opin Pediatr.* 2016;28:483–489.
17. Everett JS, Budescu M, Sommers MS. Expanding the palette of pediatric playthings: a call to action for pediatric dermatologists. *Clin Nurs Res.* 2012;21:495–516.
18. Lee MS, Lnggonegoro DW, Huang JT, Nambudiri VE. Expanding the palette of pediatric playthings: a call to action for pediatric dermatologists. *Pediatr Dermatol.* 2021;38:1601–1603.
19. Telofski LS, Morello AP 3rd, Mack Correa MC, Stamatas GN. The infant skin barrier: can we pre-serve, protect, and enhance the barrier? *Dermatol Res Pract.* 2012;2012:198789.
20. Chatrath S, Bradley L, Kentosh J. Dermatologic conditions in skin of color compared to white patients: similarities, differences, and special considerations. *Arch Dermatol Res.* 2022 Dec 1.
21. Cohen B. *Pediatric Dermatology.* 5th ed. Saunders; 2021.
22. Alexis AF, Woolery-Lloyd H, Williams K, et al. Racial/ethnic variations in skin barrier: implications for skin care recommendations in skin of color. *J Drugs Dermatol.* 2021;20:932–938.
23. He A, Okoye GA. Chemical and physical properties of hair: comparisons between Asian, Black, and Caucasian hair. In: Aguh C, Okoye G, eds. *Fundamentals of Ethnic Hair.* Springer; 2017.
24. Dehavay F, Richert B. Nails in systemic disorders: main signs and clues. *Dermatol Clin.* 2021;39:153–173.
25. Tosti A, Iorizzo M, Piraccini BA, Starace M. The nail in systemic diseases. *Dermatol Clin.* 2006;24:341–347.
26. de Berker D. Childhood nail diseases. *Dermatol Clin.* 2006;24:355–363.

CHAPTER 8

HEART AND VASCULAR ASSESSMENT

Patricia O'Brien; Julianne Evangelista

EMBRYOLOGICAL DEVELOPMENT

The heart begins to form in the fetus by the end of the third week after conception. A crescent-shaped structure is formed that fuses at the midline to create a single linear heart tube (Fig. 8.1). As the primitive heart tube elongates, it differentiates into the *atria, ventricles, bulbus cordis*, and *truncus arteriosus*. The conduction system also begins to form during this time. Valve formation begins around the fourth to fifth week after conception, and the formation of the heart is complete by the eighth week after conception. Any early changes in this process caused by genetic, maternal, or external environmental factors can lead to structural malformations of the heart.

During fetal life, the lung sacs remain collapsed and blood is oxygenated through the placenta. Oxygenated blood travels from the placenta to the heart via the umbilical veins and *ductus venosus* to the *inferior vena cava* (IVC) and into the *right atrium* (RA). Blood then streams to the *left atrium* (LA) through a *patent foramen ovale* (PFO) and into the *left ventricle* (LV), which pumps it out the *aorta* (Fig. 8.2). The less saturated venous blood traveling from the *superior vena cava* (SVC) and *coronary sinus* also flows to the RA but is directed toward the *right ventricle* (RV) and *pulmonary artery* (PA). High pulmonary vascular resistance limits blood flow into the lungs, which are not yet involved in ventilation, and redirects it through the *patent ductus arteriosus* (PDA) to the descending aorta and lower body.

With an infant's first breaths, pulmonary vascular resistance falls, causing a dramatic increase in pulmonary blood flow. The ensuing increase in pulmonary venous return to the heart raises LA pressure, causing closure of the PFO. Arterial oxygen saturation increases, resulting in improved oxygenation by the lungs. This higher saturation promotes functional closure of the PDA by 48 to 72 hours after birth, with complete anatomical closure occurring by 2 to 3 weeks of age.[1]

ANATOMY AND PHYSIOLOGY

Anatomy of the Postnatal Heart

The heart is composed of four chambers. The upper chambers (atria) are low-pressure receiving chambers, and the lower chambers (ventricles) are high-pressure pumping chambers. The heart is further divided into right and left sides. The *RA* receives deoxygenated blood from the body, and the *RV* pumps it out the pulmonary artery to the lungs to become oxygenated. The *LA* receives oxygenated blood from the lungs, and the *LV* pumps it out the aorta to the body (Fig. 8.3). The LV operates at a higher pressure than the RV. This normal circulation occurs in series, and there is no mixing of deoxygenated and oxygenated blood.

There are four valves in the heart that regulate blood flow between the atria and ventricles. The atrioventricular (AV) valves regulate blood flow between the atria and ventricles, and the semilunar valves regulate blood flow between the ventricles and great vessels. The

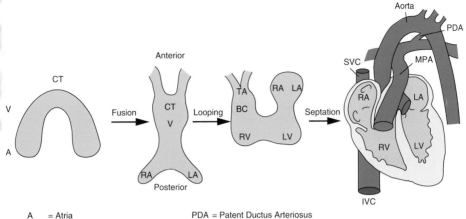

A   = Atria
BC = Bulbus Cordis
CT = Conotruncus
IVC = Inferior Vena Cava
LA = Left Atrium
LV = Left Ventricle
MPA = Main Pulmonary Artery

PDA = Patent Ductus Arteriosus
RA = Right Atrium
RV = Right Ventricle
SVC = Superior Vena Cava
TA = Truncus Arteriosus
V   = Ventricle

FIGURE 8.1 Fetal development of the heart.

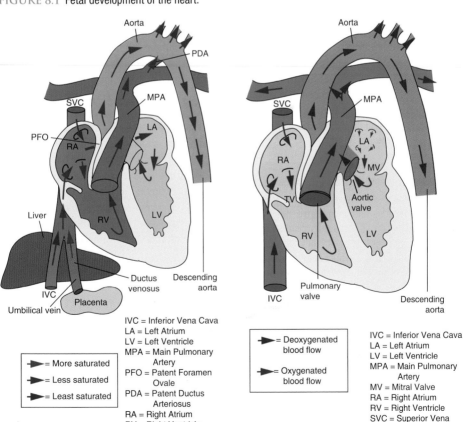

IVC = Inferior Vena Cava
LA = Left Atrium
LV = Left Ventricle
MPA = Main Pulmonary Artery
PFO = Patent Foramen Ovale
PDA = Patent Ductus Arteriosus
RA = Right Atrium
RV = Right Ventricle
SVC = Superior Vena Cava

➤ = More saturated
➤ = Less saturated
➤ = Least saturated

FIGURE 8.2 Fetal cardiac circulation.

➤ = Deoxygenated blood flow
➤ = Oxygenated blood flow

IVC = Inferior Vena Cava
LA = Left Atrium
LV = Left Ventricle
MPA = Main Pulmonary Artery
MV = Mitral Valve
RA = Right Atrium
RV = Right Ventricle
SVC = Superior Vena Cava
TV = Tricuspid Valve

FIGURE 8.3 Postnatal cardiac circulation.

tricuspid valve on the right and the *mitral valve* on the left are the AV valves (Fig. 8.3). The *pulmonic valve*, located at the base of the pulmonary artery between the right ventricle and the pulmonary artery, and the *aortic valve*, located at the base of the aorta between the aorta and LV, are the semilunar valves. Closure of these valves produces the heart sounds commonly referred to as "lub-dub" (S_1, S_2).

Physiological Variations

In preterm infants, the patent ductus arteriosus may remain open for several weeks after birth, causing hemodynamic instability and a higher mortality rate than infants without a PDA.[2]

System-Specific History

A careful and systematic history is performed at each well-child visit to monitor the overall health status of infants and children, to identify those with cardiac symptoms, and to recognize signs of cardiac disease. The Information Gathering table presents the important age-related questions to ask about the cardiovascular system and relevant questions related to maternal infections and maternal medical conditions that place infants at high risk for *congenital heart disease* (CHD).

PEDIATRIC PEARLS

Infants with CHD may have tachypnea (rapid, shallow breathing) and tachycardia but typically do not present in respiratory distress (i.e., retractions, grunting, nasal flaring) unless there is a significant increase in pulmonary blood flow or poor systemic blood flow with acidosis.

Physical Assessment

The cardiac examination is systematic and adapted to the child's developmental level (Fig. 8.4). A complete assessment of the cardiac system is key to making any conclusions about the significance of any cardiac symptoms or single abnormality. Cardiac findings should not be taken in isolation.

It is important to consistently plot height, weight, and head circumference in infants and children up to 2 years of age to evaluate whether the growth rate is proportional and to monitor for insufficient growth. For infants, any drop-off in weight percentiles as compared with length and head circumference values should raise the suspicion of CHD.[1] Temperature, heart rate, and respiratory rate are measured and assessed. Fever and respiratory distress both can elevate heart rate.

Blood pressure should be measured whenever possible during physical examinations, but once in infancy and then routinely after 3 years of age.[2] *Coarctation of the aorta* and systemic *hypertension* can go undetected if blood pressure measurements are omitted during well-child visits. If measured, blood pressure in infants should be taken in all four extremities or at a minimum in the right arm and in one leg to detect a coarctation of the aorta. In children, simultaneous palpation of the radial and femoral pulses is also important in assessing whether a coarctation may be present.

Inspection

Note general appearance and activity level and whether the child is alert, lethargic, or appears ill. Note nutritional status and the proportion of weight to height and head circumference. Also, note whether any unusual facial or other external features are present that may indicate the presence of a chromosomal syndrome or congenital anomaly. Examine for any surgical scars on the sternum and chest area that would indicate a previous surgical procedure. Note shape of chest and any presence of *pectus excavatum* or *pectus carinatum* (see Chapter 9).

Color

Note whether the child is pale or cyanotic and assess color under natural light if possible. Pallor can occur in infants who are anemic, who have vasoconstriction due to *heart failure* (HF), or who are in shock. Central cyanosis (cyanosis of the lips, mucous membranes, and tongue)

INFORMATION GATHERING FOR ASSESSING THE CARDIOVASCULAR SYSTEM AT KEY DEVELOPMENTAL STAGES

Age Group	Questions to Ask	Rationale
Prenatal, infancy, early childhood	Any family history of CHD/chromosomal abnormalities, sudden/premature death; exposure to prenatal illness/infections (both chronic and during pregnancy); exposure to prenatal medications/drug use	CHD caused by interaction between genetic and environmental factors (systemic lupus, rubella, diabetes mellitus, anticonvulsants, alcohol, etc.).
	Apgar scores if known	Usually normal with CHD except for color if cyanotic.
	Any problems with poor feeding, sweating (especially on the forehead) during feeding, poor weight gain, FTT, decreased activity level	Symptoms of CHD often occur with feeding because of increased oxygen consumption and the need for greater cardiac output.
	Any pallor or blueness in color; any changes in color, especially when crying	Infants with cyanotic heart disease turn dark blue or ruddy in color when crying due to the prolonged expiratory phase and resulting increase in right-to-left shunting. Hypercyanotic spells are often associated with extreme irritability and rapid, deep, and sometimes labored respirations.
	Any pattern of rapid breathing; frequent respiratory infections	Left-to-right shunting lesions (VSD, AVSD, PDA) cause increased blood flow to the lungs, resulting in frequent respiratory infections, FTT, and decreased exercise tolerance.
Middle childhood and adolescence	Any inability to keep up with the activity level of peers, need for frequent periods of rest, anorexia, cough, wheezing, rales, chest pain, leg cramps, syncope, light-headedness, palpitations; any history of drug use; any family history of sudden death, syncope, or arrhythmias	CHD can decrease exercise intolerance. Left ventricular outflow obstructive lesions (AS, coarctation of the aorta) can cause heart failure (HF). Undetected coarctation of the aorta can cause leg cramps. Coronary artery abnormalities (including Kawasaki disease) and cocaine use can cause chest pain. Structural and dysrhythmic heart disease can first present as syncope. Some dysrhythmias are genetic in origin and can be familial.
	Any history of recent infections, prolonged fever or malaise, recent dental work	Untreated streptococcal infections, recent COVID infection, Kawasaki disease and infective endocarditis can result in HF or acquired heart disease.

AS, Aortic stenosis; *AVSD*, atrioventricular septal defect; *CHD*, congenital heart disease; *HF*, heart failure; *FTT*, failure to thrive; *PDA*, patent ductus arteriosus; *VSD*, ventricular septal defect.

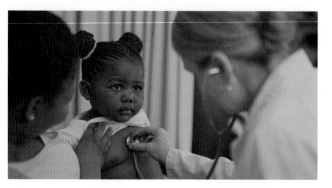

FIGURE 8.4 Cardiac examination of the infant.

occurs when arterial oxygen saturation falls below 85% in patients with normal hemoglobin levels. In patients with less skin pigmentation, cyanosis presents as a dark bluish tint to the skin and mucous membranes (which reflects the bluish tint of unoxygenated hemoglobin). In patients with greater skin pigmentation, cyanosis may present as gray or whitish (not bluish) skin around the mouth, and the conjunctivae may appear gray or bluish. In patients with yellowish skin tone, cyanosis may cause a grayish-greenish skin tone.[3]

Clubbing

Clubbing occurs when arterial desaturation has been present for at least 6 months or longer. The fingers and toes become red and shiny and progress to wide, thick digits with eventual loss of the normal angle between the nails and the nail beds (Fig. 8.5).[2] With early surgical treatment of cyanotic heart defects in infancy, severe clubbing is an unusual finding.

Palpation

Pulses are evaluated for their presence or absence, intensity, timing, symmetry, and whether the pulse is regular or irregular, weak, or bounding. A comparison also should be made as to right and left symmetry and quality of pulses in the upper and lower extremities. A pulse that is absent or weaker in the lower extremities compared with the upper extremities is diagnostic of *coarctation of the aorta*. A strong pedal pulse is a good indication that

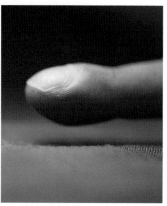

FIGURE 8.5 Clubbing of nails resulting from arterial desaturation. (Modified from Hochberg MC, Silman AJ, Smolen JS, et al. *Rheumatology*. 3rd ed. St. Louis: Mosby; 2003.)

there is no coarctation. Irregular pulses may be due to an *arrhythmia*. Weak and thready pulses may indicate poor perfusion or shock, whereas bounding pulses are usually noted with PDA, AV malformation, or aortic insufficiency.[2] *Peripheral perfusion* is also important to assess, especially in infants. Normally, extremities should be warm to the touch and have a brisk capillary refill time (CRT) of less than 3 seconds—a quick measure of cardiac output. Older children with cardiac conditions may have weak distal pulses on one side or the other because of previous cardiac catheterizations or cardiac surgeries.

Normal liver size is usually 1 to 2 cm below the right costal margin. In conditions of abnormal cardiac position, or situs (positional abnormalities), the liver edge is midline or on the left side of the abdomen. *Hepatomegaly*, or liver engorgement, is a consistent indicator of right heart failure when noted in conjunction with other cardiac findings.

Palpate the anterior chest wall over the heart, the *precordium*, to determine the location of the *point of maximal impulse*, or PMI. The PMI is important in determining ventricular overload, cardiomegaly, and the presence or absence of thrills. Normally, the PMI is felt at the apex in the left midclavicular line, indicating LV dominance. However, it is normal for newborns and infants to have a greater RV impulse, with the PMI felt at the left lower sternal border (LLSB). A PMI that is diffuse and rises slowly is called a *heave*, and a PMI that is sharp and well localized is known as a *tap*.[2]

A *thrill* indicates turbulent blood flow and is never normal. It is felt as a vibratory sensation on palpation and should be examined not only on the *precordium* but also in the suprasternal notch and over the carotid arteries. Precordial thrills are best felt with the palm of the hand, whereas thrills in the suprasternal notch and over the carotid arteries are best felt with the fingertips.[2]

PEDIATRIC PEARLS

Palpation of the liver for enlargement is a critical indicator of overall fluid status in infants and children with HF.

Auscultation

Auscultation of heart sounds in children should be performed in a stepwise fashion, using both the diaphragm and the bell of a stethoscope to elicit both high (diaphragm) and low (bell) frequency sounds (Fig. 8.6). Children with a thin chest wall have heart sounds that are louder than in adults. However, the faster heart rate can make it difficult to accurately distinguish the heart sounds from other adventitious sounds, particularly in early infancy. In children who are overweight or obese, heart sounds are softer due to the increase in adipose tissue. It is recommended that the individual heart sounds be identified first and then analyzed before identifying murmurs.

Heart Sounds

The *first heart sound* is called S_1 and is created by the closure of the tricuspid and mitral valves. It is usually heard best at the LLSB or at the apex. A split S_1 can be a normal but uncommon finding in children.[2]

The *second heart* sound is called S_2 and is created by the closure of the aortic and pulmonic valves. It is usually heard best at the left upper sternal border (LUSB). Evaluation of S_2 is critical in children because it provides important clues as to the presence of structural defects and to the pressures in the heart. S_2 normally varies with respiration—split with inspiration and single or narrowly split in expiration. A fixed split, single S_2, or loud S_2 warrants referral and further evaluation

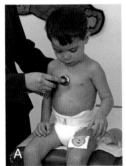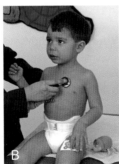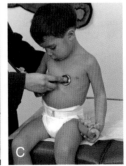

FIGURE 8.6 Stethoscope positioning for auscultation of the heart sounds (**A**) Right upper sternal border, (**B**) Left upper sternal border, (**C**) Left lower sternal border.

by a cardiologist. Abnormal splitting of the S_2 may indicate increased pulmonary blood flow, pulmonary valve abnormality, or a cyanotic heart condition. A loud single S_2 may indicate pulmonary hypertension or malposition of the great arteries.[2]

A *third heart sound* (S_3) can be a common finding in children and young adults. S_3 can be heard at the apex and is caused by vibrations in the ventricle as it fills rapidly during diastole.

A *fourth heart sound* (S_4 or *gallop rhythm*) is rare in infants and children. An S_4 is an abnormal finding and suggests decreased ventricular compliance in conditions such as congestive heart failure (CHF).[2]

Ejection clicks are extra heart sounds that occur between S_1 and S_2. They are heard best at the upper sternal border and are usually associated with stenotic semilunar valves or dilated great arteries.[2]

Murmurs

Murmurs are produced when blood flows across the chambers of the heart and has a pressure difference that causes turbulence or disturbed flow. Murmurs should be assessed and evaluated according to their timing in the cardiac cycle, location, transmission, intensity, frequency, and quality. It is always important to note whether a murmur radiates the sound to the lung fields, axillae, clavicles, or neck. A normal grading scale is used to describe a murmur's intensity (Table 8.1).

Murmurs are described in relation to their timing during the cardiac cycle—systolic, diastolic, or continuous. Systolic murmurs occur between S_1 and S_2, and diastolic murmurs are heard after S_2. Systolic murmurs are further described as *ejection* crescendo-decrescendo or *regurgitant* long systolic-decrescendo.

Systolic ejection murmurs begin shortly after the first heart sound, are due to semilunar valve or great vessel stenosis, usually vary in intensity, and are diamond shaped. They can be short or long in duration but usually end before S_2. Regurgitant murmurs typically begin with S_1. Although they usually do not obscure the first heart sound, they are the result of mitral or tricuspid valve insufficiency and can be long or short in duration. Holosystolic murmurs obscure S_1 at their maximal or loudest point and are usually caused by a *ventricular septal defect* (VSD).[2]

Diastolic murmurs occur between S_2 and S_1 and are described as early, mid, or late. Diastolic murmurs are usually caused by aortic or pulmonic regurgitation or mitral stenosis and are never normal.[2]

Continuous murmurs begin in systole and continue without interruption through S_2 and into diastole. They are usually caused by conditions in which vascular shunting occurs throughout the cardiac cycle, such as in PDA or a surgical aorta-to-pulmonary shunt. A continuous murmur from a PDA has a machinery-like quality, is best heard in the left clavicular area or back, and has a crescendo-decrescendo shape.[2]

The origin of a murmur is usually found at the point where the murmur is heard the loudest. The location of the murmur provides valuable information regarding the

TABLE 8.1	Grading Scale for Cardiac Murmurs
Grade	Sound
1	Barely audible and softer than usual heart sounds
2	Still soft, but about as loud as usual heart sounds
3	Louder than usual heart sounds, but without a thrill
4	Louder than usual heart sounds, and with a thrill
5	Can be heard with stethoscope barely on chest (rare)
6	Can be heard with stethoscope off chest, or with naked ear (extremely rare)

Data from Park M. *Pediatric Cardiology for Practitioners.* 7th ed. St. Louis: Mosby/Elsevier; 2021.

cardiac malformation. If a murmur is heard throughout the chest, the area of highest frequency will define its origin. For example, a systolic ejection murmur that radiates to the axillae and back is usually pulmonary in origin, and one that radiates to the neck and carotid arteries is typically aortic in origin. The frequency or pitch of a murmur is a good indicator of the pressure gradient across a valve or septal defect. The higher the pressure gradient, the higher the frequency of the murmur.

TABLE 8.2	PHYSIOLOGIC OR INNOCENT MURMURS	
Murmur	Characteristics/Evaluation	Age of Occurrence
Still's murmur	Localized between LLSB and apex Grade 1-3/6 systolic ejection (outflow murmur), decreasing with inspiration, when upright, or disappearing with Valsalva maneuver Low frequency, vibratory, musical in quality Often confused with VSD murmur	Most often heard at 2–7 years old
Peripheral pulmonic stenosis (PPS)	Also known as newborn pulmonary flow murmur Heard at LUSB with radiation to back, axillae Grade 1-2/6 systolic ejection, crescendo-decrescendo	Often heard in premature infants, infants with low birth weight, and infants up to 4 months of age Need to document resolution by 4–5 months of age to rule out organic cause or valve involvement
Pulmonary ejection	Well localized to LUSB Grade 1-3/6 systolic ejection crescendo-decrescendo Heard loudest when supine and decreases or disappears with Valsalva maneuver Does not radiate Similar to ASD murmur, but S_2 is normal	Common in 8- to 14-year-olds with greatest frequency in adolescents
Venous hum	Heard best just below clavicles at either RUSB or LUSB Grade 1-3/6 low-frequency continuous murmur Loudest when sitting, diminishes or disappears when supine; can be increased by turning patient's head away from the side of the murmur, and can be obliterated by light jugular vein compression; can be mistaken for PDA	Common in 3- to 6-year-olds
Supraclavicular carotid bruit	Heard above the right or left clavicle with radiation to the neck Grade 1-3/6 holosystolic, crescendo-decrescendo Decreases or diminishes with shoulder hyperextension Can be confused with murmur of aortic stenosis	Common at any age

ASD, Atrial septal defect; *LLSB*, left lower sternal border; *LUSB*, left upper sternal border; *PDA*, patent ductus arteriosus; *RUSB*, right upper sternal border; *VSD*, ventricular septal defect.
Data from Park M. *Pediatric Cardiology for Practitioners*. 7th ed. St. Louis: Mosby/Elsevier; 2021.

Innocent murmurs occur in up to 50% of normal children.[1] They are a common benign finding in infants and children and do not always signify heart disease.

Physiologic versus Pathologic Murmurs

It is important to distinguish physiologic, or innocent, murmurs from pathologic murmurs (Table 8.2). Innocent murmurs occur in up to 50% of normal children.[1] They are systolic ejection murmurs that are usually heard best at the LLSB and have a vibratory or musical quality (Fig. 8.7). They tend to be short and well located. They are usually no louder than grade 2 to 3 in intensity and are often accentuated during high output states such as exercise, stress, anemia, or febrile illness. Innocent murmurs are never purely diastolic except in the case of a venous hum, which is a continuous diastolic physiologic murmur heard loudest at the URSB. Innocent murmurs are usually not associated with a diastolic murmur, a thrill, abnormal electrocardiogram (ECG) or chest x-ray, cyanosis, or other symptoms of heart disease. Although innocent murmurs usually occur between 2 to 6 years of age, they also may be heard from infancy to early adolescence.

COMMON DIAGNOSTIC TESTS

Pulse Oximetry

Pulse oximetry is used to verify and document the degree of central cyanosis and is an accurate way to assess arterial oxygen saturation, especially in infants. Pulse oximetry screening for critical CHD is a component of the Recommended Uniform Screening Panel (RUSP) for newborns in the well infant and intermediate care nurseries in the United States.[4] In addition to screening for congenital heart defects, the identification of infants with other causes of hypoxia, such as infections, lung disease, or hemoglobinopathies, has been documented as an added benefit of pulse oximetry screening.[4]

Pulse oximetry readings from the right hand and one foot (together or in sequence), taken on the second day of life before discharge using a motion-tolerant pulse oximeter approved by the U.S. Food and Drug Administration (FDA) are recommended.[4] Box 8.1 presents the criteria for a positive result for pulse oximetry screening. A positive screening result is defined as any identified low oxygen level and requires follow-up with a comprehensive history and physical examination to determine the cause of hypoxia. Critical CHD is excluded using a diagnostic echocardiogram,

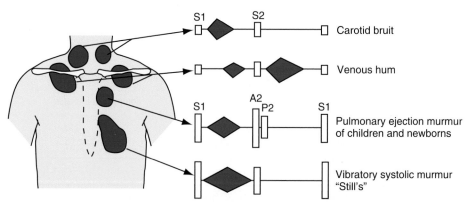

FIGURE 8.7 Anatomical locations of physiologic murmurs. (Modified from Park M. *Pediatric Cardiology for Practitioners.* 6th ed. St. Louis: Mosby/Elsevier; 2021, p. 37.)

BOX 8.1   CRITERIA FOR A POSITIVE PULSE OXIMETRY SCREENING RESULT

- Any oxygen saturation measure <89%
- Any oxygen saturation <94% in either right hand or foot on two measures taken 1 hour apart
- Greater than 4% absolute difference between readings in the upper extremity (right hand) and lower extremity (foot) on two measures taken 1 hour apart

All patients with positive screens should be referred to a pediatric cardiologist for further assessment with an echocardiogram.

Data from Martin, GR, Ewer, AK, Gaviglio, A, et al. Updated strategies for pulse oximetry screening for critical CHD. *Pediatrics* 2020;146(1):e20191650.

and it should be read and interpreted by a pediatric cardiologist.[4]

Pulse oximetry is also commonly used to monitor oxygen saturations in children with known cardiac disease. Infants and children who have complex cyanotic heart defects in which blood mixes in a common ventricle are dependent on a surgically placed aorta-to-pulmonary artery shunt or a PDA stent placed through a catheterization procedure to supply pulmonary blood flow. They normally have oxygen saturation levels between 75% and 85%. It is important to know an infant's baseline oxygen saturation to accurately assess their oxygen status. Increasingly, pulse oximeters are used at home to monitor changes in oxygen saturation in infants with hypoplastic left heart syndrome (HLHS) and other single-ventricle (SV) heart defects as part of home surveillance programs.[5]

Chest X-Ray

Chest x-rays have been the standard to assess heart size, pulmonary congestion, position of the great vessels, and abdominal situs. Although this diagnostic tool is frequently used in the inpatient or ICU setting, it is becoming less practical and valuable in the outpatient setting with advanced echocardiography, which gives more precise information of the cardiac structure and function without radiation exposure.

Heart size is determined by comparing the width of the cardiac silhouette at its widest diameter to the width of the chest at its maximal internal dimension (Fig. 8.8). This is referred to as the cardiothoracic (CT) ratio. A CT ratio greater than 0.65 is considered

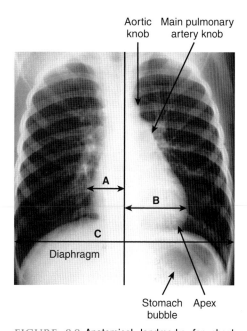

FIGURE 8.8 Anatomical landmarks for chest radiographs. (Modified from Zitelli BJ, McIntire SC, Nowalk AJ. *Zitelli and Davis' Atlas of Pediatric Physical Diagnosis.* 8th ed. Philadelphia: Elsevier; 2021; Park M. *Pediatric Cardiology for Practitioners.* 7th ed. St. Louis: Mosby; 2021, p. 66.)

cardiomegaly.[2] It is important to have a good inspiratory x-ray for diagnosis, as an expiratory film may make the heart appear larger than it is. Also, prominent *thymic tissue* in newborns is often falsely interpreted as cardiomegaly.

The position of the cardiac apex provides information about ventricular enlargement. Normally the apex points down and to the left. An upward turned apex is indicative of right ventricular enlargement, whereas an apex that is pushed more downward and leftward than normal is caused by left ventricular enlargement. The *main pulmonary artery* (MPA) is normally seen as a small knob at the LUSB (Fig. 8.8). The prominence or absence of this shadow provides clues about the size, position, and presence of the MPA.[2] Pulmonary vascular markings provide important information about the degree of pulmonary blood flow and should be noted as normal, increased, or decreased.

Chest x-rays can also determine *abdominal situs.* The location of the cardiac apex is normally on the left and should be on the same side as the stomach bubble and opposite the liver shadow. When these structures are misaligned (with the stomach bubble on the right and the apex on the left), or the liver is midline, then *heterotaxy* or situs abnormality is present, which is often associated with serious heart defects.

Electrocardiogram

An ECG is a screening tool that provides information about heart rate, heart rhythm, conduction, and forces of contraction in the heart. It is particularly useful in the diagnosis of arrhythmias and ventricular hypertrophy. However, ECG patterns can vary within diagnostic groups. Therefore, except for arrhythmias, ECGs are most often used to confirm a diagnosis of structural CHD as opposed to establishing one.

Echocardiogram

Cardiac ultrasound, or *echocardiogram*, has become the primary diagnostic tool for patients suspected of having CHD. An echocardiogram can be done safely and noninvasively in the outpatient setting or at the bedside and provides accurate information for all age groups including premature infants. The addition of Doppler ultrasound and three-dimensional

TABLE 8.3	OVERVIEW OF COMMON DIAGNOSTIC TESTS IN CHD
Test	**Applications/Specific Modalities**
Chest x-ray	Information on heart size and shape, enlargement of cardiac chambers, size and position of the great vessels, degree of pulmonary blood flow, position of abdominal organs
Electrocardiogram (ECG)	Graphic measure of electrical activity with information on rhythm, conduction, and force of contraction, chamber hypertrophy **Holter:** 24-hour continuous ECG recording used to assess arrhythmias
Echocardiogram	Noninvasive imaging using high-frequency ultrasound to assess cardiac structures and ventricular function **Transthoracic echocardiogram (TTE):** Transducer is on the chest, most common. Infants and toddlers may need sedation for full study. • *M-mode:* One-dimensional graphic display to estimate chamber size and ventricular function, assess valve motion and pericardial fluid • *2-D:* Real-time cross-sectional images to assess cardiac anatomy • *3-D:* Imaging primarily to assess valve anatomy • *Doppler:* Demonstrates blood flow patterns and pressure gradients **Transesophageal echocardiogram (TEE):** Transducer placed in esophagus to obtain images of posterior cardiac structures, used in patients with poor thoracic imaging. Widely used in the operating room after cardiac surgical repairs. Patient must be sedated or under general anesthesia. **Fetal:** Images fetal cardiac structures in utero.

TABLE 8.3	OVERVIEW OF COMMON DIAGNOSTIC TESTS IN CHD—CONT'D
Test	**Applications/Specific Modalities**
Cardiac MRI	Provides 3D imaging and measurement of intracardiac structures and extracardiac vascular anatomy, assesses function. • Often used in adolescents or young adults with limited imaging by echocardiogram. • Children younger than 8 years of age or those with claustrophobia or anxiety may need anesthesia or sedation.
Cardiac computerized tomography (chest CT, cardiac CT)	Computer-processed x-rays to obtain detailed images of the heart and chest structures. • Recent improvements in technology (decreased image acquisition time and decreased radiation exposure) have increased the use of chest CT. • Used to evaluate aortic arch abnormalities, vascular rings, coronary arteries, and pulmonary veins
Exercise (stress) test	Monitors heart rate, blood pressure, ECG, oxygen saturation, oxygen consumption, and presence of symptoms (i.e., chest pain, dizziness) at rest and with progressive exercise on bicycle or treadmill • Done with physician supervision and emergency equipment available • 6-minute walk test: Assess maximum distance walked in 6 minutes while monitoring heart rate and oxygen saturation; used in patients with severe exercise limitations or those with pulmonary HTN.
Cardiac catheterization	Invasive imaging modality using radiopaque catheters placed in peripheral vessels (femoral access most common) and advanced into the heart to visualize cardiac structures, measure chamber pressures and oxygen levels, and assess blood flow patterns. **Hemodynamics:** Assessment of pressures and oxygen levels in cardiac chambers. **Angiography:** Injection of contrast material to image heart structures and flow patterns under fluoroscopy. **Biopsy:** Bioptome catheters used to obtain tiny samples of heart muscle for microscopic examination; used to assess for infection, inflammation, or muscle dysfunction disorders, and posttransplant rejection. **Electrophysiology:** Special catheters with electrodes used to record electrical activity from inside the heart and assess rhythm abnormalities.

CHD, Congenital heart disease; *HTN*, hypertension; *MRI*, magnetic resonance imaging.

(3D) images makes it possible to evaluate valve anatomy, function, and flow patterns throughout the heart and proximal vessels. This is particularly useful in quantifying degrees of shunting and obstruction. Advanced fetal cardiac echocardiography has become a standard prenatal evaluation tool for families with a history of CHD or other cardiac risk factors. Echocardiogram testing is best ordered by a cardiologist, after a thorough evaluation and examination has been done to determine need and suspicion of heart disease.

Referral to a cardiologist should be as complete as possible and include data about the history, physical examination, ECG, chest x-ray if indicated, and oxygen saturation that have raised suspicion of CHD. Table 8.3 presents the common tests used to diagnose CHD.

CARDIAC SYMPTOMS

Arrhythmias and Palpitations

It is not unusual for children to complain of skipped heartbeats, a fast heart rate, or extra heartbeats. Most complaints are benign in origin, but a history of chest pain, light-headedness, or syncope can be indicative of a serious arrhythmia.[2]

Family history should be directed toward any structural heart disease or history of sudden death, and the patient history should include any association of symptoms with exercise, food intake (especially caffeine), medications (especially cough preparations, and stimulants or opioids), or specific positioning. Physical findings, except the arrhythmia, are usually not present. Evaluation begins with an ECG. Documentation of the cardiac rhythm on an ECG is essential for determining diagnosis and treatment; however, obtaining this documentation can be challenging, especially if the symptoms are infrequent. For a complete evaluation, referral to a pediatric cardiologist or electrophysiologist is essential. To properly identify the heart rate and rhythm during subjective complaints of irregular heartbeats or palpitations, home monitoring devices are quite useful. There are several new devices available including continuous monitors, event recorders, external patch recorders, mobile cardiac outpatient telemetry, and even implantable cardiac monitors.[6] Many heart rhythms can now be assessed by smartphone applications that can be transmitted directly to the health care team. Additionally, even personal fitness trackers, such as those available in smartphone applications, are helpful in measuring heart rates in older children and adolescents.

Syncope

Syncope is a common complaint in older children and adolescents (especially adolescent females).[2] *Vasovagal syncope*, also called *simple syncope, simple faint or neurocardiogenic syncope*, or *vasodepressor syncope* is the most common cause of syncope in children and adolescents. It is usually characterized by a loss of consciousness, falling, and then a quick recovery once the child or adolescent is lying down. Most episodes have the same characteristics including visual disturbances, light-headedness, pallor, generalized weakness, and often nausea and diaphoresis. Most syncopal events are benign, but a careful evaluation is always warranted, because it may be the first symptom of serious cardiac, neurologic, or metabolic disease. Syncope is uncommon in children less than 6 years of age unless it is related to seizures, breath-holding, or cardiac arrhythmias.[2] The most common neurological cause is a seizure disorder, and possible metabolic causes include hypoglycemia, electrolyte imbalance, or profound anemia. In early childhood, the causes include breath-holding, and in adolescents, hyperventilation techniques.

Arrhythmias, long QT syndrome, and *hypertrophic cardiomyopathy* (HCM) are other potential cardiac causes of syncope. Information gathering should include careful details of the event and a family history of similar events or sudden cardiac death. Medication history and past medical history are important to elicit. Often, the only evidence of HCM on physical examination may be the increased intensity of a cardiac murmur from supine to standing. If the neurological examination is negative, an ECG should be obtained. Referral to a cardiologist is warranted if a murmur is heard on physical exam, or if there is an abnormal ECG, a family history of sudden death, or cardiomyopathy.[2]

Chest Pain

Chest pain in children is a common complaint, causing anxiety in both patients and their parents. However, chest pain due to a cardiac cause is rare in children, occurring in fewer than 5% of cases.[7] The most common cause of chest pain is musculoskeletal in origin, including muscle strain, trauma, and costochondritis, which accounts for close to 70% of cases of chest pain in children.[7] *Costochondritis* is an inflammation of the chest wall, causing sharp,

---

BOX 8.2   INFORMATION GATHERING FOR PRESENTING CHEST PAIN IN CHILDREN

Questions to Ask
- Has the child had a fever or recent illness?
- Is the pain related to breathing or activity? Does it occur with exercise or at rest?
- Any sports activities or injuries that may have preceded the onset of chest pain?

- Is the chest pain accompanied by palpitations, dizziness, or fainting?
- Anything improve the pain? Anything make the pain worse?
- Any illicit drug use or use of caffeine supplements or drinks?

---

short, and well-localized pain that can be reproduced with pressure on palpation. Other causes of chest pain in children are pulmonary (especially asthma or illnesses associated with coughing), gastrointestinal (esophagitis or gastroesophageal reflux), or psychogenic (less often in children less than 12 years of age but more frequent in adolescent females).[2]

A careful history is important in assessing the cause of chest pain in children (Box 8.2). It is important to elicit the onset and duration of the pain and how long the child has been experiencing pain, if the chest pain occurs at rest or only with exercise and sports participation. Document the severity, location, and radiation of the chest pain. A family history of sudden death, CHD, cardiomyopathy, or a clotting disorder is concerning for cardiac disease. Chest pain associated with fever may have an infectious cause. Illicit drug use, particularly cocaine, can cause myocardial ischemia with chest pain as a presenting symptom.

The physical exam should note the child or adolescent's color, perfusion, pulses, respiratory effort, and degree of pain evaluated on a pediatric pain rating scale (Chapter 2). Auscultation includes the evaluation and quality of breath sounds bilaterally, as well as the identification of abnormal heart sounds, murmurs, rubs, gallops, or muffled heart sounds.

Cardiac origins of chest pain include ischemic causes (coronary artery abnormalities or cardiomyopathies), inflammatory conditions such as pericarditis or myocarditis, arrhythmias, aortic dissection, or pulmonary embolus.[7] *Pericarditis*, an inflammation of the pericardium, is characterized by chest pain

that is worse lying down and improves with sitting and leaning forward.[2] Careful cardiac history, family history, physical examination, and selected use of the ECG can identify potentially life-threatening or other nonemergent causes of cardiac chest pain, which require further evaluation.[7] If acute chest pain of cardiac origin is suspected, an ECG should be obtained, with immediate referral to a pediatric cardiologist.

PEDIATRIC PEARLS

Chest pain with exertion, or if associated with dizziness, syncope, palpitations, or radiation of pain to the back, jaw, or left arm could be indicative of cardiac disease and requires prompt evaluation by a cardiologist.[7]

CARDIOVASCULAR DISEASE

Cardiovascular disease in children is divided into two broad categories: congenital or acquired. CHD comprises most cardiovascular disorders in the pediatric population. CHD is not a singular entity, but rather a myriad of structural anomalies in the heart that develop during fetal life and thus present at birth. *Acquired heart disease* (such as Kawasaki disease, some cardiomyopathies, myocardial infections, rheumatic fever, hypertension, and dyslipidemia) occurs after birth and develops during an individual's lifetime. These conditions usually occur in children with structurally normal hearts but can be seen in those with CHD as well. The COVID-2019 pandemic led to the identification of a new syndrome, multisystem inflammatory syndrome in children (MIS-C), that usually presents 2 to 6 weeks after COVID infection with common symptoms of fever, GI symptoms, rash, conjunctivitis, headache, and lethargy.[8] Cardiac involvement is common with depressed left ventricular function on echocardiography, possible coronary abnormalities, and symptoms of shock. Inflammatory markers and troponins are elevated.[8]

Congenital Heart Disease

CHD is prevalent in at least 10 per 1000 live births, close to 1% of all births in the United States.[9] Forty percent of CHD malformations are diagnosed during a child's first year of life. Adults now account for two-thirds of patients with severe and other chronic forms of CHD in the general population.[9] Maternal infections such as parvovirus, enterovirus, rubella, adenovirus, and commonly coxsackie B virus or other viruses contracted during pregnancy can be associated with CHD or myocarditis. Medications, alcohol, and other drugs may act as teratogens on the developing fetus. Maternal medical conditions associated with an increased risk of the fetus developing CHD include diabetes mellitus (cardiomyopathy, transposition of the great vessels) and systemic lupus erythematosus (congenital heart block).[2] Table 8.4 reviews common presentations of CHD in children.

CHD is caused by the interaction between genetic and environmental factors. Single gene mutations account for 3% of CHD, gross chromosomal anomalies account for 5%, environmental factors (rubella, fetal alcohol syndrome, other maternal illness/infections) account for 3%, and multifactorial genetic random event mediation for the remainder.[1] Genetic etiologies include genetic syndromes, deletion/duplication syndromes, and both syndromic and nonsyndromic single-gene disorders. At least one or more additional congenital malformations in other body systems can be found in 20% to 30% of infants with CHD.[1] Although knowledge and understanding of the role of genetics in CHD have advanced significantly, the science is evolving. Table 8.5 presents some examples of the more common syndromes associated with CHD diagnoses.

TABLE 8.4	COMMON PRESENTATIONS OF CONGENITAL HEART DISEASE		
Presentation	**Physiology**	**Signs and Symptoms**	**Potential Diagnoses**
Cyanosis (infants)	• Central, arterial (vs. peripheral) desaturation • Desaturated blood mixes with saturated blood in the heart due to right-to-left shunting	• Bluish or deeply ruddy color around mouth/lips • Usually not visible unless O_2 saturations are <85% • O_2 saturations for infants with cyanotic heart disease are normally 75%–85% • Supplemental O_2 will not raise saturations to normal levels of 95%–100% • Hct usually higher than normal • Cyanosis not evident if patient is anemic and will be greater with polycythemia • Can be tachypneic without respiratory distress	• TOF • PA

TABLE 8.4	COMMON PRESENTATIONS OF CONGENITAL HEART DISEASE—CONT'D		
Presentation	**Physiology**	**Signs and Symptoms**	**Potential Diagnoses**
HF	• Heart is unable to meet metabolic demands (output) of the body • Etiologies can be both cardiac and non-cardiac-related	• Tachycardia • Tachypnea with or without respiratory distress (grunting, wheezing, rales) • Cough, wheezing, rales (older children) • Gallop rhythm • Hepatomegaly (liver palpable >2 cm below right costal heart margin) • Peripheral edema plus hepatomegaly (older children) • Pallor due to vasoconstriction • Poor feeding, failure to thrive (infants) • Sweating, especially on forehead, during feeding (infants) • Anorexia, somnolence (older children) • Frequent respiratory infections • Fatigue, exercise intolerance, inability to keep up with peers	• VSD • HCM • Decreased ventricular function post-CHD surgical repair or intervention • Arrhythmia • Myocardial infection • Anemia
Shock	• Severe obstruction of blood flow out of the heart • Can occur suddenly in newborn infants with undetected coarctation of the aorta or interrupted aortic arch when the PDA closes at 2–3 weeks of age	• Hypotension • Extreme pallor • Poor ventricular function, circulation • Hypovolemia • Weak pulses • Poor urine output	• Coarctation of the aorta • Interrupted aortic arch

CHD, Congenital heart disease; *HCM*, hypertrophic cardiomyopathy; *HF*, heart failure; *PA*, pulmonary atresia; *PDA*, patent ductus arteriosus; *TOF*, tetralogy of Fallot; *VSD*, ventricular septal defect.

Common Presentations of Congenital Heart Disease

Cyanosis in Infants

Cyanosis indicative of CHD is due to arterial desaturation and may not be visible unless the oxygen saturation is 85% or less.[1,2] Central cyanosis (cyanosis of the lips, mucous membranes, and tongue) occurs when arterial oxygen saturation falls below 85% in patients with normal hemoglobin levels. Central cyanosis should be distinguished from peripheral cyanosis, which can occur in a cold environment,

TABLE 8.5	COMMON PEDIATRIC SYNDROMES ASSOCIATED WITH CONGENITAL HEART DISEASE		
Type	**Clinical Entity**	**% CHD**	**Associated CHD Diagnosis**
Chromosomal	Trisomy 21 (Down syndrome)	40–50	AVSD, VSD, ASD, PDA, TOF
	Deletion 22q11 (DiGeorge syndrome; VCFS)	75	IAA-B, TA, aortic arch abnormalities, TOF, VSD
	Deletion 7q11.23 (Williams-Beuren syndrome)	50–85	Supravalvar or supravalvular AS (SVAS) and PS, PPS
	Deletion 20p12 (Alagille syndrome)	85–94	PPS, pulmonary artery hypoplasia, PS, TOF
	Turner syndrome (45 XO)	25–35	CoA, BAV, valvar or valvular AS, aortic dissection, mitral atresia, HLHS
Single gene disorders	CHARGE (Hall-Hittner syndrome)	60–90	Conotruncal malformations, ASD, VSD, PDA
	Holt-Oram syndrome	75	Secundum ASD, VSD, progressive AV conduction delay
	LEOPARD syndrome	85	PS, HCM, rhythm abnormalities
	Marfan syndrome and other connective tissue disorders	80	Aortic dilation/dissection, MVP, MPA dilation, TVP

AS, Aortic stenosis; *ASD*, atrial septal defect; *AV*, atrioventricular; *AVSD*, atrioventricular septal defect; *BAV*, bicuspid aortic valve; *CoA*, coarctation of the aorta; *HCM*, hypertrophic cardiomyopathy; *HLHS*, hypoplastic left heart syndrome; *IAA-B*, interrupted aortic arch type B; *MPA*, main pulmonary artery; *MVP*, mitral valve prolapse; *PDA*, patent ductus arteriosus; *PPS*, peripheral pulmonic stenosis; *PS*, pulmonic stenosis; *TOF*, tetralogy of Fallot; *VCFS*, velocardiofacial syndrome; *VSD*, ventricular septal defect.

Data from Ruppel K. Disorders of the cardiovascular system. In Rudolph C, et al., eds: *Rudolph's Pediatrics*. 23rd ed. New York: McGraw-Hill; 2018.

and *acrocyanosis*, which in newborns is due to sluggish circulation in the fingers and toes.[1]

PEDIATRIC PEARLS

The intensity of cyanosis is dependent on the concentration of desaturated hemoglobin and not on the actual arterial oxygen saturation.

An infant who has *polycythemia*, an abnormal increase in circulating erythrocytes, will appear more cyanotic than an infant who is anemic in the presence of the same degree of arterial desaturation. Therefore, it is important to follow a cyanotic infant's hemoglobin (Hgb) and hematocrit (Hct) levels, particularly at 2 to 3 months of age, the time of normal physiological anemia.

Heart Failure

HF (previously called CHF) is the inability of the heart to adequately meet the metabolic demands of the body. It is a progressive clinical syndrome caused by cardiac and noncardiac abnormalities that result in characteristic signs and symptoms including edema, respiratory distress, growth failure, and exercise intolerance.[10] In the United States today, the most common cause of pediatric heart failure is CHD.[10] Heart failure can be a presenting symptom for some congenital heart defects such as VSD, AV septal defect, aortic stenosis, or coarctation of the aorta or a late sequelae following surgical repairs. Cardiomyopathy is the most common cause in structurally normal hearts.[10] Noncardiac diseases such as anemia, sepsis, hypoglycemia, and renal failure can also cause heart failure. The multiple causations of HF manifest in a variety of clinical presentations that are usually age specific. Infants most commonly present with tachypnea, poor feeding, diaphoresis with feeds, tachycardia, pallor, and growth failure. Older children are often unable to keep up with their peers (exercise intolerance) and may exhibit peripheral edema, abdominal pain, anorexia, and respiratory symptoms such as cough, wheezing, rales, and dyspnea.

Acquired Heart Disease

Hypertension

The incidence of *hypertension* (HTN) is increasing in children and adolescents in the United States, largely related to the increase in childhood obesity.[11] There is now evidence that blood pressure in childhood tracks into adulthood, so children who are hypertensive in middle childhood are frequently hypertensive as adults.[12] Screening for HTN in childhood and effective management is aimed at decreasing the risk of cardiac disease in adulthood. The definition of HTN is derived from blood pressure percentiles based on sex, age, and height (Table 8.6).[12] Chapter 2 reviews the proper

method for obtaining blood pressure measurements, and both the systolic and diastolic values are of equal importance.

HTN can be classified as primary or essential (without a clear cause) or secondary to an underlying disorder (often related to renal or vascular disease). In secondary HTN, treatment of the underlying cause can cure the HTN. Secondary HTN has a higher incidence in prepubertal children and likely underlies the more severe or stage 2 HTN. Primary or essential HTN is more often seen in older school-age children and adolescents and is often associated with excess weight gain, obesity, and/or a positive family history of HTN.[12,13]

The goal of HTN screening is to identify children and adolescents with HTN and distinguish between primary and secondary causes. Evaluation of HTN includes a comprehensive history and physical examination, as well as baseline laboratory studies including complete blood count, serum electrolytes, blood urea nitrogen, creatinine, lipids, glucose, and urinalysis. Renal and cardiac ultrasounds are performed to assess for secondary causes or to document end-organ involvement such as increased left ventricular mass. Additional diagnostic tools include a 24-hour ambulatory

TABLE 8.6	CLASSIFICATIONS OF BP AND HYPERTENSION
Classification	**Criteria**
Normal	Both systolic and diastolic BP are <90th percentile
Elevated hypertension	Systolic and/or diastolic BP ≥90th percentile but <95th percentile OR BP exceeds 120/80 mm Hg
Stage 1 HTN	Systolic and/or diastolic BP measures ≥95th percentile measured on three separate occasions OR BP exceeds 130/80 mm Hg
Stage 2 HTN	Systolic and/or diastolic BP ≥95th percentile OR BP exceeds 140/90 mm Hg

Data from Flynn JT, Kaelber DC, Baker-Smith CM, et al. Subcommittee on Screening and Management of High Blood Pressure in Children: Clinical practice guidelines for screening and management of high blood pressure in children and adolescents. *Pediatrics* 2017;140:1–72.

BP, Blood pressure; *HTN*, hypertension.

blood pressure monitor that measures blood pressures every 20 to 30 minutes over a 24-hour period during normal daily activities and uses an oscillometric technique to document mean systolic and diastolic blood pressure measurements. Blood pressure can now be assessed by smartphone applications that can be transmitted directly to the health care team. Additionally, personal fitness trackers are helpful in measuring blood pressure during daily activities.

It is also important to identify other risk factors associated with HTN such as premature atherosclerosis, smoking, overweight/obesity, dyslipidemia, family history of premature cardiovascular disease, diabetes, and chronic renal disease. The target blood pressure for children with other cardiovascular risk factors is a systolic and diastolic blood pressure less than 90% (Table 8.6).[11]

EVIDENCE-BASED PRACTICE TIP

Both blood pressure and lipid levels track from childhood to adulthood. Elevated blood pressure and elevated lipid levels in childhood frequently remain elevated in adulthood.[11,12]

Dyslipidemia

Recent evidence supports the correlation between lipid disorders in childhood and the onset and severity of atherosclerosis in children and young adults.[11] Like HTN, elevated lipid levels track from childhood to adulthood. In the past, targeted screening for lipid disorders was recommended for children with a strong family history of lipid disorders (familial hypercholesterolemia) or premature cardiovascular disease or HTN. The increase in childhood obesity has contributed to a larger population of children at risk for dyslipidemia. Dyslipidemia, genetic factors, and childhood obesity are contributing factors to coronary artery atherosclerosis along with diabetes, nephrotic syndrome, chronic renal disease, postcardiac transplant, history of Kawasaki disease with aneurysms, and chronic inflammatory disease.

There is continued controversy about universal lipid screening with those opposed contending that most patients are already identified with targeted screening, preventive measures with diet and exercise are already being provided to obese children, and screening is costly. The US Preventive Services Task Force (USPSTF) recent recommendation concluded there was insufficient evidence for routine lipid screening in children and adolescents.[13] Others support universal screening as described by the Expert Panel from the National Heart, Lung, and Blood Institute (NHLBI) and endorsed by the American Academy of Pediatrics (AAP).[11] The AAP recommends universal screening for lipid abnormalities with a nonfasting lipid profile measuring total cholesterol and high-density lipoprotein (HDL) cholesterol between 9 and 11 years of age.[11] Non-HDL cholesterol (more predictive of dyslipidemia in children) is calculated by subtracting HDL cholesterol from total cholesterol. Normal values for children and adolescents are a non-HDL cholesterol value less than 145 mg/dL, with an HDL cholesterol above 40 mg/dL. If the non-HDL cholesterol is abnormal, children should have a fasting lipid profile and undergo further evaluation and follow-up.

Metabolic Syndrome

Metabolic syndrome (MetS), a combination of dyslipidemia, abnormal glucose regulation, obesity, and hypertension, has been described in obese adults and is known to significantly increase the risk for coronary artery disease and type 2 diabetes.[14] Research suggests a strong interaction between obesity, insulin resistance, and inflammatory markers that contribute to metabolic syndrome and later heart disease and diabetes. Metabolic syndrome in adults is often defined as the presence of three or more of the following risk factors: elevations in waist circumference, triglyceride levels, blood pressure, reduced levels of HDL cholesterol, and/or fasting glucose levels.[11]

With the increased incidence of obesity in children and adolescents, a similar constellation of conditions is being described as metabolic syndrome in children. While there is no agreement on the diagnostic criteria for *pediatric metabolic syndrome*, the International Diabetes Federation has proposed a pediatric definition (Table 8.7).[15] Some of the risk factors for the development of metabolic syndrome in childhood include a family history of a parent with metabolic syndrome, inactivity and sedentary lifestyle, and smoking.[15] The presence of obesity should prompt a comprehensive evaluation for other cardiovascular risk factors, including family history of premature cardiovascular disease, hypertension, dyslipidemia, diabetes, and tobacco exposure.[11] Longitudinal studies have demonstrated an increased incidence of both type 2 diabetes and cardiovascular disease when elements of metabolic syndrome are present in childhood.[15] The International Diabetic Foundation (IDF) consensus group recognizes that there are genetic, environmental, sex, and age differences, and more research is needed to establish outcomes in high-risk populations.[15] Preventive treatment for pediatric metabolic syndrome includes weight loss, diet, and exercise.

There are several clinical features of metabolic syndrome in the pediatric population. *Obesity* is a crucial component and defined as a body mass index (BMI) above the 95% for age and sex. *Body fat distribution*, assessed by

---

TABLE 8.7   DEFINITION OF METABOLIC SYNDROME IN AT-RISK CHILDREN AND ADOLESCENTS[A]

Age Group (years)	Obesity (WC)	Triglycerides	HDL-C	Blood Pressure	Glucose (mmol/L) or Known T2DM
6–10 years	≥90th percentile	Metabolic syndrome cannot be diagnosed, but further measurements should be made if there is a family history of metabolic syndrome, T2DM, dyslipidemia, cardiovascular disease, hypertension, and/or obesity.			
10–16 years— Metabolic syndrome	≥90th percentile or adult cutoff if lower	≥1.7 mmol/L (≥150 mg/dL)	<1.03 mmol/L (<40 mg/dL)	Systolic ≥130/ diastolic ≥85 mm Hg	≥5.6 mmol/L (100 mg/dL) (If ≥5.6 mmol/L [or known T2DM], recommend an OGTT)
16 years— Young adult metabolic syndrome[a]	≥90th percentile or adult cutoff if lower	≥1.7 mmol/L (≥150 mg/dL)	<1.03 mmol/L (<40 mg/dL) in males and <1.29 mmol/L (<50 mg/dL) in females	Systolic ≥130/ diastolic ≥85 mm Hg	Glucose (FPG) = 5.6 mmol/L (≥100 mg/dL), or known T2DM

Use existing IDF criteria for adults including waist circumference central obesity and any two of the four factors listed previously.

Data modified from Zimmet P, Alberti KGMM, Kaufman F, et al. IDF Consensus Group. The metabolic syndrome in children and adolescents—an IDF consensus report. *Pediatr Diabetes* 2007;8:299–306.
[a]*HDL-C*, High-density lipoprotein cholesterol; *IDF*, International Diabetes Federation; *OGTT*, oral glucose tolerance test; *T2DM*, type 2 diabetes mellitus; *WC*, waist circumference.

waist circumference, is often associated with increased insulin resistance.[14] *Dyslipidemias*, defined as an increase in triglycerides or a decrease in HDL cholesterol, can be detected on cholesterol screening. Blood pressure measurements should be done annually to screen for *hypertension. Insulin resistance* is often found in obese children, and some may progress to glucose intolerance and diabetes. *Inflammatory markers* such as c-reactive protein (CRP) may be elevated, but the relationship between increased CRP and metabolic syndrome has not been well defined in children.[14] *Nonalcoholic fatty liver disease (NAFLD)* (characterized by intrahepatic fat accumulation) and *polycystic ovary syndrome* (characterized by hyperandrogenism) are both associated with insulin resistance and are more prevalent in obese children and adolescents.[14] Physical examination includes pulse, blood pressure, calculation of BMI, assessment for obesity, increased waist size, hepatomegaly, and *acanthosis nigricans* (Chapter 7).

Telehealth Tips

Telehealth has increased significantly in pediatric cardiology as it has in other pediatric specialties since the COVID-19 pandemic occurred. In addition to addressing licensing, insurance reimbursement, and other legal and regulatory issues, limited access to the internet or access to a smartphone can limit patient access in some populations. Many assessment technologies commonly used in cardiology such as echocardiography, EKG, and arrhythmia assessment can be performed remotely and evaluated by a cardiologist in a distant location. Some chief complaints that depend heavily on obtaining a history such as the evaluation of palpitations, chest pain at rest, dizziness or syncope, dyslipidemias, HTN, and genetic disorders can be initially evaluated via telehealth.[16] Many follow-up visits for repaired congenital heart disease can also be done via telehealth with remote testing. Some issues that require a physical exam and in-person assessment include infants and toddlers with a murmur or cyanosis and older children with exertional chest pain or syncope.[16] Home equipment to assess oxygen saturation and heart rate by pulse oximetry, ambulatory blood pressure monitoring, and weight can provide vital signs to augment visual assessment.[16]

SUMMARY OF EXAMINATION

- Obtain a thorough history, including gestational history, birth history, family history, and any presenting symptoms.
- Routine cardiac assessment begins with evaluation of weight, height, BMI, and head circumference in infants.
- Assess temperature, heart rate, respiratory rate, color, activity level, and oxygen saturation *when indicated*.
- Accurately assess blood pressure in all children whenever possible, and routinely once in infancy, and beginning at 3 years of age (Table 8.6).
- Approach the inspection systematically, starting from the periphery and moving inward and upward toward examination of the chest assessing perfusion and pulses in upper and lower extremities.
- Palpate cardiac area for any heaves and presence of a thrill.
- Palpate liver edge for enlargement and position. Note: 1 to 2 cm below the right costal margin is normal in infants.
- Inspect head and neck for signs of abnormal facial features or asymmetry; inspect the chest for scars, signs of respiratory distress, and pectus excavatum or pectus carinatum.
- Auscultate lungs for quality of breath sounds, wheezing, grunting, or rales.
- Auscultate systematically through the four precordial areas moving from LLSB to apex listening for *first heard sound* to the LUSB listening for *second heart sound*, noting variation with respiration and any *third* or *fourth heart sounds* or *ejection clicks*.
- Findings of tachypnea, respiratory distress, tachycardia, bradycardia, low oxygen saturation with pallor or hypoperfusion,

hepatomegaly, and syncope require immediate further evaluation and consultation.

- Diagnostic chest x-ray and ECG are performed *as indicated.*
- Telehealth has increased significantly in pediatric cardiology and many assessment technologies commonly used in cardiology can be used remotely and assessed by a cardiologist.
- Refer to cardiology for further evaluation *as indicated* by examination findings,

diagnostic results, or parental anxiety/concern, and before echocardiogram.

DOCUMENTATION

1-Month-Old Infant With Murmur
Cardiac: Increased RV (right ventricular) impulse, normal S1, split S2, Grade 2-3/6 low-frequency SEM (systolic ejection murmur) nonradiating heard best at LLSB. No diastolic murmur, extra heart sounds, thrill, or clicks.

REFERENCES

1. Teitel DF. The neonate and infant with cardiovascular disease. In: Kline MW, ed. *Rudolph's Pediatrics, 23e.* McGraw-Hill Education; 2018.
2. Park MK, Salamat M. *Park's Pediatric Cardiology for Practitioners. E-Book.* Elsevier Health Sciences; 2020.
3. Sommers MS. Color awareness: a must for patient assessment. *Am Nurse Today.* 2011;6:6.
4. Martin GR, Ewer AK, Gaviglio A, et al. Updated strategies for pulse oximetry screening for critical congenital heart disease. *Pediatrics.* 2020;146:e20191650.
5. Rudd NA, Ghanayem NS, Hill GD, et al. Interstage home monitoring for infants with single ventricle heart disease: Education and management: A scientific statement from the American Heart Association. *J Am Heart Assoc.* 2020;9:e014548.
6. Kusumoto FM, Schoenfeld MH, Barrett C, et al. 2018 ACC/AHA/HRS guideline on the evaluation and management of patients with bradycardia and cardiac conduction delay: A Report of the American College of Cardiology/American Heart Association Task Force on Clinical Practice Guidelines and the Heart Rhythm Society. *Heart Rhythm.* 2019;16:e128–e226.
7. Friedman KG, Alexander ME. Chest pain and syncope in children: a practical approach to the diagnosis of cardiac disease. *J Pediatr.* 2013;163:896–901. e1-3.
8. Feldstein LR, Rose EB, Horwitz SM, et al. Multisystem Inflammatory Syndrome in U.S. Children and Adolescents. *N Engl J Med.* Jul 23 2020;383(4):334–346. https://doi.org/10.1056/NEJMoa2021680.
9. Marelli AJ, Ionescu-Ittu R, Mackie AS, Guo L, Dendukuri N, Kaouache M. Lifetime prevalence of congenital heart disease in the general population from 2000 to 2010. *Circulation.* 2014;130:749–756.
10. Watanabe K, Shih R. Update of pediatric heart failure. *Pediatr Clin North Am.* 2020;67:889–901.
11. Expert Panel on Integrated Guidelines for Cardiovascular Health and Risk Reduction in Children and Adolescents; National Heart, Lung, and Blood Institute Expert Panel on Integrated Guidelines for Cardiovascular Health and Risk Reduction in Children and Adolescents: summary report. *Pediatrics.* 2011;128(Suppl 5):S213–256.
12. Flynn JT, Kaelber DC, Baker-Smith CM, et al. Clinical practice guideline for screening and management of high blood pressure in children and adolescents. *Pediatrics.* 2017;140:e20171904.
13. Bibbins-Domingo K, Grossman DC, Curry SJ, et al. Screening for lipid disorders in children and adolescents: US Preventive Services Task Force recommendation statement. *JAMA.* 2016;316:625–633.
14. Wittcopp C, Conroy R. Metabolic syndrome in children and adolescents. *Pediatr Rev.* 2016;37:193–202.
15. Christian Flemming GM, Bussler S, Körner A, Kiess W. Definition and early diagnosis of metabolic syndrome in children. *J Pediatr Endocrinol Metab.* 2020;33:821–833.
16. Chowdhury D, Hope KD, Arthur LC, et al. Telehealth for pediatric cardiology practitioners in the time of COVID-19. *Pediatr Cardiol.* 2020;4:1081–1091.

CHEST AND RESPIRATORY ASSESSMENT

Concettina (Tina) Tolomeo

EMBRYOLOGICAL DEVELOPMENT

Knowledge of lung development is critical when performing a respiratory assessment in early childhood, especially in a newborn infant who is born preterm. This information, along with an understanding of respiratory anatomy and physiology, will provide you with a foundation for assessing and interpreting pulmonary symptoms.

Lung development begins in utero at approximately 3 weeks gestation. It occurs in five stages: embryonic, pseudoglandular, canalicular, saccular, and alveolar. During the embryonic phase (weeks 3 to 7), the lungs form from a sac on the ventral wall of the alimentary canal. Right and left branches form through budding and dividing. This is also the time when the vascular system begins to develop. During the pseudoglandular stage (weeks 7 to 17), branching of the lung bud occurs, as the trachea, bronchi, and bronchioles are formed by 16 to 17 weeks' gestation. In addition, the intrapulmonary arterial system begins to branch, and cilia and cartilage begin to form. During the canalicular stage (weeks 17 to 27), branching of the bronchioles continues and alveoli begin to form. By approximately 25 weeks, the number of bronchial generations with cartilage is the same as the adult lung. This is also the period of capillary bed expansion. Growth of the pulmonary parenchyma and *surfactant* system occurs during the saccular phase (weeks 28 to 36). By 24 weeks, the alveolocapillary membrane is ready to begin gas exchange. Maturation and expansion of the alveoli occur during the alveolar period and persist through early childhood (36 weeks to 2–3 years of age). This is when the alveolocapillary membrane matures and the gas exchange surface area increases. Alveolization is complete by about 8 years of age.[1–4]

Breathing movements occur in utero. The movements are irregular and do not open the alveoli. Fetal gas exchange occurs via the placenta. At birth, the lungs fill with air for the first time and take on the role of ventilation and oxygenation. The fluid in the lungs moves into the tissues surrounding the alveoli and is absorbed into the lymphatic system. At this point, gas exchange occurs via diffusion across the alveolar-pulmonary capillary membranes.[1,3]

ANATOMY AND PHYSIOLOGY

Thorax

The thorax is the bony cage that surrounds the heart, great vessels, lungs, major airways, and esophagus.[3] It is composed of the sternum and ribs (Fig. 9.1). The *sternum* is a flat, narrow bone made up of three parts: the *manubrium*, the body, and the *xiphoid process*.[5] The *manubrium* is somewhat triangular and attaches to the body of the sternum; the angle at which the manubrium and body meet is termed the *manubriosternal angle* or the *angle of Louis*. This angle is in line with the second rib and therefore serves as an important landmark. The *xiphoid process* is the small, thin, cartilaginous end of the

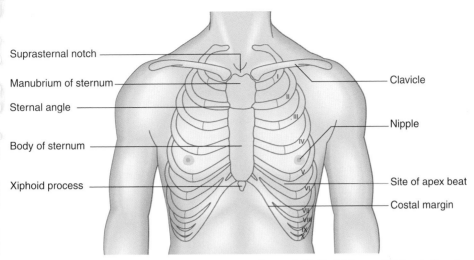

FIGURE 9.1 Anatomy of the rib cage and thorax. (From Revest P. *Medical Sciences*. Edinburgh: Saunders Ltd.; 2009.)

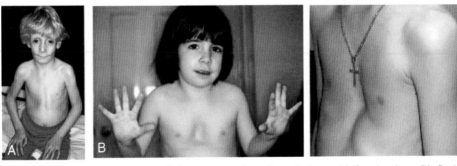

FIGURE 9.2 **A,** Pectus carinatum. **B,** Pectus excavatum. (From Graham, JM, Sanchez-Lara, PA. Pectus excavatum and pectus carinatum. In *Smith's Recognizable Patterns of Human Deformation*. 4th ed. Philadelphia: Elsevier; 2016.)

sternum, which varies greatly in shape and prominence in infants and children because of the influence of heredity, intrauterine environment, and nutrition. It sits at the level of T9.[3,5] *Pectus carinatum*, pigeon breast, is the abnormal protrusion of the xiphoid process and sternum, and *pectus excavatum*, funnel chest, is the abnormal depression of the sternum (Fig. 9.2).[3,5,6] The chest cavity is divided, with the middle portion known as the *mediastinum*.

There are 12 pairs of ribs; the first 7 pairs attach anteriorly via their corresponding costal cartilages to the sternum. Ribs 8, 9, and 10 are attached to the costal cartilage on the rib above them; ribs 11 and 12 do not attach anteriorly and are known as floating ribs. All 12 pairs of ribs attach posteriorly to the thoracic vertebrae. The diaphragm sits at the bottom of the rib cage and is the major muscle of respiration. There are 11 intercostal muscles anteriorly and posteriorly and 8 thoracic muscles, all of which

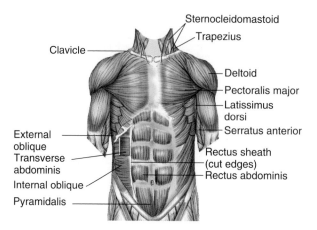

FIGURE 9.3 Anterior thoracic muscles.

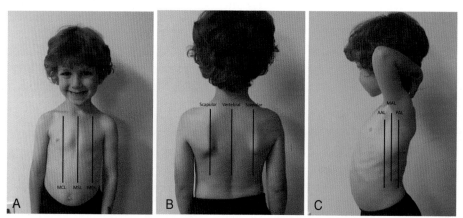

FIGURE 9.4 Anatomical landmarks of the chest. **A,** Anterior chest. **B,** Posterior chest. **C,** Lateral chest. (From Ball JW, et al. Chest and lungs. In Ball JW, et al., eds. *Seidel's Guide to Physical Examination.* 10th ed. St. Louis: Elsevier; 2023.)

help to increase the volume of the rib cage with inspiration and decrease the thoracic volume with expiration (Fig. 9.3).[3]

The following landmarks are often used in describing the location of physical findings of the chest: the midsternal line (MSL), which runs down the middle of the sternum; the midclavicular line (MCL), located on the right and left sides of the chest, runs parallel to the MSL and through the middle of the clavicles (midway between the jugular notch and acromion) bilaterally. Laterally there are three lines on each side, the anterior axillary line (AAL), the midaxillary line (MAL), and the posterior axillary line (PAL). The AAL begins at the anterior axillary folds, the MAL begins at the middle of the axilla, and the PAL begins at the posterior axillary folds. Posteriorly is the vertebral line that runs down the middle of the spine and the scapular line, which runs down the inferior angle of each scapula (Fig. 9.4).[3–5]

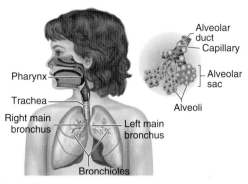

Alveolar duct
Capillary
Pharynx
Alveolar sac
Trachea
Alveoli
Right main bronchus
Left main bronchus
Bronchioles

FIGURE 9.5 Lower respiratory tract.

Lower Respiratory Tract

The respiratory system is divided into two parts: the *upper respiratory tract* and the *lower respiratory tract*. The upper respiratory tract consists of the nasal cavity, pharynx, and larynx and is reviewed in Chapter 12. The *lower respiratory tract* consists of the trachea, bronchi, bronchioles, alveolar ducts and sacs, and alveoli (Fig. 9.5). The *trachea* is a tube that lies anterior to the esophagus. The distal end of the trachea splits into the right and left mainstem/primary *bronchi*. This bifurcation occurs at the level of T3 during infancy and childhood. By the time the child is an adult, this bifurcation occurs at T4 or T5. The right mainstem bronchus is shorter and more vertical than the left and, therefore, more susceptible to aspiration of foreign bodies in the young child. Beyond the bifurcation, the bronchi continue to branch into lobar/secondary bronchi. There are three branches on the right and two on the left, each branch supplies one of the lung lobes. These branches further divide into segmental/tertiary smaller bronchi to supply each segment of the lungs and finally the terminal *bronchioles*. Ultimately, the respiratory tract terminates with the alveolar ducts, alveolar sacs, and alveoli, where gas exchange takes place. The bronchial arteries branch from the aorta and supply blood to the lung parenchyma. The blood supply is returned primarily by the pulmonary veins.[1,3]

Lungs

The lungs are positioned in the lateral aspects of the thorax, separated by the heart and the mediastinal structures. The right lung has three lobes (upper, middle, and lower), and the left lung has two lobes (upper and lower). The *apex* is the top portion of the upper lobes, which extends above the clavicles. On the right side, the minor or horizontal fissure, located at the fourth rib, divides the right upper lobe (RUL) from the right middle lobe (RML). On the left side, there is a tongue-shaped projection that extends from the left upper lobe (LUL), called the *lingula*. Laterally, the right lower lobe (RLL) and the left lower lobe (LLL) occupy most of the lower lateral chest area. Only a small portion of the RML extends to the MAL, and it does not go beyond that point. Posteriorly, the vertebral column helps in identifying the underlying lung lobes. T4 marks the inferior portion of the upper lobes and the superior portion of the lower lobes. The *base* is the bottom portion of the lower lobes and is marked by T10 or T12, depending on the phase of respiration.[3] The principal function of the lungs is gas exchange between the atmosphere and the blood. Oxygen is carried into the lungs, and

TABLE 9.1   PHYSIOLOGICAL VARIATIONS OF THE CHEST AND LUNGS

Age Group	Physiological Variation
Preterm infant	Respiratory muscles are weak, poorly adapted for extrauterine life; periodic breathing occurs that is similar to fetal breathing; preterm infants become easily hypoxic, and apnea occurs
Newborn	Diaphragm is flatter, more compliant; paradoxical breathing occurs in the neonate with inward movement of chest during inspiration due to the compliance of the chest wall; predominantly nose breathers until 4 weeks of age; chest circumference very close in size to head circumference at birth
Infancy	Smaller airways with increased resistance to airflow; rapid respiratory rate; minimal nasal mucus causes mild to moderate upper airway obstruction
Early childhood (1–4 years of age)	Rapid growth and maturation of alveoli improve ventilation; respiratory rate decreases dramatically from newborn period
Middle childhood (5–10 years of age)	Alveoli continue to increase in number
Adolescence	Alveolar size matures to adult capacity

Data from Nakra N. Pediatric pulmonary anatomy and physiology. In Tolomeo C, ed. *Nursing Care in Pediatric Respiratory Disease.* Ames: Wiley-Blackwell; 2012; Ball JW, Dains JE, Flynn JA, Solomon BS, Stewart RW. Chest and lungs. In Ball JW, Dains JE, Flynn JA, Solomon BS, Stewart RW, eds. *Seidel's Guide to Physical Examination.* 10th ed. St. Louis: Elsevier; 2023.

carbon dioxide is eliminated. The lungs play a significant role in acid-base balance.

PHYSIOLOGICAL VARIATIONS

Table 9.1 presents variations in growth and development that impact the function of the respiratory system in the infants and young children.

SYSTEM-SPECIFIC HISTORY

Complete and accurate information gathering is essential when assessing an infant, child, or adolescent with respiratory symptoms. Physical examination findings and test results should always be interpreted within the context of the past and current health history. The health history should be approached in a nonjudgmental manner. The environment should be welcoming and culturally sensitive to ensure communication is open and responsive to parent or caregiver.[7,8] Ask the child's preferred name and pronoun and include this information in the medical record. For transgender individuals undergoing social and medical affirmation, it is important to ask about and note on physical examination if breast binding is utilized (see Chapter 16 for further information). Breast binding can result in reduced lung expansion, which can lead to dyspnea and lung infections.[8] The Information Gathering table presents respiratory-focused questions based on developmental stages. Questions should be open ended and age specific to allow the parent or caregiver the opportunity to give a full explanation of past and present concerns. In addition, always obtain information directly from the older child or adolescent when possible. Table 9.2 presents a symptom-focused assessment of respiratory conditions for children and adolescents. Box 9.1 presents two examples of validated questionnaires that are useful for information gathering related to asthma symptoms in children.[9]

TABLE 9.2	SYMPTOM-FOCUSED ASSESSMENT OF RESPIRATORY CONDITIONS
Symptom	**Questions to Ask**
Cough	History: Onset of cough symptoms, was it sudden or gradual? How long has the cough been present? Is cough worsening or changing character? Is cough wet, dry, hacking, barking, whooping? Worse during day or at night? Worse with feeding, sleeping, running? Any other symptoms: Shortness of breath, chest pain/tightness, or wheeze? Choking episodes? History of aspiration (small toy, food, etc.)? Rhinorrhea or nasal congestion? In the older child/adolescent: Is cough productive with sputum or nonproductive? If productive, what color is the sputum?
	Pattern: Occasional, persistent, or coughing spasms?
Wheeze	History: Onset of wheezing, was it sudden or gradually worsening? Any other symptoms: Cough? Shortness of breath? Chest pain/tightness? Is it associated with upper respiratory infection symptoms? Where is wheezing heard—nose, neck, chest? History of aspiration (small toy, food, etc.)?
	Pattern: Occasional, increase with exercise?
Shortness of breath	History: Onset of shortness of breath—was it sudden or gradual? Does it occur with activity or rest? Is it difficult to get air in, out, both? History of aspiration (small toy, food, etc.)? Accompanying symptoms of cough, wheezing? Any diaphoresis?
Chest pain	History: Onset of chest pain—was it sudden or gradual? Does it occur on inspiration, expiration, or both? Chest pain occurs with movement or rest? Type of pain (sharp, dull)? Ask verbal child to point to area of pain. History of trauma or recent sports injury or weightlifting? Any other symptoms—cough, wheezing, shortness of breath, syncope?
	Pattern: Occasional with respirations or persistent?

BOX 9.1 VALIDATED TOOLS FOR ASSESSMENT OF ASTHMA SYMPTOMS

Test for Respiratory and Asthma Control in Kids (TRACK)[9]
- children less than 5 years of age
- five-item questionnaire to assess asthma symptoms and the use of bronchodilators or oral steroids
- score of 80 or more indicates good control
- available at https://getasthmahelp.org/documents/track.pdf
  Childhood Asthma Control Test (C-ACT)[9]
- children 4 to 11 years of age (ACT is the version for children 12 years and older)

- seven-item questionnaire to assess day and nighttime symptoms, activity limitations, use of short-acting beta agonists, and perception of asthma control
- score of 19 or less indicates the asthma is not well controlled
- available in print and web format in several languages https://www.asthmacontroltest.com/welcome/

INFORMATION GATHERING FOR CHEST AND LUNG ASSESSMENT AT KEY DEVELOPMENTAL STAGES

Age Group	Questions to Ask
Preterm infant	How many weeks gestation? Admitted to newborn intensive care unit? Length of stay? Any episodes of apnea or tachypnea? Need for oxygen? Need for ventilation? For how long? Infant discharged to home on a ventilator/on oxygen? Infant discharged home on any medications? Any exposure to prenatal substance abuse?
Newborn	How many weeks gestation? Birth weight? Any birth complications? Meconium aspiration? Breathing problems at birth? Any episodes of apnea or tachypnea?
Infancy	History of respiratory infections as infant (respiratory syncytial virus (RSV), rhinovirus, etc.)? Frequent upper respiratory infections (URIs)? History of wheezing? History of noisy breathing? Hospitalizations? History of intubations? History of eczema/skin allergy? In childcare? Immunization status? Frequent vomiting after feeds or "choking" episodes? Arches back after feeding?
Early childhood	History of apnea/breath-holding spells? Does child's speech have a nasal, congested, or hoarse sound? History of nasal congestion, chronic URIs, allergy symptoms, tonsillitis, frequent ear infections? In childcare or preschool? Does child frequently put objects in mouth/nose? Exposure to group A streptococcal infection? Does child snore at night? Exposure to ill contacts? Recent travel or immigration from regions with endemic respiratory disease? Are symptoms associated with exercise?
Middle childhood	History of nasal congestion, chronic rhinorrhea, asthma, sinusitis, tonsillitis, chronic URIs, recurrent pneumonia? Are symptoms associated with exercise? Does child snore at night? Exposure to group A streptococcal infection? History of asthma? History of vaping? Marijuana or tobacco use? History of gastroesophageal reflux? Exposure to ill contacts? Recent travel or immigration from regions with endemic respiratory disease?
Adolescence	History of chronic URIs, allergic rhinitis, asthma, recurrent tonsillitis? Are symptoms associated with exercise? Tobacco use? How many cigarettes per day? Vaping use? Marijuana use? Any oral piercings? Does the adolescent snore at night?
Environmental risks	Year home was built? Location (inner city, suburb, rural, near highway/high traffic areas)? Is there a basement? Number of people in home? Anyone smoke in home? Pets in home? Type of heating system? Wood burning stove? Humidifier? Mold? Carpets? Drapes? Mice, rats, or roaches? Presence of chemicals/fumes in home or near home? Use of pesticides inside or outside the home?

PHYSICAL ASSESSMENT

Equipment

When auscultating breath sounds, use the diaphragm of the stethoscope. The size of the stethoscope being used is extremely important when evaluating respiratory sounds. Stethoscopes with a smaller diaphragm should be used on infants and toddlers. Isolating cardiac and respiratory sounds is difficult in small children with too large a diaphragm, and using a diaphragm that is too small on adolescents or on children who are overweight or obese causes practitioners to miss findings of cardiac and respiratory sounds on auscultation due to increased adipose tissue, which obscures respiratory sounds.

Positioning

If possible, the child should sit upright for the respiratory assessment. Young children, especially toddlers, may be more relaxed sitting on their parent's lap during the examination of the chest. Children should be allowed to help as much as possible during the exam. Have them hold the stethoscope in place once you position it in the appropriate location. Other techniques include letting children role-play by allowing them to listen to their parent, a doll, or a stuffed animal. School-age children are very curious. Therefore, explain what you will be doing during the exam and why, using developmentally appropriate vocabulary. Taking a few extra minutes to incorporate the child's developmental level into your exam will result in more thorough and reliable findings. In addition, pictures of lungs in the exam room can be helpful with older children when you are explaining what you are looking for and listening to during the examination.

PHYSICAL EXAMINATION

Astute physical examination skills are important when making a diagnosis. Missed diagnoses have been associated with failure to perform a physical examination, misinterpretation of physical examination findings, and missing or not eliciting a physical examination sign.[10]

Pediatric health care providers should begin the physical examination by assessing the chest. The "quieter" parts of the exam, the cardiac and respiratory exam, require sharp listening skills and less active participation of the child. Therefore, the respiratory examination is best performed first following the cardiac exam—an effective approach to assessing children among pediatric experts.

The pediatric provider must take a systematic approach to examining the chest and use all the components of physical assessment. This includes inspection, palpation, percussion, and auscultation. Examination of the chest should always include both the anterior and the posterior chest.

A thorough assessment of the chest and lungs is not complete without examination of the upper airway, head, and extremities. An examination of the nasal passages and oropharynx can reveal signs of allergy or infection that may have implications for respiratory symptoms and conditions (see Chapter 12). Examine the nasal passages to determine the size of the airway passage and the appearance of the nasal turbinates, as well as the presence of rhinitis, nasal secretions, nasal polyps, or a foreign body. When looking at the oropharynx, note tonsils that occupy greater than 75% of the oropharyngeal width.[11] An abnormal finding in any of these areas can be a cause of respiratory symptoms related to an obstructed airway. Finally, examine the extremities for signs of digital clubbing. *Clubbing* is the bulbous-shaped enlargement of the soft tissue of the distal phalanges (Fig. 9.6). To assess for *clubbing* in a simple way, ask the child to place the first phalange of each thumb together (nails facing each other). Normally this position results in a diamond shape between the two thumbs. With clubbing, the diamond shape disappears and the space between the two thumbs is decreased or absent, depending on the degree of clubbing. This is termed the *Schamroth sign*. Other methods for measuring clubbing include the phalangeal depth ratio and the *hyponychial* angle. A distal phalangeal diameter (DPD) to interphalangeal diameter (IPD) ratio of less than 1 is normal. A ratio greater than 1 is seen with clubbing. A hyponychial angle of less than 180 degrees is normal, while an angle of greater than 195 degrees is indicative of clubbing.[12,13] Clubbing can be hereditary or can be the result of cardiac disease, respiratory disease, or severe malnutrition.

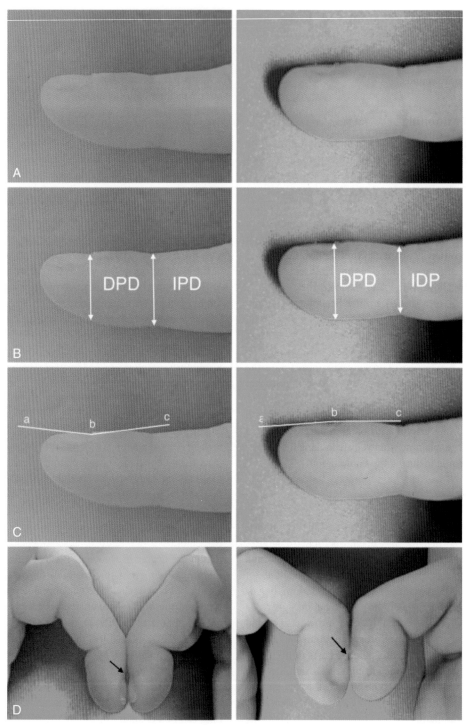

FIGURE 9.6 A) Normal and clubbed finger B) Normal and abnormal Distal phalangeal depth (DPD) and Interphalangeal finger depth (IPD) C) Normal and abnormal finger depth angle D) Schamroth sign in clubbed finger. (From Pasterkamp H, Zielinski D. The history and physical examination. In Wilmott RW, Deterding R, Li A, et al., eds. *Kendig's Disorders of the Respiratory Tract in Children*. 9th ed. Philadelphia: Elsevier; 2019.)

Inspection

Ideally, start the exam by visually inspecting the infant or child undressed from the waist up. This allows you to make general observations about the child's respiratory rate, breathing pattern, respiratory effort, accessory muscle use, inspiratory to expiratory ratio (I:E ratio), skin color, presence of noisy breathing, chest symmetry, and chest shape. In an irritable, ill, or fearful child, observation of respiratory pattern and rate may be the most helpful part of the examination if the child exhibits resistance to auscultation.

Assess the shape of the chest and note any abnormalities. The normal anterior-posterior (AP) to transverse ratio is 1:2. In the infant, the chest is round with a diameter roughly equal to the head circumference until 2 years of age and has a 1:1 AP/transverse ratio, giving a barrel chest appearance. As the child grows, the chest takes on the shape of the adult chest.[3,6] A barrel chest shape also can be seen when chronic air trapping is present, such as in advanced stages of cystic fibrosis. Other deformities of the chest that can have an impact on the child's respiratory status and decrease expansion of the lungs include pectus carinatum, pectus excavatum, or scoliosis.

Assessment of Respirations

Resting respiratory rates vary with the age of the child: the younger the child, the higher the respiratory rate (Table 9.3). The child's rhythm of breathing should be regular. Many factors can increase or decrease the respiratory rate, such as fever, pain, exercise, and medications.

PEDIATRIC PEARLS

Assess respiratory rate before the physical exam portion of the visit when the child is calm; this is best accomplished when the young child is sitting in the parent's or caregiver's lap.

TABLE 9.3	EXPECTED RANGE OF RESPIRATORY RATES FOR AGE
Age	Rate
Preterm neonate	40–70
0–12 months	24–55
1–5 years	20–30
5–9 years	18–25
9–12 years	16–22
12 years and older	12–20

Data from Hughes DM. Evaluating the respiratory system. In Goldbloom RB, ed. *Pediatric Clinical Skills.* 4th ed. Philadelphia: Elsevier/Saunders; 2011; Kleinman K, Mcdaniel L, Molloy M. *The Harriett Lane Handbook: A Manual for Pediatric House Officers.* 22nd ed. Philadelphia: Elsevier; 2021; Ball JW, et al. Chest and lungs. In Ball JW, et al., eds. *Seidel's Guide to Physical Examination.* 10th ed. St. Louis: Elsevier; 2023.

Periodic breathing is characterized by rapid breathing followed by periods of *apnea*, cessation of breathing. This is normal in the first few hours of life in healthy full-term newborns. Periodic breathing is more likely to persist in preterm infants, but the episodes of apnea should improve as infants approach term age.[3,14] *Apnea* is considered clinically significant if it lasts greater than 20 seconds or is characterized by shorter pauses associated with bradycardia (heart rate <100 beats per minute), cyanosis, or pallor.[15] *Paradoxical breathing*, or seesaw breathing, is often seen in newborns and infants because they use abdominal muscles more than intercostal muscles.[3,14] *Cheyne-Stokes breathing* is characterized by cycles of increasing and decreasing tidal volume separated by apnea. It occurs in children with congestive heart failure and increased intracranial pressure.[3,14]

Noisy breathing includes stridor, grunting, and snoring. *Stridor* is a high-pitched, loud, inspiratory sound produced by upper airway obstruction. Causes of upper airway obstruction include edema status post intubation, subglottic stenosis, laryngotracheobronchitis, and foreign body aspiration.[16] *Grunting* is a low-pitched expiratory sound present with respiratory distress and is the result of a partial closure of the glottis.[13] Snoring is a rough, snorting sound during sleep, usually on inspiration, but can also be present on expiration. It may be present during sleep in healthy children who have an upper respiratory infection. Snoring is often heard in the presence of adenoidal and tonsillar hypertrophy or congenital anomalies that involve the upper airway or facies (see Chapter 12).[6]

Inspect for nasal flaring and use of accessory muscles in the infant and toddler. Mild nasal flaring can be seen in newborns because they are obligate nose breathers in the first month of life. However, increased nasal flaring should be investigated because it is a sign of labored breathing. Other signs of increased effort and respiratory distress include retractions, bulging of the intercostal muscles, and head bobbing. Mild retractions may rarely be seen in some healthy young children; however, increased retractions can be a sign of airway obstruction. The chest wall of newborns and infants is more compliant than that of older children, making them more prone to retractions. Bulging of the intercostal spaces also may be seen with airway obstruction due to increased expiratory effort.[3,6] *Head bobbing*, the forward movement of the head, is a sign of respiratory distress due to the contraction of the *scalene* and *sternocleidomastoid* muscles.

An abnormal I:E ratio is an additional sign of respiratory distress. A normal I:E ratio in the infant is 1:2 seconds, except in the newborn, when it is variable. The inspiratory phase is greater than the expiratory phase when there is an extrathoracic (from the nose to the mid-trachea) obstruction. When there is an intrathoracic obstruction, the expiratory phase is more prolonged and accessory muscles are often used.[13] This is seen in obstructive diseases that cause air trapping, such as cystic fibrosis, or during an acute asthma exacerbation.

Assess for *cyanosis*, a bluish color to the skin or mucous membranes. *Acrocyanosis*, cyanosis of the hands and feet, is normal in the newborn and can persist for days if the infant is in a cool environment. *Central cyanosis*, which occurs in the conjunctiva, lips, mucous membranes, and nail beds, is an abnormal finding at any age and warrants immediate further evaluation. In the anemic child, it may be difficult to detect cyanosis early on because the arterial oxygen saturation at which cyanosis becomes apparent varies with the total hemoglobin level.[6] In addition, due to variations in skin tone and color, cyanosis is best assessed by looking at the mucous membranes and/or nail beds.

Auscultation

Auscultation is best performed at the beginning of the examination when the infant/child is more cooperative and attentive. This portion of the exam can also be performed while the child is sitting on the parent's lap (Fig. 9.7), on an examination table, or standing. Auscultation is performed with the diaphragm of the stethoscope placed firmly and directly on the chest. The child's chest should be bare because clothing can change the quality of the breath sounds. Remember to start at the apex, which sits slightly above the clavicles, then work down to the base. Then auscultate moving from side to side across the chest so that you can compare left to right chest sounds. Be sure to listen at each location for one full breath. Breath sounds are identified by their intensity, pitch, and duration. In children, breath sounds tend to be louder because of the thinness of the chest wall.[6] There has been much confusion about the terminology used to describe breath sounds. Table 9.4 presents the most common description of normal breath sounds in the respiratory cycle.

Transmitted voice sounds or an infant's cry can also be assessed with a stethoscope. *Vocal fremitus* is a vibration transmitted through the body and can be heard on auscultation. Voice sounds are typically muffled on auscultation. If you hear the voice sound or cry loud and clear, it is termed *bronchophony*. This technique can be used to examine an infant or uncooperative child even while he or she is crying. If the verbal

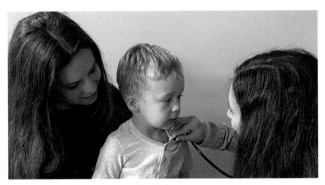

FIGURE 9.7 Auscultation of infant. *Courtsey Tina Tolomeo.*

TABLE 9.4	NORMAL BREATH SOUNDS		
Sound	Description	Duration of Inspiration and Expiration	Sound Diagram
Vesicular	Soft, low-pitched sound heard over entire surface of lungs; inspiration louder	Inspiration > expiration	
Bronchovesicular	Moderately loud and pitched sounds heard over intrascapular area; heard on inspiration and expiration	Inspiration = expiration	
Bronchial (tubular)	Loud and high-pitched sounds heard over trachea near suprasternal notch; louder on expiration	Inspiration < expiration	
Tracheal	Loudest and highest pitched sounds heard over the trachea; heard on inspiration and expiration	Inspiration = expiration	

Data from Hughes DM. Evaluating the respiratory system. In Goldbloom RB, ed. *Pediatric Clinical Skills.* 4th ed. Philadelphia: Elsevier/Saunders; 2011; Wick RM. Respiratory system. In Willis LM, ed. *Health Assessment Made Incredibly Visual.* 3rd ed. Philadelphia: Wolters Kluwer; 2017; Ball JW, et al. Chest and lungs. In Ball JW, et al. eds. *Seidel's Guide to Physical Examination.* 10th ed. St. Louis: Elsevier; 2023.

child speaks the sound "ee" and it sounds like "ay," it is called *egophony*. If the child whispers a word and it is heard loud and clear, it is called *whispered pectoriloquy*. If any of these signs are positive, it is evidence of a consolidation indicated by fluid or exudate in the alveolar spaces.[5]

Abnormal Lung Sounds

In addition to normal lung sounds, you may hear adventitious or abnormal breath sounds (Table 9.5). Adventitious lung sounds are sounds that are superimposed on normal breath sounds.

Palpation

Palpation is performed to identify anatomical landmarks, respiratory symmetry, and areas of tenderness or abnormalities. Begin by counting the ribs, locate the *angle of Louis*, and move your fingers laterally to feel the second rib and

TABLE 9.5	ABNORMAL BREATH SOUNDS
Sound	Description
Crackles	Discontinuous sounds, bubbly, heard primarily on inspiration, do not clear with cough; associated with pneumonia, pulmonary edema, cystic fibrosis
	• Fine crackles—soft and higher in pitch, generally indicative of fluid in smaller airways in infants and children
	• Coarse crackles—loud and lower in pitch, usually signify fluid in larger airways
Wheezes	Continuous, high-pitched musical sounds heard primarily on expiration; associated with foreign body aspiration, bronchiolitis, asthma
Rhonchi	Continuous low-pitched sounds; clears with coughing; caused by secretions/mucus in larger airways as in bronchitis and lower respiratory tract infections
Stridor	High-pitched, harsh sounds; heard primarily with inspiration but can be biphasic; associated with laryngotracheobronchitis, laryngomalacia, subglottic stenosis, and vocal cord dysfunction; can be heard without a stethoscope
Stertor	Noisy breathing heard on inspiration and expiration. Caused by the echoing of soft structures at the level of the nasopharynx and pharynx. Can occur with stridor, especially when there is external compression of the larynx and supraglottis

Data from Hughes DM. Evaluating the respiratory system. In Goldbloom RB, ed. *Pediatric Clinical Skills.* 4th ed. Philadelphia: Elsevier/Saunders; 2011; Wick RM. Respiratory system. In Willis LM, ed. *Health Assessment Made Incredibly Visual.* 3rd ed. Philadelphia: Wolters Kluwer; 2017; Ball JW, et al. Chest and lungs. In Ball JW, et al., eds. *Seidel's Guide to Physical Examination.* 10th ed. St. Louis: Elsevier; 2023; Cox LC. Examination of the respiratory system. In Cox LC, ed. *Physical Assessment for Nurses.* West Sussex: Wiley-Blackwell; 2010; Kleinman K, Mcdaniel L, Molloy M. *The Harriett Lane Handbook: A Manual for Pediatric House Officers.* 22nd ed. Philadelphia: Elsevier; 2021; and Ida JB, Thompson DM. Pediatric stridor. *Otolaryngol Clin N Am.* 2014;47:795–819; Bertrand P. Clinical history and physical examination of the respiratory system. In: Bertrand P, Sanchez I, eds. *Pediatric Respiratory Diseases. A Comprehensive Textbook.* Switzerland: Springer Nature; 2020.

corresponding costal cartilage. Directly below this rib is the second intercostal space. From there, count downward to the other ribs and their respective intercostal spaces.[3,5]

To assess chest excursion, place your hands along the lateral rib cage and squeeze the thumbs toward each other so that you gather a small amount of skin in between your thumbs. As the child inhales, note the symmetry of the chest excursion. Again, this should be done both anteriorly and posteriorly. Asymmetry is an abnormal finding. In the newborn period, asymmetrical chest excursion may be a sign of a diaphragmatic hernia. Other possible abnormalities associated with asymmetrical chest excursion during the newborn period or later include diaphragmatic dysfunction, pneumothorax, mass, foreign body, or abnormal chest wall shape. An important part of the exam that should not be ignored is palpation of the trachea

to assess for a mediastinal shift. To perform this exam on toddlers and older children, place fingers in the suprasternal notch on both sides of the trachea (Fig. 9.8). The distance between the trachea and the sternocleidomastoid tendons should be equal on both sides. A shift in the trachea occurs when there is a difference in volume or pressure between the two sides of the chest, as is seen in a pneumothorax or pleural effusion.[3]

To complete the palpation portion of the exam, assess for *tactile fremitus.* To do this, place your palms, the ulnar surface of your hands, or your fingers, depending on the size of the chest wall, on the child's back (right and left side), and ask the verbal child to say "1-2-3." With an infant or uncooperative child, this technique can be performed while the child is crying. Perform this exam both anteriorly and posteriorly. Vibrations or fremitus should be of equal intensity bilaterally. A pneumothorax or

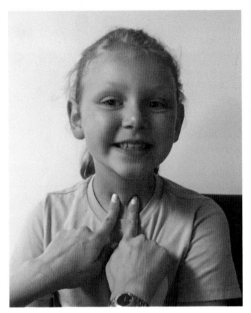

FIGURE 9.8 Palpation of trachea.

TABLE 9.6	PERCUSSION SOUNDS			
Tone	**Intensity**	**Pitch**	**Quality**	**Clinical Implication**
Tympanic	Loud	High	Drumlike	Air collection (i.e., large pneumothorax)
Resonant	Loud	Low	Hollow	Normal lung
Dull	Moderate	Moderate	Dull thud	Solid area (i.e., mass)
Flat	Soft	High	Very dull	Consolidation (i.e., pneumonia)

Data from Wick RM. Respiratory system. In Willis LM, ed. *Health Assessment Made Incredibly Visual*. 3rd ed. Philadelphia: Wolters Kluwer; 2017; Ball JW, et al. Chest and lungs. In Ball JW, et al., eds. *Seidel's Guide to Physical Examination*. 10th ed. St. Louis: Elsevier; 2023; and Bertrand P. Clinical history and physical examination of the respiratory system. In: Bertrand P, Sanchez I, eds. *Pediatric Respiratory Diseases. A Comprehensive Textbook*. Switzerland: Springer Nature; 2020.

hyperinflation can decrease fremitus; a mass or pneumonia can increase fremitus.[5]

Percussion

Percussion is used to determine the sounds of the underlying organs and tissues and may be particularly useful for providers in areas without easy access to imaging centers. It helps distinguish whether the tissue is air filled, fluid filled, or solid. There are five sounds that are produced with percussion: *resonance, hyperresonance, dull, flat,* and *tympany*. The sounds are distinguished by their intensity, pitch, and duration. In infants and toddlers, the sound produced is more resonant because the chest wall is thinner than in older children and adolescents (Table 9.6). To perform percussion, hyperextend the middle finger of your nondominant hand and press the distal interphalangeal joint firmly on the chest. With the middle finger of your dominant hand, strike down on the hyperextended interphalangeal joint. The movement must be sharp and quick, and the only portion of the nondominant finger that should be touching the chest should be the hyperextended joint. Strike each area two

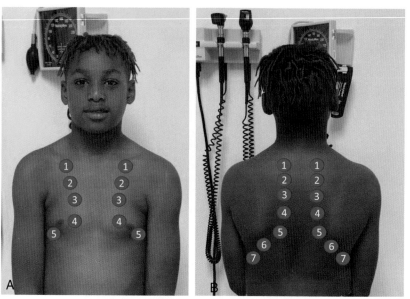

FIGURE 9.9 Sequence for percussion of the thorax. A, Anterior percussion. B, Posterior percussion.

or three times and then move to the opposite side for comparison (Fig. 9.9). Lastly, it may be necessary to repeat auscultation to confirm findings that were revealed during palpation and percussion. Percussion is often deferred in infants and young children because the examiner often cannot discriminate between sounds that originate from organs that are proximate to each other.[5,15]

DIAGNOSTICS

Pulse Oximetry

For a discussion on pulse oximetry, see Chapter 8.

Chest Radiograph

Chest radiography is often used to identify pulmonary pathology in the presence of pulmonary symptoms such as coughing, wheezing, shortness of breath, and chest pain. A comparison of inspiratory to expiratory radiographs may be useful when evaluating a child with a suspected foreign body. If a localized area of the lung does not empty on the expiratory view, it is indicative of a bronchial obstruction.[13] A finding of hyperinflation is indicative of air trapping and is frequently seen in children with bronchiolitis or an acute asthma exacerbation. Atelectasis or collapse may indicate mucus retention and can be present in children with bronchiolitis, asthma, or bronchomalacia. Consolidation can be caused by pneumonia, and an area of hyperlucency without normal lung markings is indicative of a pneumothorax or other air-containing pathology such as a cyst.

Pulmonary Function Testing

Pulmonary function testing is performed to evaluate pulmonary symptoms and assess for obstructive and/or restrictive lung disease. It is also used to monitor disease progression and response to therapy. Although infant pulmonary function testing is available at specialized Pediatric Pulmonology Centers, pulmonary function tests are generally reserved for children ≥5 years of age. Predicted values are based on a reference population and are dependent upon age, height, and sex. There are specific guidelines for the performance of lung function testing; an experienced technician is of paramount importance in the testing process. An assessment of patient technique and effort is necessary when interpreting results; in addition, acceptability criteria must be met before a test can be considered interpretable.[17] Severity of lung dysfunction is categorized as normal, mild, moderate, severe.[18] There are many types of pulmonary function tests available, and the details are beyond the scope of this chapter. As such, this chapter will provide a general overview of the most common tests performed in the pediatric population.

Spirometry

The most common pulmonary function test is spirometry. Portable spirometers are available for office use. *Spirometry* is defined as "a physiological test that measures how an individual inhales or exhales volumes of air as a function of time."[19] Measures to be reported include (1) forced vital capacity (FVC), which is the maximum volume of air forcefully exhaled after a maximal inhalation; (2) forced exhaled volume (FEV$_1$) in the first second, which is the maximum volume of air exhaled in the first second of FVC; and (3) FEV$_1$/FVC, which is the ratio of air exhaled in the first second to the total volume of air exhaled. The forced expiratory flow 25-75 (FEF 25-75), which is the forced expiratory flow between 25% and 75% of FVC, has not demonstrated added value in identifying airway obstruction.[18] A reduced FEV$_1$ and FEV$_1$/FVC is indicative of an obstructive pattern, as seen in asthma. A reduced FVC and FEV$_1$ and a normal FEV$_1$/FVC are indicative of a restrictive pattern as seen in chest wall abnormalities. A mixed pattern may be seen in someone with advanced cystic fibrosis. The *Expert Panel Report 3: Guidelines on the Diagnosis and Management of Asthma* recommends performing spirometry at the initial assessment after treatments have been initiated and symptoms have stabilized, during periods of loss of asthma control, and at least every 1 to 2 years.[20] Updated asthma guidelines also include the measurement of fractional

exhaled nitric oxide (FENO) to evaluate the diagnosis of asthma if the diagnosis is uncertain or if spirometry cannot be performed.[21]

Evaluation of the spirogram is as important as the evaluation of the spirometry values. The spirogram is a graphic depiction of the spirometry values. The flow-volume curve and the time volume curve provide the expiratory phase of the maneuver. The flow volume loop provides both the inspiratory and the expiratory phases of the maneuver (Fig. 9.10). An evaluation of the curve shapes can provide you with a sense of the quality of the test, as well as whether an obstructive or restrictive pattern is present.[22] If the expiratory curve has a concave shape, it is indicative of an obstructive pattern. If the expiratory curve has a steep slope, it is indicative of a restrictive pattern (Fig. 9.11). If the inspiratory loop is blunted, it is indicative of vocal cord dysfunction.

Lung Volumes

A restrictive pattern on spirometry must be confirmed with *lung volume testing*. Common lung volume measures include (1) total lung capacity (TLC), which is the volume of air in the lungs after a maximal inspiration; (2) functional residual capacity (FRC), which is the volume of air in the lungs at the end of expiration during tidal breathing; and (3) residual volume (RV), which is the volume of air in the lungs at the end of a maximal expiration. A decreased TLC is indicative of a restrictive pattern. An increased RV is indicative of an obstructive pattern.[18]

Bronchodilator Response Testing

Bronchodilator response testing is used to assess for the presence of reversible airflow limitation. To perform the test, the patient should first undergo baseline spirometry. This is followed by the administration of a short-acting beta agonist and repeat spirometry after medication administration. Each facility should have a protocol that indicates how long after the short-acting beta agonist administration one should wait before repeating spirometry.

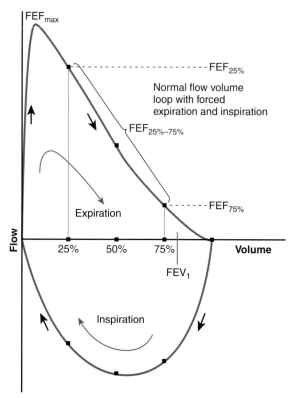

FIGURE 9.10 Normal flow volume loop. *FEF,* Forced expiratory flow; *FEV,* forced exhaled volume. (From Ryu J, Hagood JS, Haddad GG. Diagnostic approach to respiratory disease. In Kliegman RM, St Geme JW, Blum NJ, Shah SS, Tasker RC, Wilson KM, eds. *Nelson Textbook of Pediatrics.* 21st ed. Philadelphia: Elsevier, Inc.; 2020.)

A typical wait time is 15 minutes.[23] The *Expert Panel Report 3: Guidelines on the Diagnosis and Management of Asthma* considers an increase in FEV_1 of $\geq$12% from the baseline or an increase of $\geq$10% of predicted after the bronchodilator as significant reversibility.[20]

Quantitative Pilocarpine Iontophoresis Sweat Chloride Testing

The *sweat test* is the gold standard for diagnosing cystic fibrosis. The test measures the concentration of chloride in sweat after stimulation with pilocarpine. Specific guidelines for collection and analysis have been established by the Cystic Fibrosis Foundation and must be adhered to in order to ensure accuracy of results. A test is considered unlikely if the concentration of chloride is less than 30 mmol/L, intermediate if it is 30 to 60 mmol/L, and consistent with cystic fibrosis if it is greater than 60 mmol/L. Results in the intermediate range require further evaluation as patients with values of 30 to 39 mmol/L have been definitively diagnosed with cystic fibrosis.[24]

CHEST AND RESPIRATORY CONDITIONS

Table 9.7 presents respiratory conditions seen in infants, children, and adolescents by the pediatric health care provider. Diagnosing asthma during the infant and early childhood years is difficult because many children will have intermittent wheezing with respiratory infections during their first year of life. Box 9.2

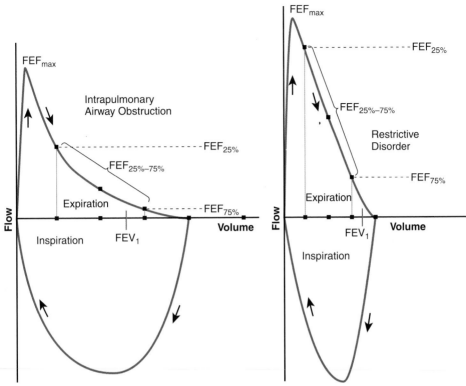

FIGURE 9.11 Obstructive and restrictive flow volume loops. *FEF*, forced expiratory flow; *FEV*, forced exhaled volume. (From Ryu J, Hagood JS, Haddad GG. Diagnostic approach to respiratory disease. In Kliegman RM, St Geme JW, Blum NJ, Shah SS, Tasker RC, Wilson KM, eds. *Nelson Textbook of Pediatrics*. 21st ed. Philadelphia: Elsevier, Inc.; 2020.)

TABLE 9.7	CHEST AND RESPIRATORY CONDITIONS
Condition	**Description**
Bronchiolitis	Inflammatory obstruction of small airways caused by edema, mucus production; occurs during first 2 years of life with peak incidence at 6 months of age
	Etiology: Viral etiology common with a large percentage caused by respiratory syncytial virus (RSV)
	Symptoms: Wheezing, crackles, cough, and rhinorrhea; when severe, nasal flaring, retractions, and tachypnea can be present
Epiglottitis	Obstructive inflammatory process of airway that is supraglottic; abrupt onset of high fever, sore throat, drooling, dysphagia, dyspnea, increasing airway obstruction; occurs between 2 and 6 years of age
	Etiology: Bacterial with marked decrease in incidence because of widespread use of *Haemophilus influenzae* vaccine; most cases post–*H. influenzae* due to streptococci and staphylococci
	Symptoms: High fever, difficulty swallowing, drooling, sore throat, rapidly progressing respiratory distress

Continued

TABLE 9.7	CHEST AND RESPIRATORY CONDITIONS—CONT'D
Condition	**Description**
Asthma	Inflammatory process characterized by airway obstruction and hyperresponsiveness; inflammation plays key role in factors leading to symptoms
	Symptoms: Cough, wheezing, tachypnea, chest tightness, and dyspnea with prolonged expiration
Croup/laryngotracheobronchitis	Acute upper airway obstruction; inflammation and edema of the airway leads to symptoms
	Etiology: 75% due to parainfluenza virus; others include influenza A and B, adenovirus, respiratory syncytial virus, and measles
	Symptoms: Hoarse, barky cough that is worse at night, stridor; respiratory distress can occur
Cystic fibrosis	A multisystem disease related to thick secretions that lead to airway obstruction
	Etiology: Inherited, autosomal recessive
	Symptoms: Chronic or recurrent cough, wheeze, recurrent pneumonia or bronchitis
Foreign body aspiration	Lodging of object in larynx, trachea, bronchi (most common site), with degree of obstruction dependent on size/location of object in respiratory tract
	Etiology: Food and small objects are the most common causes; possibility of foreign body must be considered in infants and young children with acute respiratory distress regardless of history; common in children <3 years of age
	Symptoms: Choking, prolonged cough, dyspnea, pneumonia that does not resolve
Laryngomalacia	Immature cartilage of the supraglottic larynx leads to symptoms; it slowly resolves by 12–18 months of age
	Symptoms: Inspiratory stridor with activity/feeding that improves when the child is calm
Tracheomalacia	Weakened "floppy" trachea that leads to symptoms
	Symptoms: Harsh noise/stridor on expiration caused by airway collapse; onset in early neonatal period; diagnosed by bronchoscopy.
Pneumonia	Infection of lung parenchyma or interstitium; may be primary condition or manifestation of another illness
	Etiology: Bacterial (streptococcus, staphylococcus, etc.) or viral (RSV, parainfluenza, adenovirus, etc.); most commonly caused by viral microorganisms—bacterial pneumonia is less common, *Mycoplasma pneumoniae* accounts for ~70% of all pneumonias in 9- to 15-year-olds; noninfectious causes such as aspiration should be considered
	Symptoms: Crackles, decreased breath sounds; more severe cases may also see tachypnea, nasal flaring, and retractions
Neonatal respiratory distress syndrome (Hyaline membrane disease)	A condition related to decreased number of branching airways and alveoli, surfactant deficiency (this is the main cause of the disease), atelectasis, impaired gas exchange, and hypoxemia
	Symptoms: Tachypnea, retractions, cyanosis, apnea

TABLE 9.7	CHEST AND RESPIRATORY CONDITIONS—CONT'D
Condition	**Description**
Vocal cord dysfunction	Transient obstruction of the upper airway associated with inappropriate adduction of the vocal cords during inhalation. Often mimics asthma
	Etiology: Can be psychological, physiological (hyperresponsiveness to a trigger), or exertional to name a few
	Symptoms: Can be asymptomatic; however, symptoms can range from mild dyspnea to acute respiratory distress
Primary ciliary dyskinesia	Impaired ciliary function that results in sinus disease, ear infections, and infertility
	Etiology: Typically autosomal recessive
	Symptoms: In infants can present with respiratory distress. A daily productive cough is present in young children

Data from Tolomeo C. *Nursing Care in Pediatric Respiratory Disease*. Ames: Wiley-Blackwell; 2012; Wenzel M. Gasping for a diagnosis: Pediatric vocal cord dysfunction. *J Pediatr Healthcare*. 2019;33(1):5–13; Ferkol TW. Primary ciliary dyskinesia (immotile cilia syndrome, Kartagener syndrome). In Kliegman RM, St Geme JW, Blum NJ, Shah SS, Tasker RC, Wilson KM, eds. *Nelson Textbook of Pediatrics*. 21st ed. Philadelphia: Elsevier, Inc.; 2020; and Rodrigues KK, Roosevelt GE. Acute inflammatory upper airway obstruction (croup, epiglottitis, laryngitis, and bacterial tracheitis). In Kliegman RM, St Geme JW, Blum NJ, Shah SS, Tasker RC, Wilson KM, eds. *Nelson Textbook of Pediatrics*. 21st ed. Philadelphia: Elsevier, Inc.; 2020; Bertrand P, Sanchez I, eds. *Pediatric Respiratory Diseases. A Comprehensive Textbook*. Switzerland: Springer Nature; 2020.

BOX 9.2   VALIDATED TOOL FOR ASSESSMENT OF ASTHMA RISK

Asthma Predictive Index (API) Criteria[14]
- increased risk of asthma for children with recurrent episodes of wheezing during the first 3 years of life, plus 1 major or 2 minor criteria
- major criteria
  - provider-diagnosed eczema
  - parental asthma
- minor criteria
- provider-diagnosed allergic rhinitis
- wheezing without colds
- peripheral eosinophilia $\geq 4\%$

---

presents the Asthma Predictive Index (API), a useful tool to help rule out the likelihood of asthma during the school age years in young children with wheezing.[25]

TELEHEALTH TIPS

Telehealth and specific telehealth clinics that include examination devices and on-site teams have been in existence for years, particularly for underserved areas.[26] With the emergence of the COVID-19 virus and subsequent pandemic in 2020, there was a sharp increase in the use of telehealth across the United States. Although telehealth requires an appropriate device (computer, laptop, cell phone, etc.), internet access, and training, it is a convenient method for accessing health care and has been well received by patients and providers.[27] While not all aspects of a respiratory physical assessment are possible, telehealth allows for a good portion of the examination. For example, with telehealth, the provider is still able to assess respiratory effort, chest shape and symmetry, presence of cough, skin color, skin rashes, and allergic signs such as allergic shiners and Dennie-Morgan line.[28] As with face-to-face visits, thorough questioning and good lighting are important. Although examination devices (e.g., pulse oximeter) for use with telehealth are available, most patients do not have access to them at home. As such, there are some limitations to the virtual physical examination.

However, telehealth offers the ability to detect signs and symptoms that can then be further assessed in the office or urgent care setting if necessary.

SUMMARY OF EXAMINATION

- Ensure a welcoming, nonjudgmental environment that allows for open communication.
- A thorough family and past medical history should be obtained and a detailed history of any presenting respiratory symptoms (including onset, precipitating factors, associated symptoms, etc.) from the caregiver and the child, when possible.
- Start the physical examination with inspection of the chest wall for shape and symmetry as well as respiratory rate and effort. Also assess skin for cyanosis and atopic disorders. Relate findings to child's age and symptoms.
- Systematically auscultate breath sounds bilaterally. Note any adventitious sounds and correlate findings with clinical history.
- Systematically palpate chest bilaterally. Note excursion and vocal fremitus; correlate findings with clinical history.
- Systematically percuss chest bilaterally. Note sounds; correlate findings with history.

- Telehealth has increased significantly in pediatric pulmonology and many assessment technologies commonly used in respiratory assessment can be used remotely and assessed by the pediatric primary care provider.
- Refer to pediatric pulmonology for further evaluation *as indicated* by examination findings, diagnostic results, or parental anxiety/concern.

DOCUMENTATION

7-Month-Old Infant
Chest: AP diameter 1:1. Respiratory rate 32, rate regular, respirations quiet. No nasal flaring, retractions, or intercostal bulging. I:E 1:2, Chest excursion symmetrical. Trachea midline. Vesicular lung sounds across all lung fields.

DOCUMENTATION

8-Year-Old With Acute Asthma Exacerbation
Chest: Normal AP diameter. Respiratory rate 30. Audible wheeze present. Mild nasal flaring. Coughing spasms present. I:E 1:3. Mild intercostal retractions. Symmetrical chest excursion. Breath sounds equal. Inspiratory and expiratory wheezes scattered throughout all lung fields. No crackles or stridor noted.

REFERENCES

1. Nakra N. Pediatric pulmonary anatomy and physiology. In: Tolomeo C, ed. *Nursing Care in Pediatric Respiratory Disease.* Ames: Wiley-Blackwell; 2012.
2. Davis RP, Mychaliska GB. Neonatal pulmonary physiology. *Pediatr Surg.* 2013;22:179–184.
3. Ball JW, Dains JE, Flynn JA, Solomon BS, Stewart RW. Chest and lungs. In: Ball JW, Dains JE, Flynn JA, Solomon BS, Stewart RW, eds. *Seidel's Guide to Physical Examination.* 10th ed. St. Louis: Mosby; 2023.
4. Osmeer FI, Sanchez I. Development of respiratory system. In: Bertrand P, Sanchez I, eds. *Pediatric Respiratory Diseases. A Comprehensive Textbook.* Switzerland: Springer Nature; 2020.
5. Wick RM. Respiratory system. In: Willis LM, ed. *Health Assessment Made Incredibly Visual.* 3rd ed. Philadelphia: Wolters Kluwer; 2017.
6. Hughes DM. Evaluating the respiratory system. In: Goldbloom RB, ed. *Pediatric Clinical Skills.* 4th ed. Philadelphia: Elsevier/Saunders; 2011.
7. Hadland SE, Yehia BR, Makadon HJ. Caring for LGBTQ youth in inclusive and affirmative environments. *Pediatr Clin North Am.* 2016;63:955–969.
8. Silverberg B. Best practices for LGBTQ—Friendly urgent care. *Journal of Urgent Care Medicine.* Available at https://www.jucm.com/best-practices-for-lgbtq-friendly-urgent-care/. Accessed December 28, 2021.
9. Voorend-van Bergen S, Vaessen-Verberne AA, de Jongste JC, Pijnenburg MW. Asthma control questionnaires in the management of asthma in children: a review. *Pediatr Pulmonol.* 2015;50:202–208.
10. Verghese A, Charlton B, Kassirer JP, Ramsey M, Ioannidis JPA. Inadequacies of physical examination as a cause

of medical errors and adverse events: a collection of vignettes. *Am J Med.* 2015;128:1322–1324.

11. Kumar DS, Valenzuela D, Kozak FK, et al. The reliability of clinical tonsil size grading in children. *JAMA Otolaryngol Head Neck Surg.* 2014;140:1034–1037.

12. Bertrand P. Clinical history and physical examination of the respiratory system. In: Bertrand P, Sanchez I, eds. *Pediatric Respiratory Diseases. A Comprehensive Textbook.* Switzerland: Springer Nature; 2020.

13. Ryu J, Hagood JS, Haddad GG. Diagnostic approach to respiratory disease. In: Kliegman RM, St Geme JW, Blum NJ, Shah SS, Tasker RC, Wilson KM, eds. *Nelson Textbook of Pediatrics.* 21st ed. Philadelphia: Elsevier, Inc; 2020.

14. Tolomeo C. Pediatric respiratory health history and physical assessment. In: Tolomeo C, ed. *Nursing Care in Pediatric Respiratory Disease.* Ames: Wiley-Blackwell; 2012.

15. Eichenwald EC. AAP Committee on Fetus and Newborn. Apnea of prematurity. *Pediatrics.* 2016;137:e20153757.

16. Ida JB, Thompson DM. Pediatric stridor. *Otolaryngol Clin N Am.* 2014;47:795–819.

17. Culver BH, Graham BL, Coates AL, et al. Recommendations for a standardized pulmonary function report. *Am J Respir Crit Care Med.* 2017;196:1463–1472.

18. Stanojevic S, Kaminsky DA, Miller MR, et al. ERS/ATS technical standard on interpretive strategies for routine lung function tests. *Eur Respir J.* 2022;60:2101499.

19. Lamb K., Theodore D., Bhutta B.S. Spirometry. [Updated 2022 Jul 18]. In: StatPearls [Internet]. Treasure Island (FL): StatPearls Publishing; 2022 Jan. Available from: https://www.ncbi.nlm.nih.gov/books/NBK560526/

20. National Heart, Lung, and Blood Institute. Expert Panel Report 3: Guidelines for the Diagnosis and Management of Asthma. Available at https://www.nhlbi.nih.gov/sites/default/files/media/docs/EPR-3_Asthma_Full_Report_2007.pdf. Accessed December 29, 2021.

21. National Heart, Lung, and Blood Institute. 2020 Focused Updates to the Asthma Management Guidelines. Available at https://www.nhlbi.nih.gov/health-topics/all-publications-and-resources/2020-focused-updates-asthma-management-guidelines. Accessed December 29, 2021.

22. Banasiak NC. Spirometry in primary care for children with asthma. *Pediatr Nurs.* 2014;40:195–198.

23. Graham BL, Steenbruggen I, Miller MR, et al. Standardization of spirometry 2019 update. *Am J Respir Crit Care Med.* 2019;200:963–971.

24. Farrell PM, White TB, Ren CL, et al. Diagnosis of cystic fibrosis: consensus guidelines from the Cystic Fibrosis Foundation. *J Pediatr.* 2017;181S:S4–S15.

25. Huffaker MF, Phipatanakul W. Utility of the Asthma Predictive Index in predicting childhood asthma and identifying disease-modifying interventions. *Ann Allergy Asthma Immunol.* 2014;112:188–190.

26. Weinstein RS, Krpinski EA, Doarn CR. Clinical examination component of telemedicine, telehealth, mHealth, and connected health medical practices. *Med Clin North Am.* 2018;102:533–544.

27. Davis J, Gordon R, Hammond A, et al. Rapid implementation of telehealth services in a pediatric pulmonary clinic During Covid-19. *Pediatrics.* 2021;148e2020030494.

28. Benziger CP, Huffman MD, Sweis RN, Stone NJ. The telehealth ten: a guide for a patient-assisted virtual physical examination. *Am J Med.* 2021;134:48–51.

CHAPTER 10

EYES

Karen G. Duderstadt

The eye is the most remarkable organ in the body as it is underdeveloped at birth and undergoes dramatic development in the first year of life. Although the eyes are anatomically complete, the sense of vision begins to develop over the first weeks and months of life. The development of normal vision depends on the reception of light rays that stimulate the internal eye during the early critical period of development after birth. Visual acuity is also determined by an infant's genetic predisposition, as well as physical and environmental health factors. Eye conditions that limit or occlude the process of visual development in the first year of life may affect the long-term visual health of the infant and child.

The eye is the window to the health of the body and can often assist the pediatric health care provider in diagnosing congenital genetic syndromes as well as many chronic health conditions that impact the eye at the onset of the illness. A complete and thorough eye examination by the pediatric health care provider is critical to early detection and treatment of visual problems to assure optimum visual development for infants and children.

EMBRYOLOGIC DEVELOPMENT

The development of the eye begins in the third week of embryonic development, with the optic grooves forming in the neural tube, and by the end of the fourth week the optic vesicle is formed and lies close to the ectoderm surface. The surface of the ectoderm thickens and forms the lens placode. By the fifth week of gestation the optic cup and the lens cavity are formed, and by the sixth week, invagination of the optic vesicles occurs, forming the choroid layer and vasculature of the eye. The formation of the cornea, lens, and anterior chamber proceeds during the seventh and eighth week, and the eyelid folds develop and begin to cover the palpebral fissure. It is during this period of gestation that exposure to prenatal infections, such as rubella and varicella, cause the development of congenital cataracts. The development of the retina proceeds peripherally from the head of the optic nerve during gestation.[1] Development of the retinal tissue continues with the differentiation of the nerve fiber layer, proliferative layer of the macula, and the pigmented layer of the retina. That precedes the development of the iris and the ciliary body, which occurs between the 9th and 12th weeks of embryonic development. The ciliary body gives rise to the ciliary muscles, which control the accommodative reflex and pupillary aperture (Fig. 10.1).

Development of the structures of the eye is complete by 15 weeks of gestation. During the fourth month of gestation, the development of the retinal blood vessels is initiated, and full vascularization of the retina occurs just before birth in a term infant and is incomplete in the preterm infant. The pupillary light reflex can be elicited by 30 weeks of gestation and requires an intact optic nerve and oculomotor nerve.

DEVELOPMENT OF VISION

Visual development begins at birth at the center of the *retina* in the *macula*. The macula is a circular area surrounding the *fovea*. The fovea,

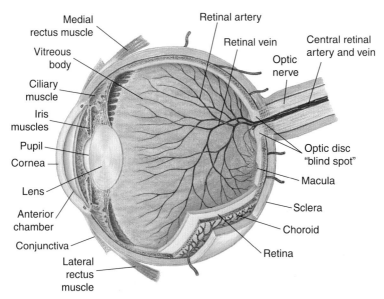

FIGURE 10.1 Anatomy of the human eye. (From Seidel H, Ball J, Dains J, et al. *Mosby's Guide to Physical Examination.* 9th ed. American Academy of Pediatrics; 2018.)

which is the most sensitive area of the retina, is a small area that is the center of the field of vision and is fully developed by approximately 4 years of age. The outer layer of the *retina* contains photoreceptors, the rods and cones. The retina predominantly consists of rods at birth, and the cones are located near the outermost layer of the retina. As the retina is exposed to light, the cones migrate toward the center to become the anatomical macula on the *fundus* located on the posterior surface of the retina. The optical lens has a key role in focusing light on the neural layer of the retina, and the ciliary muscles assist in accommodation of the optical lens. The *optic nerve* is also developing at the same time as the retina. There are as many as 8 million cells in the optic nerve and 5 million retinal cells in the optic neuron at birth that compete for synaptic sites on the nerve. Term infants from 36 to 40 weeks of gestation can perceive shape, color, motion, and patterns at birth. Visual development in the newborn is dependent upon development of the visual pathways that link the eyes to the lateral geniculate nucleus in the thalamus and to the visual cortex located in the occipital lobe of the brain.

Exposure to light begins the synaptic development of the neurons at birth.[2]

Myelination of the optic nerves, development of the visual cortex, and growth of the lateral geniculate body occur over the first 2 years of life. Central fixation is present shortly after birth in the term infant, and the human face at a distance of 8 to 12 inches holds the most visual interest for a newborn. The term infant is *hyperopic,* or farsighted, at birth. Visual images are focused behind and not on the retina, so the visual image is blurred. For the infant to see near objects, the *ciliary muscles* of the eye must work hard to accommodate or shape the optical lens. In the first few months of life, these efforts of the *ciliary muscles* result in thickening of the lens, which makes accommodation of the image onto the retina possible. Visual stimuli are critical to the development of normal vision in the infant.

DEVELOPMENTAL AND PHYSIOLOGIC VARIATIONS

In almost all term infants, the retina and retinal vasculature are fully developed.[1] In preterm infants, the development of the retina depends on the gestational age at birth. *Hypoxia* or *hyperoxia* in preterm infants often impacts the normal development of the retina and causes a *retinopathy*, a disorder of the retinal vessels. Preterm infants have an avascular zone in the periphery of the retina that disrupts the normal proliferation of the retinal vessels and interrupts blood flow to the visual receptors. The disruption of blood flow may lead to retinal detachment from the choroid, causing visual impairment or blindness if left untreated.

All infants with a birth weight of 1500 g or less, or a gestational age of 30 weeks or younger, are at highest risk for *retinopathy of prematurity* (ROP), a disorder of the developing retinal blood vessels.[1] Infants born at 28 weeks' gestation or earlier, or weighing 1000 g or less, are also at risk for developing macular folds and retinal detachment which can lead to a loss of vision.[3] Infants with a birth weight of 1500 g to 2000 g or a gestational age of greater than 30 weeks who have received oxygen supplementation for more than a few days or had hypotension requiring treatment should also be screened or ROP. ROP is a leading cause of permanent visual impairment in infants and children.[4] Previous evidence has suggested that race or ethnicity is a risk factor for severe ROP in preterm infants; however, more recent research has demonstrated that inequities in the prevalence of ROP among children of color are likely related to gestational age, which is highly influenced by structural factors and social determinants of health.[4]

The term infant's eyes often wander or deviate in the first 6 weeks when trying to achieve visual fixation in the *central field* of vision. After 6 weeks of early visual stimulus, an infant is able to focus and visually follow an object or the parent's movements. Any inability to visually focus after 6 weeks of age in a term infant is considered suspect and at 3 months of age is considered abnormal. As the eyeball or optic *globe* grows, the hyperopia decreases and the lens hardens, but detailed visual acuity is not present until 3 to 4 months of age in the healthy eye and not until 3 to 4 months

corrected age for preterm infants (Table 10.1). Differentiation and maturation of the fovea and the retinal layers of the macula continue until 8 months of age.[2] The *fovea* is responsible for central vision, and the *macula* is responsible for seeing colors and contrasts, and normal development of both is required for precise visual acuity. The critical window for normal development of full visual acuity is from birth to 5 to 6 years of age, and the synaptic development of the neuronal pathways in the visual cortex continues until approximately 10 years of age. After 10 years of age, conditions of the eye that affect early visual development cannot be completely corrected (Table 10.2).

TABLE 10.1	VISUAL DEVELOPMENT
Age	Developmental Stage of Vision
Birth	Awareness of light and dark
Neonatal	Rudiments of fixation on near object
2 weeks	Intermittent fixation
4 weeks	Follows moving objects
6 weeks	Fixates and follows moving objects
8 weeks	Convergence beginning to stabilize
4 months	Inspects hands and small held objects; vision 20/300
6 months	Retrieves small objects; hand-eye coordination appears
9 months	Binocular vision clearly established, beginning of depth perception
12 months	Vision 20/180; looks at pictures with interest; fusion is established
18 months	Convergence established; visual localization peripherally poor
2 years	Accommodation well developed; vision 20/40 to 20/50 in normal eyes

TABLE 10.2	PHYSIOLOGIC VARIATIONS OF THE EYE
Age Group	Variations
Preterm infant	• 24 weeks: Partially fused eyelids • 24–28 weeks: Eyelids open spontaneously • 28–30 weeks: Eyes have membranous embryonic vascular network over iris to protect lens, producing dull retinal or red light reflex • 36–40 weeks: Membrane over iris normally resolves; persistent membrane may result in anterior cataracts
Newborn	• Macula not fully developed, eyes tend to drift in initial newborn period • Benign scleral hemorrhage often present after birth • Definite ability to follow object not developed until 4–6 weeks • Lacrimation present at 6 weeks of age
Infancy	• 3–4 months: Fully fixates and follows object • Sucking often stimulates infant to open eyes and focus attention on surroundings • 3–5 months: Color discrimination present • 6 months: Eye color generally established • Sclera may be visible above and below cornea • Intermittent convergent strabismus common until 4 months of age
Early childhood	• 2 years of age: Binocular vision and depth perception are developed in healthy eye • Visual acuity should be 20/40 to 20/50 • >3 years of age: Visual acuity should be 20/30 • Accommodation and convergence are smooth and well-established
Middle childhood	• Refractive error is common beginning at 9 years of age • Visual concerns about near vision in school-age child may be related to learning differences
Adolescence	• Hormonal changes during early and middle adolescence often cause change in visual acuity

ANATOMY AND PHYSIOLOGY

External Eye

The *bony orbit* is the structure surrounding the eye in the cranium. Only one-third of the optic *globe* in the infant and child is exposed, and the cranium protects the remainder of the optic *globe* in the orbital cavity. The *optic foramen* is the opening in the cranium that allows the passage of the optic nerve, ophthalmic artery, and ophthalmic vein to pass from the globe to the brain and visual cortex. The upper eyelid is shaped by connective tissue containing *tarsal plates*. The *meibomian glands* are located in the tarsal plates near the hair follicles of the eyelashes in the upper and lower lids. The *meibomian glands* are one of the oil-producing sebaceous glands in the body. In infants and children with atopic or allergic reactions, they can exude a whitish or yellowish sebaceous material onto the base of the eyelids.

The *lacrimal gland* is located in the lateral aspect of the frontal bone in the orbital cavity (Fig. 10.2). It is a peanut-sized gland similar to the salivary glands. In each eyelid, the *lacrimal duct* opens onto the eyelid margin, and the *nasolacrimal duct* opens into the *lacrimal sac*, which is buried in the frontal process of the maxillary bone. The *lacrimal puncta* are noted at the edge of the upper and lower eyelids at the *medial* or *inner canthus* and allow the drainage of tears into the *nasolacrimal duct* and the *lacrimal caruncle*. The *lacrimal caruncle* is the elevated area of tissue bordering the upper and lower medial canthus and assists in drainage of tears. Tear production is normally present by 6 weeks of age in the term infant. The eyelashes add further protection to the surface of the eye and assist in lubricating the exterior surface of the eye.

The *sclera*, the outermost layer of the exterior structure of the *globe*, is the firm collagenous layer that protects the intraocular structures (Fig. 10.1). The *conjunctiva* is a thin mucous membrane lining the anterior surface of the sclera and inner eyelids and acts along with the tear film as a protective covering for the cornea (Fig. 10.2). The conjunctiva has two surfaces: the palpebral and bulbar. The *palpebral conjunctiva* lines the inner eyelids, is vascular, and is covered by papillae. The *bulbar conjunctiva* is clear and contains no papillae and very few blood vessels. The *bulbar conjunctiva* covers the sclera up to the *limbus*, the juncture of the sclera and the cornea.

The *cornea*, the most anterior aspect of the external eye, is a lens-like structure that acts as a refractory surface for the eye and connects with the sclera at the limbus. The cornea is transparent and contains no blood vessels.

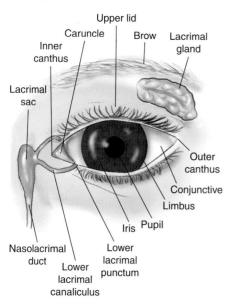

Upper lid
Caruncle   Brow   Lacrimal
Inner   gland
canthus
Lacrimal
sac
                              Outer
                              canthus
                           Conjunctive
                           Limbus
                    Iris Pupil
Nasolacrimal   Lower
duct   lacrimal
       Lower   punctum
       lacrimal
       canaliculus

FIGURE 10.2 External eye and lacrimal apparatus.

The transparency allows light to be focused on the retina. It derives oxygen from the aqueous humor and from tears. The *anterior chamber* is directly behind the cornea, and the *posterior chamber* is the thin area between the lens and the posterior iris. The anterior and posterior chambers contain *aqueous humor*, a clear nutrient fluid that circulates around the lens and the cornea and provides nutrition and oxygen. *Glaucoma* is increased intraocular pressure resulting from abnormalities in the ocular drainage of the aqueous humor, which damages the optic nerve. *Congenital glaucoma* may result from the abnormal development of the ocular drainage system at birth that causes clouding or enlargement of the cornea. It may be present at birth or develop during the first year of life and may result in blindness if undetected and untreated.

The *iris* is the pigmented structure containing the sphincter and dilator muscles, connective tissue, and pigmented epithelium. An absence of color in the iris may indicate *albinism*. The center of the iris is controlled by the *ciliary body* and *iris muscles* and forms the aperture, or pupil. The *pupil* constricts or dilates depending on the amount of light entering the eye. The ciliary body produces aqueous humor and controls accommodation. The iris lies behind the anterior chamber and in front of the *crystalline lens* and is protected by a thin clear capsule attached by small filaments to the ciliary body. A *cataract* is an opacity that occurs in the crystalline lens and obscures vision. The prevalence of *congenital cataract* is 2 per 10,000 births in the United States.[3]

The upper eyelid is elevated by the *levator muscle*, which inserts into the tarsal plate in the upper eyelid and is innervated by cranial nerve III.

Extraocular Muscles and Internal Eye

The six *ocular muscles*, inserted into the scleral surface, control the movement of the eye (Fig. 10.3). The four *rectus* muscles—the *superior, inferior, medial,* and *lateral recti*—originate at the top of the *globe* deep in the cranium

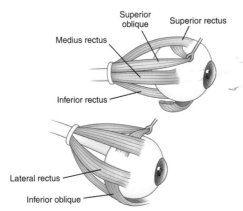

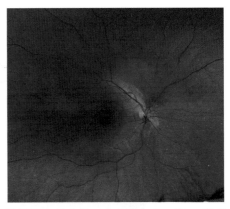

FIGURE 10.3 Four extraocular recti muscles and two oblique extraocular muscles. (From Newman NJ, ed. *Bradley and Daroff's Neurology in Clinical Practice.* 8th ed. Philadelphia, PA: Elsevier; 2022.)

FIGURE 10.4 Normal right fundus. (From Zitelli BJ, McIntire SC, Norwalk AJ, Garrison J. *Zitelli & Davis' Atlas of Pediatric Physical Diagnosis.* 8th ed. Philadelphia, PA: Elsevier; 2023.)

and extend from the anterior to the posterior *globe* and insert at the back of the *globe*. The medial rectus muscle is responsible for the movement of the eye toward the midline, and the lateral rectus muscle, which is innervated by cranial nerve VI, moves the eye away from the midline. The inferior and superior rectus muscles move the eye up and down and also have overlapping functions with the oblique muscles. The two *oblique* muscles—the *superior* and *inferior oblique*—insert at the anterior and posterior *globe*. The superior oblique tendon passes through the *trochlea*, the small, cartilaginous pulley on the frontal bone. The *superior oblique* muscles are responsible for movement of the eye downward and inward, and the *inferior oblique* moves the eye upward and inward. The *superior oblique* muscle is also innervated by cranial nerve IV, and paralysis of the cranial nerve IV causes a head tilt or torticollis in children to compensate for the weakened muscle.

The *vitreous body* is the large interior cavity of the *globe* and contains a clear gel or *vitreous humor*. The *choroid* is the interior layer of the eye between the sclera and the retina and is continuous with the iris and ciliary body. It is highly vascular and nourishes the receptor cells of the retinal epithelium. The rods and cones

in the retina are stimulated by light focused by the lens and translate light energy or impulses into neuronal activity. The neurons activate the nerve fiber layer of the retinal epithelium and synaptic activity and transmit through the optic nerve to the brain, which perceives the visual image.

The retinal vessels and optic nerve fibers enter and exit through the *optic cup* and divide into two branches on the surface of the *optic disc*. The *optic disc*, the anterior aspect of the optic nerve, is pink to orange-red or pale to dark with a yellow cup at its center (Fig. 10.4). There are no photoreceptors in the *optic disc*, which creates a blind spot of 5 degrees in the visual field.[2] The *macula* lies medial to the optic nerve on the *fundus*, the posterior surface of the retina. The *fovea* or *fovea centralis* is a central depression in the macula without vessels and has darker pigmentation than the retina. This is the area where vision is most perfect, and the ciliary body works to accommodate the lens to focus an image on the fovea.

The *arteries* on the fundus appear thinner and more orange-red or pale than the *veins*, which are larger and darker (see Fig. 10.4). The normal arterial-to-venous ratio (A:V) is approximately 2:3 in the healthy individual. Vascular changes that present in the retina may

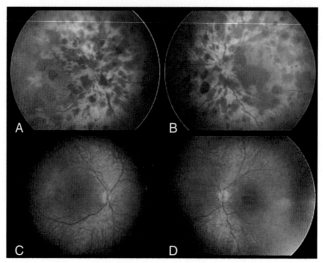

FIGURE 10.5 Extensive retinal hemorrhages in a shaken infant. (**A and B**) Retinal hemorrhages. (**C and D**) Normal right and left fundus. (From Wang L, Petrak M, Holz FG, Müller A, Krohne TU. Retinal hemorrhages in shaken baby syndrome. *J Pediatr.* 2019;207:256.)

reflect abnormal conditions in the systemic vasculature such as diabetes and hypertension. *Papilledema*, bilateral optic disc edema, is also associated with increased intracranial pressure. *Retinal hemorrhage* is associated with acute traumatic brain injury and inflicted traumatic brain injury in infants and children. *Retinal hemorrhages* associated with *inflicted traumatic brain injury* in children involve deeper layers of the retina and are found more on the periphery of the retina (Fig. 10.5).[5]

Variations in Eye Development

Thick epicanthal folds can be seen in some infants and young children, and they often partially or completely cover the inner canthus at birth and diminish by middle childhood. Retinal pigment or melanin is often found on the scleral surface of children with greater skin pigmentation. The pigmented area on the sclera usually becomes evident in early or middle childhood and persists into adulthood. This is within the range of normal variations of the eye and does not impact visual health. The *retinal light reflex* varies in color from red in individuals with less pigmentation to pale yellow in individuals with

Oculodermal melanocytosis

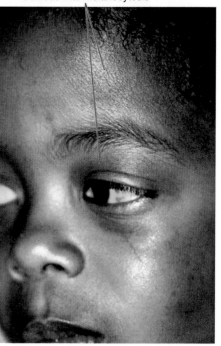

FIGURE 10.6 Scleral melanocytosis. (From Kaiser PK, Friedman NJ, Pineda R. *The Massachusetts Eye and Ear Infirmary Illustrated Manual of Ophthalmology.* 4th ed. London: Saunders; 2014.)

greater pigmentation. The *fundus* appears pale yellow or beige because of the increased melanin in the skin, and the optic disc is also often a pale yellow. *Scleral melanocytosis* is a pediatric condition that characteristically features black or gray-blue pigmentation in the scleral tissue and becomes more prominent with increasing age. It is a benign condition seen in individuals with greater skin pigmentation and it usually occurs bilaterally (Fig. 10.6).

SYSTEM-SPECIFIC HISTORY

Detecting vision problems early is critical to the healthy development of the visual system in infants and young children and critical to timely referral and intervention. Obtaining a complete history is key to early identification of visual problems or visual changes in infants, children, and adolescents. The Information Gathering table reviews the pertinent areas of

INFORMATION GATHERING FOR EYE ASSESSMENT AT KEY DEVELOPMENTAL STAGES

Age Group	Questions to Ask
Preterm infant	History of oxygen exposure in early neonatal period? History of retinopathy of prematurity? History of intraventricular insult? History of exposure to prenatal substance or alcohol abuse?
Newborn	Significant neonatal or exposure to prenatal infections? Does infant focus on face of caregiver when alert? Any eye discharge or swelling? Family history of congenital cataracts or glaucoma? History of exposure to prenatal substance or alcohol abuse?
Infancy	When did infant begin visually following caregiver? Does infant blink/react to bright light? Any *rapid* involuntary movement of eyes? Persistent discharge or tearing on one or both sides? Any caregiver concern about visual development? Significant jaundice in neonatal period? History of exposure to prenatal infection? Neonatal meningitis? History of abusive head trauma?
Early childhood	Does child sit close to TV or screen? Amount of screen time? Able to see birds/plane in sky? Any clumsiness/bumping into objects? Holds books or cell phone close to face? Abnormal head positioning? Appropriate response to visual cues? Frequent eye rubbing? History of frequent stye or *hordeolum*? Repeated blinking? Difficulty with color recognition? Family history of color vision deficit? History of abusive head trauma?
Middle childhood	Amount of screen time? History of visual problems? Headache? Family history of myopia (nearsighted), strabismus? Is the child squinting? Does child have corrective lenses or refuse to wear them? Date of most recent eye exam? Where is child seated in classroom? Any difficulty reading? Does child learn at grade level? Protective eyewear for sports? Eye pain or strain?
Adolescence	History of eye trauma? Screen time? Any difficulty with eyestrain with increased screen time or when studying? Headache? Wears corrective lenses or refuses to wear them? Contact lens wearer? History of corneal abrasion? Date of most recent eye exam? Protective eyewear for sports? History of concussion or head trauma? Driver's license? Restricted license due to limited vision?
Environmental risks	Exposure to eye irritants? Contact with chemical cleaning agents, hazardous chemicals, or tobacco/vaping smoke?

information gathering for each pediatric age group and developmental stage of childhood.

PHYSICAL ASSESSMENT

Equipment

The health care provider can use a traditional ophthalmoscope to perform all necessary screening of the internal eye structures in the pediatric population. The PanOptic ophthalmoscope, if available, provides a larger view of the internal eye structures (Fig. 10.7). A penlight may be used for screening the corneal light reflex and testing the pupillary reflex in a darkened environment. The Snellen E, Tumbling E, Lea symbols, Allen vision cards, photoscreening instruments, color vision, and near vision testing cards may be used in the clinical or school setting for vision acuity testing for the young child through young adulthood. An eye cover will assist in proper vision screening testing. Testing of cranial nerves is presented in Chapter 19.

Inspection of the External Eye

Begin the inspection of the eyes with a general inspection of the periorbital region, globe

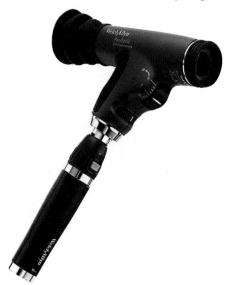

FIGURE 10.7 PanOptic ophthalmoscope. (Copyright Welch Allyn. Used with permission.)

position, and lid margins. Note any asymmetry in the eyelids or eyebrows and whether the eyelashes are normally distributed. Note the size and shape of the periorbital cavity. The *palpebral fissure* or opening of the eye can be on a horizontal plane between the medial and lateral canthus in infants or slant upward laterally. The upper eyelids should appear symmetrical. Inspect the *conjunctiva* for erythema or irritation, and the lid margins for erythema, crusting, lash distribution, and cysts or lesions. The eyelashes should be carefully examined for possible nits or lice. Observe for *entropion* (eyelashes curl inward) or *ectropion* (lower eyelid appears droopy and eyelashes curl under).

Conditions such as *ptosis*, an eyelid that droops or has an absent or faint lid crease unilaterally, are most often associated with the absence or reduced function of the palpebral superioris muscle (Fig. 10.8). It can be the result of a brachial plexus injury or third nerve palsy, or Horner syndrome, which produces a lighter colored iris on the affected side that requires imaging studies and referral.[6] Also, *ptosis* extending partially over the pupil and causing the child to tilt the head to see constitutes an impact on the visual field and requires prompt referral to a pediatric ophthalmologist. When closed, the upper eyelid should meet the lower eyelid and completely cover the cornea and sclera.

Inspection of the Upper Eyelid

Inspection of the inside of the upper eyelid may be necessary when a child or adolescent

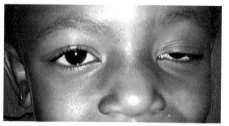

FIGURE 10.8 Congenital ptosis. (From SooHoo JR, Davies BW, Allard FD, Durairaj VD. Congenital ptosis. *Surv Ophthalmol.* 2014;59:483–492.)

presents with conjunctival irritation, infection, trauma, foreign body, or possible injury or abrasion of the cornea. To evert the upper eyelid for examination in the cooperative child or adolescent, give the child a toy and ask the child to look down at the object or have an adolescent look down at an object such as their cell phone. Grasp the upper eyelashes at the base and *gently* pull out and up while pushing in and down with a cotton applicator on the upper *tarsal plate* (Fig. 10.9). Gently remove the cotton applicator and hold the eyelid while inspecting the *adnexa*. The palpebral conjunctiva should have a pink and glossy appearance and the adnexa should be clear. To return the lid to a normal position, have the child look up as the lid is released. This procedure is well tolerated by middle childhood and in cooperative school-age children. In early childhood, administration of a topical anesthetic, such as proparacaine, may be necessary, or referral to an ophthalmologist or urgent care setting may be made if indicated to ensure a thorough assessment of the eye. Newborn infants will occasionally have an inverted eyelid, which is within the normal range of variations.

Assessment of Visual Fields and Visual Alignment

Sight is the most complex of the senses, and any insult to the eye along the visual pathway during development of the sensory organ can impact vision. The alignment and position of the *pupil* in the visual field and the clarity of the cornea is determined by the *corneal light reflex*, or *Hirschberg test*. It can be performed with a penlight or otoscope light without the speculum (Fig. 10.10). Focus the light source towards the bridge of the nose from about 12 inches from the infant or young child and note the reflection of the light from the cornea at the center of the pupil. The light should be symmetrical in the center of each pupil. Any asymmetry of the light reflex could indicate ocular misalignment and could impact visual development.

Next, evaluate the six extraocular muscles (EOMs) by having the child or adolescent hold their head still and follow a penlight or the examiner's finger through the six cardinal fields of gaze in the visual field (Fig. 10.11A). This testing evaluates the normal function of the oculomotor (cranial nerve III), trochlear (cranial nerve IV), and abducens (cranial nerve VI) nerves (see Fig. 10.11B–D). In infancy and early childhood, the examiner should focus the light approximately 12 inches from the eyes. A cooperative infant should normally be able to follow the light on horizontal and vertical planes by 6 months of age.

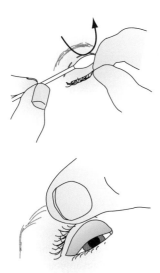

FIGURE 10.9 Examination of the upper eyelid.

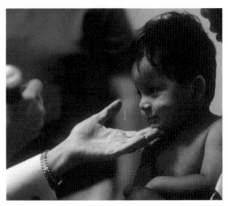

FIGURE 10.10 Testing corneal light reflex.

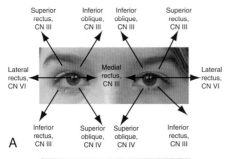

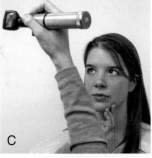

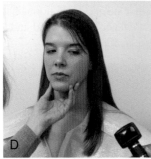

FIGURE 10.11 **(A)** Six cardinal fields of gaze with associated cranial nerves. **(B)** Testing lateral rectus, CN VI. **(C)** Testing superior rectus, CN III. **(D)** Testing superior oblique, CN IV. *CN,* Cranial nerve.

The *cover-uncover test* further evaluates ocular alignment and can be performed as early as 6 months of age in an alert infant. The young infant should be assessed on the examination table. The infant or toddler should be seated in the parent's lap. Begin by having the infant or child fixate on a penlight or light of the otoscope, the light of the large aperture on the ophthalmoscope, or a bright object. If the infant is alert but distracted, it is helpful to dim the lights and use a toy. Keep in mind infants will often reach for the toy but will often focus on a light. Use the nondominant hand or an occluder brought in laterally over the eye while the infant or child is fixating on the light or bright object. Observe the uncovered eye for fixation on the light or object. Remove the hand or occluder and note any deviations or movement of the covered or uncovered eye from the central gaze. Any deviation or movement of the eye from the central gaze or focus on refixation on the light by either the covered or uncovered eye may indicate abnormal alignment and should be further evaluated (Fig. 10.12).

Abnormalities in ocular alignment noted on examination may be congenital or acquired and may involve conditions affecting the muscles or nerves. An inward deviation of the eye is referred to as *esotropia* (Figs. 10.12B and 10.13A); an outward deviation is referred to as *exotropia* (Fig. 10.12C); an upward deviation is referred to as *hypertropia* (Fig. 10.12D). *Congenital esotropia* occurs in the first 6 months and *accommodative esotropia* occurs between 12 months and 7 years of age. If a *phoria* is present, the covered eye will deviate and refixate when the hand or occluder is removed. This indicates a focusing abnormality and should be referred. As visual acuity develops, the cover-uncover test should be performed with the child fixating on a distant object or wall poster and should continue to be part of the physical examination until 8 to 10 years of age.

To test for *visual accommodation* and *pupillary reaction*, shine a bright light momentarily into the eye. As the light approaches the iris, the pupil should begin to dilate. When bringing the light near the pupil from a distance, the pupils should constrict as the light nears.

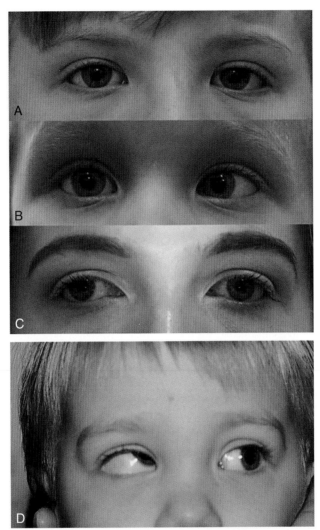

FIGURE 10.12 **(A)** Normal alignment. **(B)** Esotropia: inward movement of left eye. **(C)** Exotropia: outward movement of right eye. **(D)** Hypertropia: upward deviation of right eye. ([A–C] From: Bommireddy T, Taylor K, Clarke MP. Assessing strabismus in children. *Paediatr Child Health*. 2020;30:14–18. [D] From Zitelli BJ, McIntire SC, Norwalk AJ, Garrison, J. *Zitelli & Davis' Atlas of Pediatric Physical Diagnosis*. 8th ed. Philadelphia, PA: Elsevier; 2023.)

Conditions of Visual Alignment

The common causes of a loss of binocular vision during visual development include changes in the visual cortex due to unequal refraction in the eyes, cataracts, ptosis, congenital hemangioma of the eyelid, trauma, and untreated *strabismus. Strabismus* is nonalignment of the eyes causing the visual image to fall on the retina at a distance from the fovea. This disrupts binocular vision or visual fusion and keeps the eyes from working simultaneously. The resultant double vision and loss of depth perception from the blurred image impact normal binocular vision and visual development during the critical period of development in the first 5 to 6 years of life. Young children are often unaware

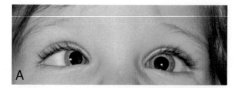

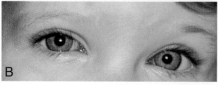

FIGURE 10.13 **(A)** Esotropia. **(B)** Shortly after corrective muscle surgery. (Note the transition of the corneal light reflex from asymmetric to symmetric.) (From Palay DA, Krachmer JH. *Primary Care Ophthalmology.* 2nd ed. St. Louis, MO: Mosby; 2005.)

of visual changes or deficits. If strabismus goes undiagnosed, amblyopia develops. A common finding in the young infant that prompts unnecessary referral to ophthalmology is *pseudoesotropia* or *pseudostrabismus*, a crossed appearance of the eyes caused by the large epicanthal folds covering the sclera (Fig. 10.14A). The corneal light reflex or Hirschberg test differentiates pseudostrabismus from strabismus,

and gentle pinching of the upper nasal bridge reduces the prominence of the epicanthal folds to allow for greater visualization (Fig. 10.14B).

Amblyopia is a monocular loss of vision during the critical period of visual development in the first 6 to 8 years of life. The visual development in one eye is suppressed due to insufficient visual stimulation and the better functioning eye becomes the dominant eye. The *cover-uncover test* and the *corneal light reflex* are both required in a complete ophthalmologic examination to detect strabismus and amblyopia.

Nystagmus is spontaneous, involuntary movement of one or both eyes and is an indication of poor visual acuity. In the preterm infant, *persistent* or *horizontal nystagmus* can indicate ROP, intracranial hemorrhage, or optic nerve tumor. In the term infant, *congenital nystagmus* can be associated with Down syndrome or trisomy 21, atrophy of the optic nerve, retinal dystrophy, congenital cataracts, abnormalities of the ocular muscles or nerves, vestibular disturbances, and decreased visual acuity. In the older child or adolescent, drug overdose or chemical toxicity is a possible cause. Slight horizontal nystagmus in the lateral fields of gaze is

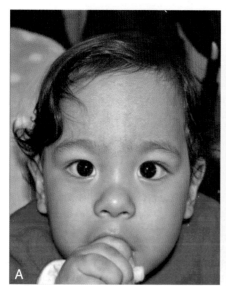

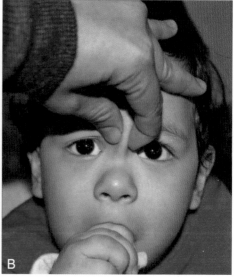

FIGURE 10.14 **(A)** Pseudostrabismus. **(B)** Examination technique for pseudostrabismus. (From Yanoff M, Duker JS. *Ophthalmology.* 6th ed. Philadelphia, PA: Elsevier Inc.; 2023.)

normal. Children with amblyopia may exhibit nystagmus because of loss of vision in the affected eye. If nystagmus is noted, a thorough neurologic examination is warranted, as well as an evaluation by a pediatric ophthalmologist.

Assessment of the Internal Eye

The *binocular retinal reflex* or *Bruckner test* assesses the *retinal light reflex* through the ophthalmoscope light reflecting simultaneously in both pupils from a distance of 18 to 30 inches. The *retinal light reflex* determines the clarity of the posterior chamber of the eye, the receptivity to light, and the sensitivity of the *retina* to visual stimulus. A symmetrical retinal light reflex should be observed in both eyes in the infant and child.[7] Any asymmetry of the light reflecting from the pupil or the presence of a white reflex indicating opacities is considered abnormal and requires referral to pediatric ophthalmology. Compare the pupil and iris in both eyes for color, size, shape, movement, and clarity. To inspect for *opacities*, dim the light and illuminate the cornea by shining the light of the ophthalmoscope obliquely approximately 15 degrees from the lateral canthus. An alert infant with normal visual development should blink at a bright light directed at the eye.

With the lights dim, use the ophthalmoscope on the "0" setting to view the fundus and the retinal light reflex. To elicit the retinal light reflex in only one eye, the examiner brings the ophthalmoscope to touch their eyebrow and positions it obliquely at a 15- to 25-degree angle lateral to the eye approximately 12 inches from the infant or child. Repeat the process from the other side of the child to examine the other eye. Inspect for symmetry and brightness, or brilliance, of the retinal light reflex. A lens that is congenitally dislocated or abruptly dislocated because of trauma appears as a darkened or asymmetrical retinal light reflex. Any asymmetry in size or color or darkness in the uniformity of the retinal light reflex indicates the need for immediate referral to an ophthalmologist (see Table 10.3).

PEDIATRIC PEARLS

To visualize the retinal light reflex in the newborn or in early infancy, hold the infant slightly upright from the exam table and, while cradling the head, gently rock the infant. As the head is lowered to the exam table, the eyes will usually open to examine the retinal light reflex.

Fundoscopic Examination

The full ophthalmoscopic exam permits the examiner to clearly visualize the internal structures of the eye in a child who is able to sit for examination and focus steadily on a distant point. This generally occurs by 5 to 6 years of age.

Using the lens selector disc, focus the ophthalmoscope on the palm at close distance before examining the child to determine the clarity of the image and accommodate for any visual deficit in the examiner. The lens indicator may read "0" or ± to produce the clearest image, depending on the visual acuity of the examiner. Resting the hand on the child or adolescent's forehead just above the eyebrow, begin with the ophthalmoscope positioned laterally approximately 2 inches from the eye to decrease *miosis*, constriction of the pupils (Fig. 10.15). The rubber pad on the face of the

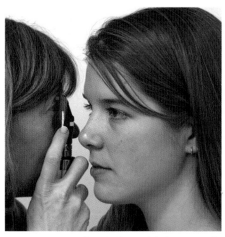

FIGURE 10.15 Positioning ophthalmoscope for exam.

TABLE 10.3   PEDIATRIC VISION SCREENING METHODS

Method	Indications for Referral	Newborn–6 mos	6–12 mos	1–3 yrs	3–4 yrs	4–5 yrs	Every 1–2 yrs after age 5 yrs
				Recommended Age			
Red reflex test	Absent, white, dull, opacified, or asymmetric	•	•	•	•	•	•
External inspection	Structural abnormality (e.g., ptosis)	•	•	•	•	•	•
Pupillary examination	Irregular shape, unequal size, poor or unequal reaction to light	•	•	•	•	•	•
Fix and follow	Failure to fix and follow	Cooperative infant ≥3 mos •	•	•			
Corneal light reflection	Asymmetric or displaced		•	•	•	•	•
Instrument-based screening*	Failure to meet screening criteria			•	•	•	•
Cover test	Refixation movement			•	•	•	•
Distance visual acuity† (monocular)	Worse than 20/50 either eye or 2 lines of differences between the eyes				•		
	Worse than 20/40 either eye					•	
	Worse than 3 of 5 optotypes on 20/30 line, or 2 lines of difference between the eyes						•

SOURCE: Hagan JF, Shaw JS, Duncan PM, eds. Bright Futures: Guidelines for Health Supervision of Infants, Children and Adolescents. 4th ed. Elk Grove Village, IL: American Academy of Pediatrics; 2017.

NOTE: These recommendations are based on panel consensus. If screening is inconclusive or unsatisfactory, the child should be retested within 6 months; if inconclusive on retesting or if retesting cannot be performed, referral for a comprehensive eye evaluation is indicated.[4]

*Subjective visual acuity testing is preferred to instrument-based screening in children who are able to participate reliably instrument-based screening is useful for some young children and those with developmental delays.

*Instrument-based screening is preferred over subjective testing for some young children.

†LEA Symbols[5] (Good-Lite Co., Elgin, IL), HOTV, and Sloan Letters[6] are preferred optotypes.

ophthalmoscope should be resting on the eyebrow of the examiner. Use a distant focal point to attract the child's attention and help them to fixate and look over the shoulder of the examiner. As the examiner moves medially toward the central field of vision, the vessels of the *fundus* should come into view. Once a vessel in the *retina* is in focus, follow along the vessel, where its "branches" will point toward the *optic nerve*. The *optic disc* should come into view in the medial aspect of the fundus. The macula is examined last to minimize miosis. Forcibly opening the eyes of a child results in a frustrated child and an incomplete examination. If examination is immediately necessary but cooperation is not achieved through verbal preparation or proper positioning of the child, then referral to a pediatric ophthalmologist is indicated.

Conditions of the Internal Eye

Any serious defect of the cornea, aqueous chamber, lens, and vitreous chamber can be detected in the infant and young child by assessing the quality of the retinal light reflex. *Leukocoria*, a whitish opacity of the pupil visible in dim light or in room light, is highly abnormal and appears as an absent retinal light reflex or a partially darkened reflex if the opacity does not cover the entire pupil (Fig. 10.16). This finding is usually *unilateral. Congenital cataracts* and *retinoblastoma* are associated with an absent or incomplete retinal light reflex and may have a presenting sign of leukocoria. A *coloboma* of the iris is an irregular or teardrop-shaped iris, which causes a deficit in the visual field and impacts visual acuity (Fig. 10.17). Most colobomas are diagnosed at birth and are associated with chromosomal syndromes. If caused by trauma, colobomas require immediate referral to a pediatric ophthalmologist.

Visual Acuity Testing

Visual acuity testing should begin with verbal children at 2 to 3 years of age, with the Allen vision cards or the LEA Symbol Distance Chart at 10 feet (Fig. 10.18A and Table 10.4).

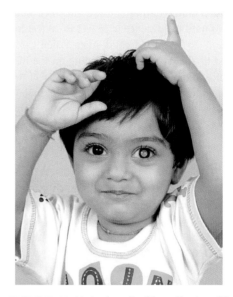

FIGURE 10.16 Leukocoria. (From Sheehan AP. Retinoblastoma: early diagnosis is crucial. *J Pediatr Health Care.* 2020;34:601–605.)

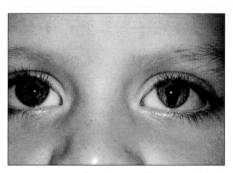

FIGURE 10.17 Coloboma of left iris. (From Femida K. Congenital and developmental abnormalities of the eye, orbit, and ocular adnexa. In: Albert DM, Miller JW, eds. *Albert & Jakobiec's Principles and Practice of Ophthalmology.* 3rd ed. Philadelphia, PA: Saunders; 2008.)

Children should be allowed to practice with a parent or caretaker to familiarize themselves with the figures. Testing should proceed starting from a near distance, testing each eye separately using an occlude held by the parent. The examiner should then show the LEA Symbols or Allen vision cards while walking backward and continue testing one eye and then both eyes until the distance is 15 feet to 20 feet for the 3- to 5-year-old child. Allen vision cards test to 20/30 or 15/30 depending on the distance from the child and the figure size of the cards. Teleophthalmology or the use of mobile applications to assess visual acuity are also convenient alternatives to vision cards and are being used in many clinical practice settings (Fig.10.18B).

Testing the eyes separately to detect a difference in refractive error is extremely important in children. Occluding the eye properly is the key to accurate testing of visual acuity. *Anisometropia*, a difference in refraction between the eyes, can lead to amblyopia. It is initially difficult to detect in the young child as the eye remains in alignment. Referral is indicated if accurate visual testing yields a greater

than 20 difference in refraction between the eyes (e.g., 20/30 in the left eye and 20/70 in the right eye) or a 20/40 refraction bilaterally.

The Snellen *Tumbling E test* is used in the prekindergarten age group and until the child knows the alphabet with accuracy. It is also used with children and adolescents with low literacy or learning differences. The examiner may ask the child which way the "legs of the table" are pointing. Using this directional approach may be difficult for children with learning disabilities, attention deficit, or behavioral conditions. The *Snellen E* distance acuity chart can be used when the child achieves literacy.

Children of school age may become *myopic* (nearsighted) as the eye matures. Variations in eye development occur as *myopia* or nearsightedness develops in children and adolescents. Myopia is a multifactorial eye condition with

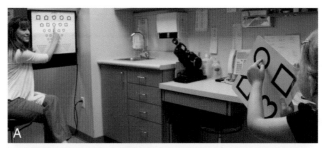

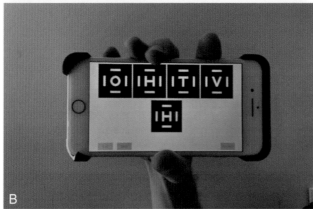

FIGURE 10.18 **(A)** Lea Chart vision screening. **(B)** HOTV visual acuity screening using a mobile application. ([A] From Lyons CJ, Lambert, SR. *Taylor and Hoyt's Pediatric Ophthalmology and Strabismus.* 6th ed. Philadelphia, PA: Elsevier Inc.; 2023. [B] From Silverstein E, Williams JS, Brown JR, Bylykbashi E, Stinnett SS. Teleophthalmology: evaluation of phone-based visual acuity in a pediatric population. *Am J Ophthalmol.* 2021;221:199–206.)

TABLE 10.4	VISUAL ALIGNMENT AND ACUITY TESTING	
Age Group	Examination at All Well Visits	Referral Criteria
Preterm infant	Retinal light reflex Penlight exam of cornea Evaluate for nystagmus	Preterm infants ≤30 weeks with birth weight of <1500 g and infants with birth weight between 1500 g and 2000 g or gestational age of >30 weeks with an unstable neonatal course
Newborn	Retinal light reflex Penlight exam of cornea Evaluate for nystagmus	Asymmetrical, absent, or white reflexes Cloudiness of cornea Presence of *rapid* involuntary ocular movement
Infancy	Retinal light reflex Penlight exam of cornea Evaluate for nystagmus Corneal light reflex Cover/uncover test Fixation to light/follow 90 degrees	Asymmetrical, absent, or white reflexes Cloudiness of cornea Presence of *rapid* involuntary ocular movement Any ocular misalignment or deviation of eye from central axis after 3–4 months of age
Early childhood	Retinal light reflex Corneal light reflex Cover/uncover test Visual acuity: Allen vision cards, Tumbling E, LEA symbols Funduscopic exam if indicated	Acuity of 20/50 to 20/40 in one or both eyes with accurate vision testing Difference of >20 between right and left eye Abnormal cover/uncover test
Middle childhood	Retinal light reflex Corneal light reflex Cover/uncover test Extraocular muscle testing Visual acuity: Tumbling E, Snellen E Funduscopic exam	Acuity of 20/40 in one or both eyes Difference of >20 between right and left eye Strabismus: Abnormal cover/uncover test Abnormal funduscopic exam
Adolescence	Visual acuity: Snellen E, Tumbling E for low literacy Extraocular muscle testing Fundoscopic exam	Visual acuity of 20/40 in one or both eyes Abnormal fundoscopic exam

both genetic and environmental influences.[8] East Asian and Southeast Asian populations have a higher prevalence of myopia, and studies examining risk factors have found that environmental influences such as near-work activity including screen time, and less outdoor time, rather than biologic differences, are significant factors driving the increased prevalence of myopia in children from these regions.[8,9] Uncorrected refractive errors from myopia contribute to poor school performance and are the leading cause of visual impairment nationally.[9] Twenty-five percent of children between the ages of 6 and 18 years in the United States would benefit from corrective lenses for refractive error yet many do not have lenses due to access to care or cost of lenses.

Instrument-Based Pediatric Vision Screening

Instrument-based pediatric vision screening uses optical images of the retinal light reflex to estimate refractive error and ocular misalignment, which put children at risk for developing amblyopia. Photoscreening instruments, which assess both eyes simultaneously, and autorefraction instruments, which screen one eye at a time, have been found to be accurate for vision screening in children 6 months to 3 years of age. The handheld infrared photorefractor instruments used in preschool and school-age children can screen for eye misalignment, unequal pupils, refractive errors, and any opacities. In a recent study, objective photoscreening instruments were found to be significantly more accurate than the LEA chart in identifying preschool children at risk for developing amblyopia.[10] Portable photoscreening and handheld autorefraction instruments may result in earlier detection of amblyopia if performed and interpreted by trained individuals. They are also useful for screening older children with developmental delay or who are unable to cooperate with routine acuity screening.[11] Recent evaluation of smartphone applications used as a photoscreening tool to detect amblyopia has demonstrated an overall sensitivity and specificity equivalent to some photoscreening instruments using manual grading of the application.[11] The use of vision charts and standard physical examination techniques to assess amblyopia in children 3 to 5 years of age remains standard practice in many clinical settings.

> ## EVIDENCE-BASED PRACTICE TIP
>
> Humans normally blink approximately 15 times a minute, but using computers and other digital screen devices, they blink half to a third that often. The American Academy of Ophthalmology recommends following the 20-20-20 rule—for every 20 minutes of screen time, users should shift their gaze to an item approximately 20 feet away for at least 20 seconds to reduce eye strain and eye dryness.[12]

Color Vision Testing

Children with difficulty or confusion when identifying colors, or a history of difficulty with color recognition, should be tested between 4 and 8 years of age for color sensitivity. Confusion with color sensitivity may be related to cognitive learning differences and should alert parents and teachers to the need for further evaluation by a learning specialist. Color sensitivity testing should be completed with the *Hardy-Rand-Rittler (HRR) test*. The HRR test uses a series of symbols rather than numbers, which allows reliable testing to be done on young children. The *Ishihara test*, which uses a series of figures and letters composed of spots of certain colors, can be used for older child. The child with a color vision deficit fails to see letters or figures of a certain color in the set of figures presented. The incidence of inherited red-green color vision deficits is 8% among males and 0.4% of females in the United States, and the incidence of inherited blue-yellow color vision deficits affect approximately 1 in 10,000 individuals and occur in equal frequency in males and females.[13] Gene therapy is currently being studied as a treatment option for color vision deficits.

EYE CONDITIONS

Table 10.5 presents the most common and chronic eye conditions seen in infants, children, and adolescents by the pediatric health care provider.

TABLE 10.5	EYE CONDITIONS

Condition	Description
Sundowning	Downward deviation of the eyes associated with hydrocephalus, intracranial hemorrhage, other pathologic brain conditions, or early sign of cerebral palsy; a sign of increased intracranial pressure when symptoms of lethargy, poor feeding, vomiting, bulging fontanel, or rapidly increasing head circumference are noted
Exophthalmos	Protrusion of the globe, also known as *exophthalmia* or *proptosis*, may be unilateral (e.g., orbital tumor, orbital cellulitis, or a retrobulbar hemorrhage) or bilateral (Graves' disease or *hyperthyroidism*)
Conjunctivitis	Acute inflammation of palpebral and bulbar conjunctiva; etiology includes viral, bacterial, corneal abrasion, allergy, or environment irritation
Blepharitis	An acute or chronic irritation of the eyelid; may be caused by allergic conditions such as seborrhea, bacterial infections (staphylococcal), inflammation of meibomian glands, or parasites
Chalazion	A cyst in the eyelid caused by inflammation of the meibomian gland; differs from a stye or hordeolum because it is usually painless. Also known as *meibomian gland lipogranuloma*
Stye or hordeolum	An infection of the sebaceous glands of Zeis at base of eyelashes; can be external or internal. Internal stye or hordeolum is an infection of the meibomian sebaceous glands lining the inside of the eyelid
Episcleritis	Inflammation of the episclera, layer beneath conjunctiva, causing acute irritation and redness of eyes. Episcleritis should be suspected in patients with IBD who present with acute redness of one or both eyes and complaints of irritation, itching, or burning.
Pterygium	Overgrowth of conjunctival tissue extending from the lateral canthus to cornea; begins in childhood with overexposure to sun and constant dust/environmental irritants
Scleral icterus	Yellowish coloration of sclera extending to the cornea; most often first indication of systemic jaundice and liver dysfunction in neonate; often first sign of liver disease in children and adolescents
Lacrimal duct obstruction	Abnormal tearing pattern; upward pressure on lacrimal sac often yields mucoid discharge; massage of nasolacrimal duct with downward pressure on lacrimal sac may open duct to normal drainage by 6 months of age
Dacryocystitis	Inflammation of nasolacrimal sac; swelling and redness occur around lacrimal sac in area of inner canthus
Retinoblastoma	Solid intraocular tumor; presents as abnormal retinal or retinal light reflex in newborn or as white pupillary reflex in infant; can be associated with proptosis, protruding eye bulb
Congenital glaucoma	Symptoms of photophobia (sensitivity to bright light), epiphora (excessive tearing), and blepharospasm (eyelid squeezing), conjunctival injection, causes ocular enlargement and visual impairment

TELEHEALTH TIPS

Telehealth has become important in maintaining continuity of care and ensuring access to routine vision testing for children and adolescents who live in remote areas or during school closures related to the global pandemic. Although telehealth visits are beneficial for some aspects of primary care, vision testing and screening generally requires face-to-face visits. As discussed earlier, smartphone applications have demonstrated equivalent accuracy to photoscreening instruments. However, any significant findings noted by the parent or caregiver require follow-up by the primary care provider in a clinical setting prior to referral to pediatric ophthalmology.

Telemedicine systems using wide-angle retinal images and clinical data may be used for preliminary ROP screening.[1] The use of digital photographic retinal images that are captured and sent for remote interpretation by a pediatric ophthalmologist is a developing alternative approach to direct ophthalmoscopic ROP screening in at-risk infants.

SUMMARY OF EYE EXAMINATION

- Begin by noting the symmetry of the eyes and the size and shape of the periorbital cavity.
- Perform the corneal light reflex to determine the clarity of the cornea, as well as the alignment and the position of the pupil in the visual field.

- Evaluate the extraocular muscles in the six cardinal fields of gaze.
- Perform the cover-uncover test for ocular alignment.
- Elicit the retinal light reflex.
- Check for pupillary accommodation.
- Perform age-appropriate visual acuity testing.
- Perform an ophthalmoscopic examination for children and adolescents.
- Telehealth visits provide limited scope for vision testing and requires complete eye examination prior to referral to pediatric ophthalmology.

CHARTING

3-Year-Old Child
Eye: Vision with Allen vision cards 20/40 bilaterally. Extraocular movements intact, sclera and conjunctiva clear, corneal reflex intact bilaterally, irides brown, pupils accommodate, symmetrical red or retinal light reflex (RLR).

CHARTING

Well Adolescent
Eye: Sclera and conjunctiva clear, extraocular movements normal (nl), irides brown, PER-RLA (*P*upils, *E*qual, *R*ound, *R*eact to *L*ight, and *A*ccommodate), fundoscopic examination—without opacities, optic disc visualized, pale yellow, disc margins clear (cl). Vessels nl, arteries/veins (A/V) ratio 2:3.

REFERENCES

1. Fierson WM. American Academy of Ophthalmology, American Association for Pediatric Ophthalmology and Strabismus, American Association of Certified Orthoptists. Screening examination of premature infants for retinopathy of prematurity. *Pediatrics*. 2018;142:e20183061.
2. Wright KW, Strube YJ. *Pediatric Ophthalmology*. 4th ed. American Academy of Pediatrics; 2019.
3. Stallings EB, Isenburg JL, Mai CT, et al. Population-based birth defects in the United States, 2011–2015: a focus on eye and ear defects. *Birth Defects Res*. 2018;110:1478–1486.
4. Karmouta R, Altendahl M, Romero T, et al. Association between social determinants of health and retinopathy of prematurity outcomes. *JAMA Ophthalmol*. 2022;140:496–502.
5. Choudhary AK, Servaes S, Slovis TL, et al. Consensus statement on abusive head trauma in infants and young children. *Pediatr Radiol*. 2018;48:1048–1065. https://doi.org/10.1007/s00247-018-4149-1.
6. Lee M.S., Brazis P.W., Wilterdink J.L. Overview of ptosis. UpToDate. Accessed December 20, 2022. https://www.uptodate.com/contents/overviewofptosis?-search=ptosis%20of%20eyelid%20in%20infant%20and%20etiology&source=search_result&selectedTitle=1~150&usage_type=default&display_rank=1#H7
7. American Academy of Ophthamology. *Pediatric Eye Evaluations Preferred Practice Pattern; Vision Screening in the Primary Care and Community Settings*. 2017. *Protective Sight Empowering Lives*.
8. Modjtahedi BS, Abbott RL, Fong DS, Lum F, Tan D, Task Force on Myopia. Reducing the global burden of myopia by delaying the onset of myopia and reducing myopic progression in children: The Academy's Task Force on Myopia. *Ophthalmology*. 2021;128:816–826. https://doi.org/10.1007/s00247-018-4149-1.
9. Killen OJ, Lee PP. Broadening access to eyeglasses in the US. *JAMA Health Forum*. 2022;3:e215236. https://doi.org/10.1001/jamahealthforum.2021.5236.
10. Vaughan J, Dale T, Herrera D. Comparison of photoscreening to chart methodology for vision screening. *J Sch Nurs*. 2022;38:310. https://doi.org/10.1177/1059840520940370.
11. Arnold RW, O'Neil JW, Cooper KL, Silbert DI, Donahue SP. Evaluation of a smartphone photoscreening app to detect refractive amblyopia risk factors in children aged 1–6 years. *Clin Ophthalmol*. 2018;12:1533–1537. https://doi.org/10.2147/OPTH.S171935.
12. American Academy of Ophthamology. Computers, Digital Devices and Eye Strain. 2020.
13. Carrol J., Conway B.R. Color Vision. In: Leff Ba, ed. *Handbook of Clinical Neurology; Neurology of Vison and Visual Disorders*. 2021.

CHAPTER 11

EARS

Adebola M. Olarewaju

The ear is a sensory organ that functions as part of a complex sensory system for hearing and vestibular equilibrium. Visual inspection of the ear is the first step in determining the normal function of this complex acoustic organ. The role of the pediatric health care provider is to maintain function of the ear to preserve hearing and balance in the child and adolescent, to detect any abnormalities early in infancy, and to refer to a specialist as needed. The goal of early detection is to promote optimum development of hearing and to support normal development of speech and language.

EMBRYOLOGIC DEVELOPMENT

External Ear

The external ear is a cartilaginous structure on the external surface of the temporal bone (Fig. 11.1). The structures of the ear evolve in the mesoderm, and development of the external ear begins during the sixth week of gestation when the six *hillocks of His* develop from the first and second branchial arches. The individual portions of the *auricle*, or flap of the ear, begin to fuse and assume the classic adult shape by the 12th week of gestation, and fusion is complete by the 20th week. The normal auricle should be no greater than 10 degrees off vertical plane or slope, and the superior portion should be in line with the outer canthus of the eye (Fig. 11.2). Minor malformations of the auricle may be normal variants, such as *preauricular skin tags*, a *preauricular sinus*, or *Darwin tubercle*, a benign slight thickening or nodule at the upper portion of the helix (Fig. 11.3).

Malformations can also be the result of intrauterine position, exposure to certain toxins or medications such as isotretinoin (Accutane) or anticonvulsants, intrauterine infection, or other intrauterine complications occurring during this early phase of fetal development. In the setting of additional congenital anomalies, minor malformations of the ear can be indicative of genetic syndromes. Some genetic syndromes such as Down syndrome, Treacher Collins syndrome, and Nager syndrome are associated with ear malformations, such as a small external ear (*microtia*), the total absence of the auricle with narrowing or absence of the external auditory opening (*anotia*), or malpositioned ears often in combination with internal ear abnormalities. Hearing loss also has viral causes (rubella, toxoplasmosis, cytomegalovirus [CMV]), and multiple genetic causes including Usher syndrome, Alport syndrome, and CHARGE syndrome (Coloboma, Heart defects, Atresia choanae [also known as choanal atresia], Growth retardation, and Ear abnormalities). Bilirubin toxicity in newborns is associated with high-frequency hearing loss.

Inner Ear

The inner and middle ear are located in the temporal bone of the skull. Although the external ear formation coincides with the gestational formation of the internal ear structures, they develop separately. The auditory placode and the acoustic facial ganglion are present the fourth week of gestation. Over the next month, the first of the three turns in the cochlea develops. Arrest in development during this phase

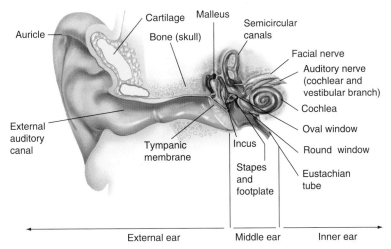

FIGURE 11.1 Anatomy of the middle and inner ear in skull.

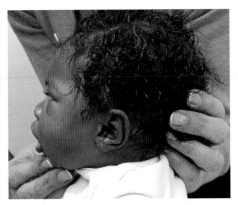

FIGURE 11.2 The normal alignment of the ear.

results in a common bony abnormality of the inner ear associated with congenital sensorineural hearing loss (SNHL) known as *Mondini dysplasia*. The final 2.5 turns of the cochlea occur by the 12th week of gestation. The *organ of Corti* develops from the epithelium of the cochlea and is responsible for transmission of sound impulses to the eighth cranial nerve, the *acoustic nerve*. Improper development of the membranous labyrinth of the organ of Corti results in a *Scheibe dysplasia*, which is the most common congenital abnormality of the cochlear duct, resulting in SNHL (see Hearing Loss). Alterations in development during this

period due to chromosomal abnormalities or other causes can lead to hearing loss of particular auditory tones. The semicircular canals first appear in the sixth week of gestation with differentiation of canal structures being complete by the 16th week. The sensory cells needed for equilibrium attain adult size by the 23rd week of gestation.

Middle Ear

Simultaneous with the early development of the inner ear is the formation of the first pharyngeal pouch, Meckel cartilage, in the oropharynx. The proximal portion of the pharyngeal pouch develops into the *eustachian tube*, and the distal portion becomes the tympanic cavity and supporting structures. The eustachian tube lies 10 degrees off the horizontal plane and the tympanic cavity separates the external ear from the inner ear. The development of the tympanic cavity with the three ossicles, the malleus, incus, and stapes, starts at the fourth week of gestation.[1] Development is not complete until the eighth month of gestation, but the malleus and incus reach adult size and shape by the 18th week of gestation and the stapes by the 20th week of gestation.[2] *Meckel cartilage* forms the *incus* and *malleus*

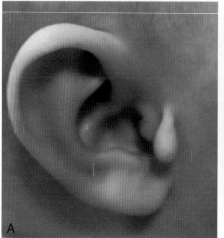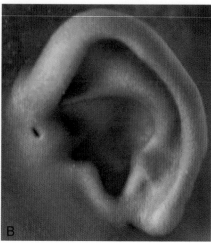

FIGURE 11.3 **(A)** Accessory tragus. (From Gupta, K, Sidbury, R. Cutaneous congenital defects. In Gleason, CA, Juul, SE, eds. *Avery's Diseases of the Newborn*. 10th ed. Philadelphia: Elsevier; 2018.) (B) Preauricular pit. (From Liaw J, et al. Congenital anomalies of the external ear. *Oper Tech Otolaryngol Head Neck Surg*. 2017; 28(2):72–76.)

of the middle ear, and the second pharyngeal pouch, the *Reichert cartilage*, forms the *stapes*. Failure of these structures or their supporting ligaments to form properly results in a conductive hearing loss[3] (see Hearing Loss). Any malformation, dysfunction, or damage of the middle ear structures can result in *conductive hearing loss* (CHL).

DEVELOPMENTAL VARIATIONS

Table 11.1 presents variations in the pediatric age group from the preterm infant to the school-age child.

ANATOMY AND PHYSIOLOGY

External Ear (Pinna)

The external ear, the *pinna*, is divided into sections: the outer portion is called the *helix*, just medial and parallel to the helix is the *antihelix*, and the *concha* is the cavity leading to the *external auditory meatus* or opening of the external canal (Fig. 11.4). A firm protuberance on the anterior portion of the ear just at the entrance to the auditory canal is the *tragus*, and across from the tragus on the border of the antihelix

is the *antitragus*. Beneath the tragus is the soft fold of skin that forms the ear lobe or *lobule*. Although the shape of the auricle varies slightly from person to person, the ears should be comparable bilaterally in size, shape, position, and appearance. Infants with malformed external ear structures require close monitoring.

The external auditory canal is an S-shaped canal that connects the outer ear to the middle ear and funnels sound waves to the tympanic membrane. The auricular muscles are innervated by the seventh cranial nerve, or *facial nerve*. The medial portion of the canal is innervated by the fifth cranial nerve, or *trigeminal nerve*, and the posterior canal is innervated by the 10th cranial nerve, or *vagus nerve*. The distal third of the ear canal contains hair follicles, ceruminous glands, and sebaceous glands. The *cilia* (specialized hair) are extremely sensitive to tactile stimulation and assist in sensing sound. The *ceruminous* gland, a modified apocrine sweat gland, secretes a milky substance that forms cerumen when exposed to the secretions of the sebaceous glands and air. *Cerumen* lubricates the skin of the canal, acts as a barrier to foreign objects entering the interior canal, and has protective antibacterial properties

TABLE 11.1	DEVELOPMENTAL VARIATIONS OF THE EAR
Age Group	**Physiologic Variations**
Preterm	Vulnerable to hearing loss, particularly before 33 weeks, from noise exposure, hypoxia, ototoxic drugs, hyperbilirubinemia, persistent pulmonary hypertension
Newborn	At birth, tympanic membrane is almost adult size but lies in a more horizontal plane compared to the adult ear, which alters visual assessment Intrauterine positioning may result in disfiguring of the pinna, which will usually resolve after birth with proper positioning because of the elastic quality of the ear cartilage Whitish material including vernix caseosa may be present in external auditory canal Canal is narrow and curved making assessment of the middle ear difficult Determining patency of canal is critical
Infancy	Fluid easily trapped in the middle ear due to eustachian tube dysfunction, particularly common in infants with Down syndrome, preterm infants, and any infant with craniofacial abnormalities
Early childhood	External auditory canal ossifies by 2 years of age, straightening the canal and improving visualization of tympanic membrane The pinna is approximately 80% of the adult size in the 4- to 5-year-old
Middle childhood	In a 9-year-old, the pinna and external auditory canal have attained adult size The canal measures 2.5 cm and has become somewhat S shaped

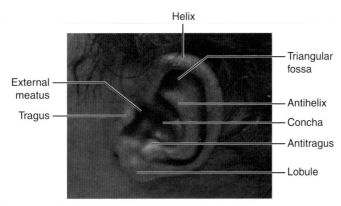

FIGURE 11.4 Anatomy of the external ear of small child labeled with anatomy.

to reduce the incidence of skin infection in the external canal. Mucociliary clearance occurs as the natural lateral movement of skin and hair cells in the external canal facilitates drainage of cerumen and other debris from the external ear canal.

Middle Ear

The mastoid cavity is part of the temporal bone and opens up into the middle ear. The middle and inner ear are located deep in the temporal bone. The middle ear consists of the ossicles, round window, oval window, eustachian tube, and tympanic membrane. The tympanic membrane is a thin, oval-shaped layer of skin attached to the wall of the external canal and is approximately 0.1 mm thick and 10 mm in diameter (Fig. 11.5).[4,5] It is concave, being pulled in by its attachment to the malleus, and sits at an oblique angle in the external canal. It is surrounded by a fibrous band called the *annulus*, which becomes sclerotic later in life,

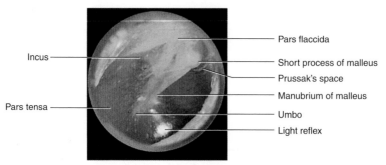

FIGURE 11.5 Normal left tympanic membrane. (From Ball JW, et al. *Seidel's Guide to Physical Examination: An Interprofessional Approach.* 10th ed. St. Louis: Elsevier; 2023.)

diminishing movement of the tympanic membrane and often resulting in conductive hearing loss. The tympanic membrane is attached to the malleus along the manubrium, conducting sound waves to the incus, stapes, and oval window of the inner ear. The tympanic membrane has a resonance frequency of 800 to 1600 Hz, approximating the normal speech frequency of 500 to 2000 Hz found in humans.

The tympanic membrane is divided into sections: (1) the *pars flaccida* is superior to the lateral process of the malleus, (2) the *pars tensa* comprises the majority of the tympanic membrane inferior to the lateral process of the malleus, and (3) the *Prussak space*, which lies medial to the pars flaccida in the anterior superior quadrant of the tympanic membrane (Fig. 11.5).[6] The *Prussak space* is the most common location of retraction pockets and congenital or acquired *cholesteatoma* (Fig. 11.6), an initially asymptomatic white mass (sometimes described as a pearl) in the middle ear that is thought to arise from repeated infections or pulling inward of the eardrum due to eustachian tube dysfunction. Histologically, it is the build-up of squamous keratinizing cells.[4] Over time, this keratin mass can increase in size and impair or destroy the ossicular chain of the middle ear and nearby structures, leading to CHL.[2,4,7] Although rare, a cholesteatoma in the external auditory canal should be considered in a child with complaints of otalgia and otorrhea but no middle ear disease.[7] Tympanosclerosis, thickening and scarring of

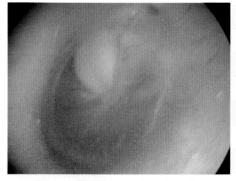

FIGURE 11.6 Cholesteatoma. (Reproduced from Nevoux J, Lenoir M, Roger G, Denoyelle F, Ducou Le Pointe H, Garabédian EN. Childhood cholesteatoma. Eur Ann Otorhinolaryngol Head Neck Dis. 2010 Sep;127(4):143–150. doi: 10.1016/j.anorl.2010.07.001. Epub 2010 Aug 11. PMID: 20860924. published by Elsevier Masson SAS. All rights reserved.

the tympanic membrane, is commonly seen after chronic infections of the middle ear or traumatic injury or surgery to the tympanic membrane (Fig. 11.7). Scarring can cause CHL due fixation of the ossicles. *Myringosclerosis*, scarring isolated to the tympanic membrane, is a result of previous inflammation and can be asymptomatic acoustically.

The three *ossicles* of the inner ear, the smallest bones in the body, transmit the movement of the tympanic membrane to the oval window and subsequently to the vestibular and cochlear branches of the eighth cranial nerve, the *acoustic nerve* (Fig. 11.8). The head of the *malleus* articulates with the body of the *incus* at the incudomalleolar joint. The long crus, or leglike structure of the incus, articulates with the head of the *stapes* at the incudostapedial joint. These joint areas are the most vascular regions of the *ossicles* and, therefore, are the most susceptible to trauma or infection and can lead to CHL.[1] The footplate of the stapes sits upon the oval window of the inner

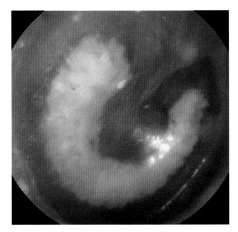

FIGURE 11.7 Endoscopic view of typical appearing tympanosclerosis in a right ear. (From Barry JY, et al. Tympanosclerosis presenting as mass: Workup and differential. *Case Rep Otolaryngol.* 2016; 2016:9821493.)

ear at the fibrous stapediovestibular joint. With typical development of the stapes, the mechanical function of the three ossicles and transmission of sound waves from the larger surface area of the tympanic membrane to the smaller surface area of the oval window produce a net increase of 22 times the radiation of sound energy. A defect in the stapes position can result in abnormal hearing.

The eustachian tube opens into the oropharynx just behind the nasal cavity and is the drainage and ventilatory structure for the middle ear. The motor division of the fifth cranial nerve, or trigeminal nerve, innervates the musculature that controls the function of the eustachian tube. The middle ear is a pressurized air-filled space and has the same air pressure as the outside air when patent. Equalization of pressure in the middle ear is critical for normal sound wave vibration of the tympanic membrane. Swallowing, yawning, and sneezing all open the eustachian tube and restore and equalize the pressure between the middle ear and outside air. Changes in altitude or ambient pressure as during airplane travel can cause decreased air pressure in the middle ear. This results in pain

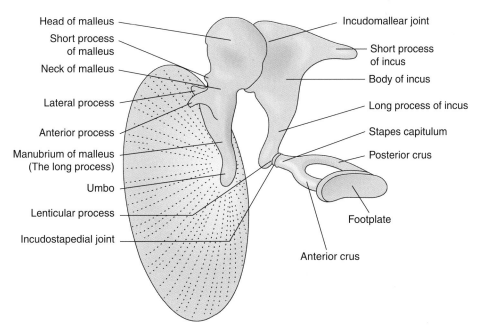

FIGURE 11.8 Anatomy of the inner ear.

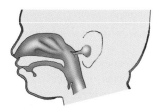

Infant–horizontal position
of eustachian tube

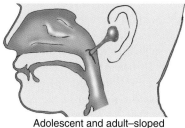

Adolescent and adult–sloped
position of eustachian tube

FIGURE 11.9 Position of eustachian tube in infant and in adult.

or discomfort if the eustachian is swollen or blocked. Repeated swallowing can often open the eustachian tube, equalizing pressure and reducing the associated pain. Encouraging an infant to suck on the bottle or breast can, therefore, reduce this discomfort in flight.

In infancy, the eustachian tube averages half the length of the adult and lies in a more horizontal plane. This allows bacteria and viruses to migrate more easily from the oropharynx to the middle ear (Fig. 11.9). In infants and children with cleft palate or other craniofacial anomalies such as Down syndrome, structural or functional abnormalities of the eustachian tube interfere with normal ventilation and clearance of the middle ear, increasing the risk for otitis media (OM). Muscle maturation, elongation of the eustachian tube, and a more vertical position all contribute to the decreased incidence of OM and middle ear effusions in middle childhood, adolescence, and young adulthood.

Inner Ear

The inner ear is the sensory end organ and is directly responsible for hearing and balance. The inner ear contains the *vestibule, semicircular canals*, and *cochlea* (Fig. 11.1). Fluid in the inner ear facilitates the transmission of sound

waves to the auditory nerve and sensations of balance in the *semicircular canals*. The sound waves pass over approximately 30,000 innervated hair cells in the cochlea, which are the primary receptors, transducers, and conveyers of sound energy to the brain.

HEARING LOSS

There are more than 400 known causes of genetic hearing loss.[8] Autosomal recessive nonsyndromic SNHL accounts for approximately 70% to 80% of all genetic forms of hearing loss in children. The most common form of recessive hearing loss is due to one gene, connexin 26 (CX26). Autosomal dominant nonsyndromic SNHL accounts for 10% to 15% of genetic hearing loss.[1] Approximately 15% of congenital hearing loss occurs with other clinical findings as a result of genetic syndromes, such as Usher syndrome, Pendred syndrome, Branchio-Oto-Renal syndrome, Stickler syndrome, Waardenburg syndrome, or Jervell and Lange-Nielsen syndrome.[8] Infants identified with nonsyndromic hearing loss (hearing loss without additional clinical findings) may be missed and are harder to diagnose.

Many genetically determined causes of hearing loss do not present at birth and may not be identified through newborn screening. Radiographic imaging such as a computed tomography (CT) scan or magnetic resonance imaging (MRI) can identify up to 40% of middle and inner ear abnormalities, but imaging is used infrequently for infants and young children due to the concern for long-term risks of exposure to radiation and anesthesia in the developing brain. Genetic testing is now often the first investigative tool to identify the cause of hearing loss.[3]

Acquired causes of hearing loss are numerous, and risk factors must be identified (Box 11.1). Prenatal risk factors include maternal metabolic disorders (diabetes and renal or liver failure) congenital infections (CMV, rubella, toxoplasmosis, herpes, syphilis, varicella), and fetal exposure to teratogens (alcohol, methyl mercury, thalidomide, cocaine).[9] Prematurity, birth hypoxia, hyperbilirubinemia, sepsis, and administration of ototoxic medications (aminoglycosides, loop diuretics, quinine) are risk factors for acquired hearing loss in the perinatal period. Otoxicity causes the destruction of the cochlear hair cells. Postnatal risk factors include being underimmunized or unimmunized and exposure to secondhand smoke.

Head trauma, infections (mumps, measles, varicella, meningitis, Lyme disease), recurrent OM, and excessive noise exposure are risk factors for hearing loss at any developmental stage.[3] Children and adolescents should be screened for exposure to loud sounds in their home, school, or recreational environments. Children living in industrial areas with heavy traffic or near loud machinery are at risk for a hearing loss in the decibel range associated with the environmental exposure.[3]

SYSTEM-SPECIFIC HISTORY

The Information Gathering table presents the important information to be gathered for each age group and developmental stage. Table 11.2 presents the important information for a symptom-focused history for children or adolescents presenting with ear symptoms.

BOX 11.1   RISK FACTORS FOR HEARING LOSS IN INFANTS AND CHILDREN

- Congenital syndromes (Alport, Jervell, Lange-Nielsen, Usher, Down, Treacher Collins)
- Congenital infections: cytomegalovirus, rubella, toxoplasmosis, herpes, syphilis, and varicella
- Premature birth
- Very low birth weight (VLBW)
- Persistent pulmonary hypertension of the newborn
- History of extracorporeal membrane oxygenation (ECMO) therapy
- History of meningitis
- Exposure to ototoxic drugs (aminoglycosides, platinum-containing chemotherapy) and cranial radiation
- Cholesteatoma
- Chronic or recurrent acute otitis media (AOM) and otitis media with effusion (OME)
- Osteogenesis imperfecta
- Trauma, intentional, and nonintentional child maltreatment

INFORMATION GATHERING FOR EAR ASSESSMENT AT KEY DEVELOPMENTAL STAGES

Age Group	Information to Gather
Preterm infant	History of prenatal infection? Exposure to prenatal drug use or diabetes? Perinatal antibiotic treatment with aminoglycosides, other ototoxic antibiotic use, or salicylates? Is there a family history of hearing deficit or loss, congenital or acquired?
Newborn	Newborn hearing screening results? ABO incompatibility? Elevated bilirubin level >20 mg/100 dL of serum? Premature infant? History of anoxia, pulmonary hypertension, ECMO therapy, or meningitis? Any craniofacial abnormalities noted? Family history of hearing deficit, congenital or acquired?
Infancy	Does infant react to sound with startle response or change in activity? Turn head or body toward sound or when name is called? Does the infant make cooing or babbling noises? Is the infant breastfed? Up to date on immunizations? Does the infant drink with the bottle propped while in bed? Does infant have frequent colds? History of recurrent ear infections or ruptured tympanic membrane? Ear drainage? Parental concerns regarding infant hearing or verbalizing? Are there any concerns regarding the child's motor development?

Continued

Information Gathering for Ear Assessment at Key Developmental Stages—cont'd

Age Group	Information to Gather
Early childhood	Do you have any concerns about child's ability to hear or speak?
	How many words does child use? Does child combine words into meaningful sentences? Does the child stutter while trying to speak?
	How clear is child's pronunciation?
	How many languages are spoken at home or by care providers?
	Does child play with his/her ears? Has he/she ever put small objects in his ears or nose?
	Has child ever had a hearing test done? Were the results normal?
	History of ear infection, ear pain, or ear drainage? Was it treated with antibiotics?
	Does child have frequent colds or respiratory allergies? Does the child attend daycare?
	If in daycare or preschool, do care providers have any concerns about child's hearing, speech, or balance?
	Is the child up to date with all recommended immunizations?
	Has the child had any serious infections, head trauma, or concussion?
	Does the child use headphones or ear buds for activities and how is the volume monitored?
	Is the child exposed to loud environmental noises at home, school, in the community?
	Is the child walking, running, climbing as well as his/her peers? Does the child fall or appear clumsy more than other children?
Middle childhood	Does child have frequent colds or respiratory allergies? Has child had any drainage from ears? Frequent ear pain?
	Do you or child's teachers have any concerns about child's hearing, speech, gross motor, reasoning, or learning ability?
	Does child have difficulty following directions in school?
	Has child been exposed to repetitive environmental loud noises? Does child use headphones or ear buds to listen to music, play video games? Is the volume loud?
	Has child ever complained of ringing in ears, dizziness?
	Does child spend a lot of time in the water, play water sports?
	Is there a history of concussion, injury/trauma to head, ears, or mouth? What type of sports does the child play and what safety precautions are used? Is the child exposed to firearm sounds? Wear protective earplugs?
	Is the child clumsy, have poor coordination or balance, fall frequently, or complain of dizziness?
	History of meningitis?
	History of cancer therapy?
Adolescence	History of frequent colds, nasal allergies, or ear infections or ear pain?
	Does adolescent use headphones/earbuds to listen to music? Is the volume audible to others? Has adolescent had frequent exposure to unusually loud music or noises?
	Has adolescent ever complained of ringing in ears, dizziness?
	Does adolescent spend a lot of time in the water, playing water sports?
	Any recreational activities potentially affecting ear (e.g., swimming, scuba diving, flying, boxing, hunting) or work activities (construction work, machinery use)?
	Has the adolescent complained of clumsiness, poor coordination, dizziness, poor balance, or frequent falls?

INFORMATION GATHERING FOR EAR ASSESSMENT AT KEY DEVELOPMENTAL STAGES—CONT'D

Age Group	Information to Gather
Environmental risks	Crowded living conditions?
	Exposure to secondhand smoke?
	Exposure to loud noises?

ECMO, Extracorporeal membrane oxygenation.

TABLE 11.2	SYMPTOM-FOCUSED HISTORY FOR EAR ASSESSMENT
Symptom	**Questions to Ask**
Ear pain	Onset, duration, and intensity of pain? Location? Unilateral or bilateral?
	Associated symptoms (e.g., fever, rhinorrhea, cough, drainage from eyes, ear drainage, hearing loss, vertigo, ringing in ears, swelling or redness around ear, mouth sores, dental pain, sore throat, difficulty sucking or swallowing, vomiting, neck swelling, tenderness)?
	Concurrent illness (e.g., upper respiratory infection, mouth infection, skin infection, conjunctivitis)?
	Home management of pain (e.g., medications/home remedies/complementary and alternative therapies): type, how much, how often, how effective?
	Changes in activities of daily living (e.g., loss of sleep, change in appetite, ability to attend daycare, school, or work)? Changes in activity level, balance, dizziness/vertigo, talking, or movement of temporomandibular joint? Change in interaction with others (e.g., playful, withdrawn, irritable)?
	What makes the pain feel better, worse?
	Others at home, daycare, school, or work with similar symptoms?
	What do you think might be the cause of the pain?
	In infancy: is infant pulling at ear, showing increased irritability, feeding poorly, or waking more frequently at night?
Ear drainage	Onset, duration, color, and intensity of discharge?
	Associated symptoms (e.g., fever, rhinorrhea, cough, ear pain, hearing loss, vertigo, ringing in ears, swelling or redness around ear, vomiting)?
	Concurrent illness (e.g., upper respiratory infection, mouth infection, skin infection, conjunctivitis)?
	Changes in activities of daily living (e.g., loss of sleep, change in appetite, ability to attend daycare, school, or work)? Changes in activity level, balance, dizziness/vertigo, interaction with others (e.g., playful, withdrawn)?
	Home management of drainage (e.g., medications/home remedies/complementary and alternative therapies): type, how much, how often, how effective?
	Injury caused by pressure or trauma (e.g., laceration or barotrauma)? Any foreign body in ear canal?
	Others at home, daycare, school, or work with similar symptoms?
	How do you care for/clean your child's ears?
	What do you think might be the cause of the ear drainage?

Continued

TABLE 11.2   SYMPTOM-FOCUSED HISTORY FOR EAR ASSESSMENT—CONT'D

Symptom	Questions to Ask
Hearing difficulty relevant in school-age child and adolescent	Gradual or sudden onset? Progressive? Bilateral or unilateral? Associated with other symptoms (e.g., ear pain, sense of fullness, drainage, balance problems or dizziness, systemic symptoms of illness)? Concurrent illness (e.g., otitis media, otitis media with effusion, respiratory allergies, developmental delay)? Trauma or exposure to loud noises? Changes in activities of daily living (e.g., difficulty hearing in school, at home, watching television, talking on phone. Difficulty walking)? Home management of hearing difficulty (e.g., sitting closer to television or in front of classroom, increasing visual cues for communicating)? What conditions make hearing better or worse? What do you think might be the cause of the hearing difficulty?
Dizziness or vertigo relevant in school-age child and adolescent	Gradual or sudden onset? When does it occur? With activity? Position change? Associated with other symptoms (e.g., nausea, vomiting, tinnitus, ear pain, ear drainage, hearing loss, systemic symptoms of illness)? Concurrent illness (e.g., viral illness, gastroenteritis, respiratory allergies/illness)? Use of medications or recreational drugs? Changes in activities of daily living (e.g., ability to attend school and work)? Any sports activities? Home management of dizziness? Others in home with similar symptoms? What makes dizziness better or worse? What do you think might be the cause of the dizziness?

PHYSICAL ASSESSMENT

Equipment

Equipment for examining the ear includes an otoscope with halogen light and speculum, pneumatic bulb attachment, and gloves for proper infection control practices. MacroView otoscopes (Fig. 11.10B) offer improved images of the ear canal and tympanic membrane, and computer-aided and cell phone software is also available for advanced viewing and education in the clinical setting.

Positioning

Proper positioning of the infant and young child will ensure the least discomfort during the examination, prevent injury to the canal or tympanic membrane during examination, and ensure the health care provider has sufficient opportunity to visualize the canal and tympanic membrane. Letting the young child become familiar with the otoscope by touching the light of the otoscope on the finger or hand often decreases the anxiety of the ear exam (Fig. 11.11A). Demonstration on the accompanying caregiver can also be comforting for the young child. The young infant is best positioned lying on the examination table with head securely held by the examiner and the arms restrained by a comforting parent. Older infants who are able to sit securely and young children are best positioned in the parent's lap with the arm and head secured by the parent or examiner (Fig. 11.11B). Distraction may work for some older infants and young children while examining the ears. The curve of the pediatric ear canal can be lessened by pulling the auricle inferiorly and posteriorly (down and back) in the infant and young child, as compared with superiorly and posteriorly (up and back) in

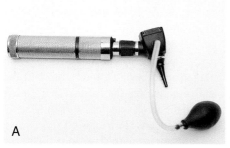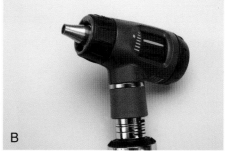

FIGURE 11.10 **(A)** Insufflator or pneumatic attachment to otoscope. **(B)** Advanced MacroView otoscope. (From Wilson S, Giddens J. *Health Assessment for Nursing Practice*. 5th ed. St. Louis: Mosby; 2013.)

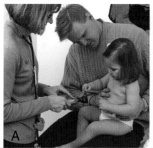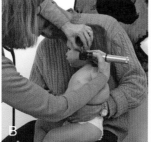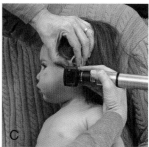

FIGURE 11.11 **(A)** Preparing the young child for the ear exam. **(B)** Positioning of the toddler for ear exam. **(C)** Positioning of tragus forward with hand above the ear.

middle childhood and adolescence. Be sure not to hold the auricle too firmly because this can cause pain when attempting to straighten the ear canal. Another examination technique that is very useful in the pediatric patient is for the examiner to position the hand above the ear, supporting the ear with the forefingers, and pulling the tragus forward or anteriorly with the thumb or forefinger (Fig. 11.11C). This position effectively opens the external canal in young children to improve visualization of the tympanic membrane and causes less discomfort. The handle of the otoscope can be held horizontally or vertically, with the examiner's hand resting on the child's head (Fig. 11.12). This provides a stable platform and prevents movement of the otoscope during the examination. If the child moves unexpectedly, your hand and otoscope will move with the child in order to prevent ear canal trauma.

PEDIATRIC PEARLS

The technique of pulling the tragus forward straightens the auditory canal for ease in examination and causes less discomfort than pulling on the pinna in young children.

If the child is complaining of ear pain in one ear, examine that ear last.

Do not attempt to examine the tympanic membrane unless the child can be securely positioned and held still for the examination.

External Ear

Inspection

Before examining the ear, inspect the head, face, and neck for any asymmetry or indication of craniofacial abnormality, defect, or infection. The superior portion of the auricle should be equal in height to the outer canthus of the

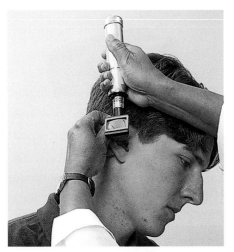

FIGURE 11.12 Holding the otoscope handle in the upright position. (From Wilson S, Giddens J. *Health Assessment for Nursing Practice*. 3rd ed. St. Louis: Mosby; 2005.)

eye and vertical with no more than a 10-degree tilt (Fig. 11.2). An ear that is set lower than an imaginary horizontal line drawn from the outer canthus of the eye or tilted greater than 10 degrees may indicate chromosomal abnormality or congenital abnormalities in other body systems or structures.

Inspect the auricles for size, shape, deformity, placement, discharge, and color. The size and shape of the ears should be similarly symmetrical and may have familial characteristics. In the newborn, the cartilage should have instant recoil but in the premature infant the cartilage may appear flattened and have less prominent incurving of the helix or concha. Grossly misshapen external ears are often associated with anomalies of the middle and inner ear structures and with SNHL. There should be no discharge from the external ear canal, although cerumen may be evident near the opening to the canal. Serous or purulent drainage may indicate a ruptured tympanic membrane, the presence of patent myringotomy tubes, inflammatory response to a foreign object in the ear, or a cholesteatoma. A white cheesy drainage may indicate an infection in the external auditory canal. The color of the auricle should be similar to the facial skin. Redness or swelling of the auricle may indicate inflammation or trauma, and bruising is of particular concern as an indication of possible head injury or nonaccidental trauma. Redness and swelling over the mastoid bone, located behind the auricle, can indicate a more serious infection such as mastoiditis.

The common normal variations of the auricle include *auricular* or *preauricular sinus, preauricular skin tags*, and *Darwin tubercle* (see Fig. 11.3). Occasionally, an infection can occur in the preauricular sinus, resulting in inflammation, redness, or discharge from the sinus. Ear piercings should be examined for signs of infection, excessive scar tissue, or trauma.

Palpation

Palpate the auricle for any masses or areas of tenderness. Scar tissue may be palpable around ear piercings but is generally nontender. Sebaceous cysts may occur around the auricle or in the external canal and are often mildly inflamed and tender. If movement of the auricle results in pain, the examiner should suspect *otitis externa*, or other inflammation of the auditory canal. A foul-smelling cheesy discharge is commonly found with otitis externa and often is caused by the bacterium *Pseudomonas*. The mastoid process, posterior to the auricle, should be palpated for swelling or pain. *Mastoiditis* is a less common finding in immunized children, but a serious complication of OM. If undiagnosed and untreated, it can lead to meningitis and hearing loss.

External Canal

Inspection

Inspect the external auditory canal for patency, color, discharge, odor, and foreign bodies. The largest speculum that will fit comfortably into the external canal should be used to increase the field of vision and create an airtight seal for pneumatic otoscopy. The smallest ear speculum (2.5 mm) is often used for the infant and young child and the larger speculum (4.5 mm) is often used in the older child and adults. During the initial newborn examination, patency or atresia of the external auditory canal must be determined. If the canal is not patent or is abnormally narrow or curved, additional abnormalities of the auditory system should be suspected and referral to otolaryngology and genetics for further evaluation should be made immediately. Children with Down syndrome have external canals that are narrower than normal, so the tympanic membrane may be difficult to visualize in early infancy. Vernix caseosa, a whitish cheesy debris, can often be seen in newborn ear canals and can obstruct visualization of the tympanic membrane. It also can be a contributing factor in failed newborn hearing screening or *evoked otoacoustic emission* (OAE) testing in the newborn. Because of the normally curved S shape of the canal, visualization is improved with minimal discomfort if the tragus is pulled forward to visualize the auditory canal and the tympanic membrane. The tympanic membrane of the newborn infant lies on a more horizontal plane, making visualization more difficult.

Internal Ear

Inspection

Inspect the tympanic membrane for contour (normally concave), intactness (no perforations or tympanostomy tubes), color (normally gray or silver but may be pink or red after crying), translucency (normally translucent without scarring or opacity), and presence of visible landmarks (umbo, handle of malleus, and light reflex; Fig. 11.5). The light reflex is usually found between the 4 and 6 o'clock positions on the right tympanic membrane and 6 to 8 o'clock on the left tympanic membrane. The tympanic membrane in newborn infants is thicker, grayer, and less translucent than in older children. The examiner should also look for the appearance of fluid bubbles behind the tympanic membrane or a fluid line, indicating the eustachian tube is not properly draining the middle ear (Fig. 11.13). If present, tympanostomy

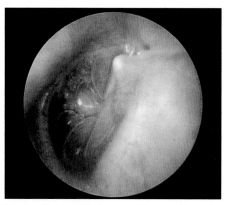

FIGURE 11.13 Middle ear with eustachian tube dysfunction and fluid bubbles. (From Zitelli BJ, et al. *Zitelli and Davis' Atlas of Pediatric Physical Diagnosis*. 8 th ed., Philadelphia: Elsevier; 2023.)

tubes should be located at the inferior aspect of the tympanic membrane (Fig. 11.14). The tubes should be patent to allow drainage of the middle ear. If the tube is blocked by cerumen or sitting in the ear canal, then it is no longer functional.

PEDIATRIC PEARLS

Color of the tympanic membrane is less important in diagnosing middle ear infections than identifying bony landmarks and the movement and quality of the tympanic membrane. A red or pink tympanic membrane may occur as a result of crying, irritation, or fever and may not be an indication of an acute otitis media.

Mobility of the tympanic membrane, an important indication of middle ear pressure, can be assessed with a pneumatic attachment to the otoscope (Fig. 11.10A). If the middle ear pressure is equalized, the tympanic membrane will move or flutter in response to air pressure from the *pneumatic insufflator* in the external canal. The speculum should be inserted deep into ear canal to create a seal but not cause pain. Squeeze and release the pneumatic bulb gently several times to assess the movement of the tympanic membrane. This can be visualized through the otoscope as movement of the light

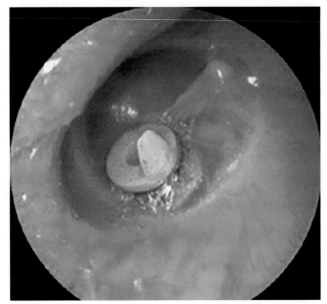

FIGURE 11.14 Presence of a tympanostomy tube in the TM. (From Schilder AGM, et al. Acute otitis media and otitis media with effusion. In Flint PW, et al., eds, *Cummings Otolaryngology: Head and Neck Surgery.* 7th ed. Philadelphia: Elsevier; 2021.)

reflex. Complete immobility of the tympanic membrane is not necessary to diagnose otitis media with effusion. Movement that is sluggish or restricted is a positive finding. Middle ear pressure can also be recorded on a tympanometer, as an equal rise and fall of pressure over the normal pressure setting of zero (Fig. 11.15).

Decreased or limited movement of the tympanic membrane may indicate *increased negative pressure* in the middle ear, which is associated with *eustachian tube dysfunction* and *otitis media with effusion* (OME), where the tympanic membrane is retracted and taut and the bony landmarks are accentuated. Alternatively, decreased movement may be due to fluid build-up behind the membrane, causing it to become inflamed, convex in shape, and taut. This causes an opacity in the tympanic membrane with loss of visible bony landmarks indicating infection, as in *acute otitis media* (AOM) (Fig. 11.16A,B). A ruptured tympanic membrane (perforation) related to infection or trauma, patent tympanostomy tubes, or cholesteatoma can result in discharge from the middle ear into the external canal. Ear drainage should alert the examiner to these conditions, as well as otitis externa.

EAR CERUMEN

Parents and caretakers should always be reassured that cerumen is a normal, protective ear secretion. Cerumen has two predominant types: 1) dry cerumen, which is gray and flaky; and 2) wet, honey-colored to dark brown cerumen.[2] Some infants and children naturally have more cerumen than other children. Children with allergic skin conditions often have additional cerumen, complicating the assessment of ear complaints associated with allergic symptoms or upper respiratory infections.

Parents should be encouraged to clean the child's external ears only with warm soapy water and should not use cotton-tipped applicators, which can cause injury to the ear canal or tympanic membrane or result in further impaction of cerumen. School-age children and adolescents should also be instructed not to use cotton-tipped applicators. Removal of

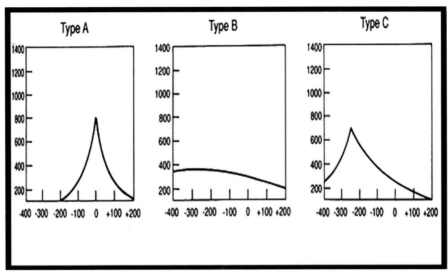

FIGURE 11.15 Sample graphs of tympanometry (Type A – Eardrum movement in normal limits, Type B – Little or no eardrum movements, Type C – Eustachian tube dysfunction due to negative pressure). (From Roy S, et al. Assessment of Eustachian tube functioning following surgical intervention of oral submucus fibrosis by using tympanometry & audiometry. *J Oral Biol Craniofac Res.* 2020; 10(2):241–245.)

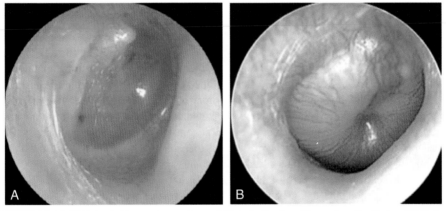

FIGURE 11.16 **(A)** Retracted tympanic membrane (TM) indicative for otitis media with effusion. **(B)** Red and bulging TM indicative for acute otitis media. (From Schilder AGM, et al. Acute otitis media and otitis media with effusion. In Flint PW, et al., eds. *Cummings Otolaryngology: Head and Neck Surgery.* 7th ed. Philadelphia: Elsevier; 2021.)

cerumen or debris from the ear canal may be necessary to visualize the tympanic membrane. If the child is cooperative, a plastic or metal cerumen spoon can be used for removal. Lighted devices for cerumen removal offer increased visualization for the examiner. An infant or young child must be positioned securely before attempting cerumen removal. If the child cannot cooperate for removal of

cerumen, when necessary, then irrigating the ear canal with warm water will usually loosen and flush out built-up cerumen. Irrigation should never be attempted if a ruptured tympanic membrane is suspected. Tympanostomy tubes inserted into the pars tensa area of the tympanic membrane for eustachian tube dysfunction are also a contraindication for irrigation of the external auditory canal (Fig. 11.14).

If the child is asymptomatic, cerumen build-up can be reduced, and the canals cleared by daily use of commercially prepared eardrops for dissolving earwax.

EVIDENCE-BASED PRACTICE TIP

Irrigation of the external ear canal should not be attempted if there is a possibility of a ruptured tympanic membrane or patent tympanostomy tubes.

HEARING ASSESSMENT

Hearing impairment in infants and children is a common disability with implications in cognitive, psychosocial, and academic development.[3] Approximately 0.9 to 1.7 per 1,000 infants screened in the universal newborn hearing screening (UNHS) program are diagnosed with hearing loss in the newborn period.[10] The goal of UNHS is to have all neonates screened for hearing loss before hospital discharge or by 1 month of age to ensure appropriate follow-up is obtained. The UNHS facilitates lower age of identifying hearing loss, lower age at initiating amplification, and lower age at starting intervention services.[11] Newborns who fail hearing screening and subsequent rescreening should be referred by 3 months of age for audiologic and medical evaluations to confirm hearing loss. All infants with hearing loss should begin receiving early intervention services before 6 months of age. Children with hearing loss and without additional disabilities who receive intervention by 6 months of age are more likely to have normal language development by 5 years of age compared to children who did not receive timely intervention.[12] Early Hearing Detection and Intervention programs are working to ensure all newborns are screened for hearing loss, receive follow-up diagnostic testing if they fail the screening, and are enrolled in deaf and hard of hearing (DHH) early interventions services if diagnosed with permanent hearing loss.[5] The pediatric health care provider must continue to track infants who fail the newborn screening to ensure these infants are retested, diagnosed by a pediatric otolaryngologist, and initiate hearing augmentation in a timely manner.[13] The health care provider should not assume if the newborn hearing screen is normal that the growing infant or child's hearing is normal and no further hearing screening is necessary. One to two per one thousand children acquire hearing loss after birth.[13] It is important to routinely screen for hearing deficits, assess language development, and inquire about any changes noted in the home or school setting that may be pertinent to hearing loss when gathering the health history.

It is recommended that all children and adolescents be screened annually via conventional pure tone audiometry starting at age 3 years. Any child under 3 years of age with speech and language delays, or a history indicating high risk for hearing loss, or whose caregivers have concern regarding the child's hearing should be referred to an audiologist or otolaryngologist for testing (Box 11.1). If significant concerns about hearing are present at any age, generated either from the health history or initial screening, then referral is indicated. Most primary care practices have access to conventional pure tone audiometry, but a variety of other screening tests are available for infants and young children (Table 11.3).

Behavioral audiometry determines the weakest intensity at which a child shows behavioral awareness of the presence of sound. Behavioral audiometry with reliable responses can be performed in children as young as 8 months old who have appropriate development. Normal sound fields include 250 Hz to 6000 Hz, but hearing screening is often performed at 25 decibels between 500 Hz and 4000 Hz. Physiologic measures of hearing determine the infant's physiologic response to stimulation of the auditory system (Table 11.4). Speech audiometry determines the child's response to speech stimuli and tests the clarity of sound received and perceived (Table 11.5).

TABLE 11.3	BEHAVIORAL AUDIOMETRY IN INFANTS AND YOUNG CHILDREN	
Test	**Age**	**Method**
Conventional audiometry	4–5 years	Child is instructed to listen quietly for the test tone and to raise a hand or give a verbal response when it is heard
Bone-conduction testing	5 years	Calibration standards have not been established on infants and children; responses to bone-conducted stimuli may be inferred by head-turn response or as in conventional testing; young children may object to wearing oscillator
Hear test	Infants	Infant reaction to different frequency sounds is observed; elicited with standardized toys (e.g., bell, squeak toy) that make noises at different frequencies
Conditioned play audiometry	Developmental age 2–5 years	Child performs a repetitive play task (e.g., places block in dish or peg in pegboard) in response to transmitted tone
Visual reinforcement audiometry	Developmental age 5 months–2 years	Loudspeakers, earphones, or bone-conduction oscillator is used to observe child's ability to hear and localize sound (by turning head or body); visual reward (e.g., lighted toy) provided for accurate responses
Behavioral observation	Developmental age birth to 5 months	Similar to visual reinforcement audiometry but used for infants or children unable to move head or eyes reliably; any repeatable response to sound may indicate hearing

TABLE 11.4	PHYSIOLOGIC MEASURES OF HEARING
Screening Test	**Response**
Auditory brainstem response (ABR)	Measures electrical activity via scalp electrodes in the entire hearing pathway to determine the presence and type of hearing loss. Headphones or ear probes administer sounds and electrodes on the head measure the waveform response to sound. Can be used for UNHS with pass/fail reading or as diagnostic test. Results can give frequency range and decibel response level information. Recommended after failed newborn hearing screen. Test can also be used for children of all ages that are unable to participate in behavioral tests.
Otoacoustic emissions (OAE)	Measures function of the external auditory canal, tympanic membrane, middle ear, and outer hair cells of the cochlear but not the inner hair cells or cochlear nerve. Failure may indicate a nonpatent ear canal, nonaerated middle ear, or lack of normal outer hair cell function needed for auditory nerve function. Test is appropriate for infants and children of all ages.
Tympanometry	Measures the function of the tympanic membrane and the middle ear as air pressure in the ear canal is systematically varied. It is routinely used as a component of the hearing evaluation. An abnormal peak pressure pattern may indicate middle ear dysfunction. Test is appropriate for infants and young children.

UNHS, Universal newborn hearing screening.

TABLE 11.5 SPEECH AUDIOMETRY

Screening Test	Response
Speech detection threshold	Speech stimulus used to determine the ability to hear at varying decibels and frequencies via sound field, earphones, or bone conduction. Threshold is the lowest hearing level that the infant or child can detect the presence speech 50% of the time. Test is appropriate for developmental age 5 months to 2 years.
Speech reception threshold	Word stimulus given and child repeats word or points to picture to indicate word heard. Threshold is the lowest hearing level the child can repeat back two-syllable words or point to the appropriate picture. Test is appropriate for children with receptive language skills $\geq$2 years.
Central auditory processing tests	Tests evaluate school-age children with normal pure tone audiograms to determine speech perception with background noise, sounds in contralateral ear, rapid rate of presentation, or filtering

INTERPROFESSIONAL COLLABORATION

Prompt referral of infants and children identified with hearing loss, consultation and collaboration with pediatric otolaryngology and audiology specialists, and close follow-up in primary care will assure optimum development of hearing in affected children.

WEBER AND RINNE HEARING SCREENING TESTS

In older children and adolescents, the *Weber* and *Rinne* tests can be performed as additional screening tests to determine deficits in either conductive hearing or sensorineural hearing. Although these hearing screening tests are not routinely performed in the primary care setting, it remains a useful clinical tool in pediatric specialty and in health care settings in countries with low access to audiometry equipment.

The Weber test is performed by placing a vibrating tuning fork (512 Hz) midline on the skull, making sure the examiner's hand does not touch the prongs of the tuning fork or the child's head (Fig. 11.17A). The school-age child

or adolescent is then asked if he or she hears the sound of the tuning fork louder on one side or the other, or equally well on both sides. If the child/adolescent indicates the sound is heard louder on one side, this is called *lateralization* and indicates a unilateral conductive hearing deficit in the ear perceived as hearing the tuning fork louder. If the child has a unilateral sensorineural hearing deficit, the tuning fork is heard louder in the normal ear.

The Rinne test compares air conduction to bone conduction (Fig. 11.17B). It is used to evaluate hearing loss in one ear at a time. A vibrating tuning fork is placed on the child's mastoid bone to determine hearing via bone conduction. When the sound is no longer heard, the tuning fork should be moved to a position 1 cm to 2 cm from the external auditory canal. Sound is then being processed via air conduction in that area. Air conduction should be twice as long as bone conduction. If the bone conduction of sound is heard longer than air conduction, then a conductive hearing loss is present in the affected ear. If the ratio of air conduction to bone conduction is less than 2:1, then a SNHL is present. The Weber and Rinne tests are not reliable on children until school age.

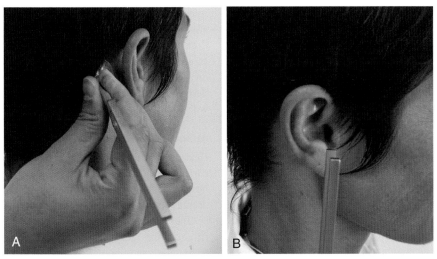

FIGURE 11.17 **(A)** Rinne test—bone conduction. **(B)** Rinne test—air conduction. (Published in Legent F, Bordure P, Calais C. *Audiologie Pratique Audiométrie.* 3rd ed. Paris: Elsevier; 2021, p 9.)

EAR CONDITIONS

Hearing Loss

Before the advent of UNHS, the average age of identification of congenital hearing loss was 2.5 to 3 years of age. Some infants with mild hearing loss will be missed in UNHS, and a proportion of children who pass the UNHS will develop acquired hearing loss that is late onset or progressive.[9] The Joint Committee on Infant Hearing has established guidelines to improve identification of children at risk for late-onset hearing impairment (Box 11.1).[2] Ongoing regularly scheduled surveillance of developmental milestones, auditory skills, speech and language development, parental concerns regarding hearing, quality of life, and objective hearing testing are needed to identify children with progressive or acquired hearing loss.[3,9,13]

Conductive Hearing Loss

Conductive hearing loss (CHL) is caused by an abnormality in the transmission of sound waves through the ear canal, the tympanic membrane, middle ear space, or middle ear ossicles. The auditory nerve system is intact, but the sound impulses do not reach the nerve.

Transient *CHL* is common during episodes of OME or AOM. Recurrent or chronic bilateral ear effusions, during the early years of rapid language development, may impede normal speech and communication development. Cholesteatoma, with its associated destruction of the middle ear, is another common cause of CHL, but this hearing loss will be permanent and progressive unless the cholesteatoma is surgically removed and middle ear reconstructed. There are no conservative treatment options for a cholesteatoma.[4] Chronic or recurrent ear infections can cause *tympanosclerosis*, visualized as white scarring and thickening of the tympanic membrane (see Fig. 11.7), but scarring alone rarely results in measurable hearing loss. Acquired ossicular fixation from chronic diseases of the ear is almost never seen in children, although it is a relatively common cause of acquired hearing loss in older adults. Children with *osteogenesis imperfecta* do develop otosclerosis and must be followed by a pediatric otolaryngologist.

Congenital Conductive Hearing Loss

Congenital CHL can occur with Down syndrome or any gestational abnormality of the craniofacial structures that disrupt the acoustic system. Isolated malformations of the external ear or *microtia, or* malformations of the ear canal, can result in *CHL*. Congenital stenosis, congenital atresia of the stapes (seen in *Treacher Collins syndrome*), or congenital fixation of the stapes in the middle ear can also result in a *CHL*.

Sensorineural Hearing Loss

SNHL is caused by abnormalities of the cochlea, auditory nerve, or the auditory pathways that traverse the brainstem ending in the auditory cortex of the brain. SNHL is often congenital and genetically acquired. Genetic predisposition is thought to play a role in 50% of those affected by SNHL. Genetic syndromes that are associated with SNHL are Alport, Jervell and Lange-Nielsen, neurofibromatosis type 2, Pendred, Stickler (incidence increases with age), Usher, and Waardenburg type II syndromes.[8]

Newborns with possible perinatally acquired infections from a variety of pathogens should be screened for SNHL based on their clinical presentation. Any newborn with a history of TORCHS (*t*oxoplasmosis and *o*ther diseases: *r*ubella, *C*MV infections, *h*erpes simplex, *s*yphilis) should also be tested and monitored for SNHL. Infants and children with symptomatic congenital CMV infection are at greater risk for hearing impairment than those with asymptomatic infection. Approximately 30% to 65% of children with symptomatic infection have subsequent SNHL compared with only 5% to 20% of the children with asymptomatic infection.[14] CMV infection at any age may result in hearing loss.

Premature infants and very low birth weight (VLBW) infants are at increased risk for hearing loss and have a higher incidence of hearing loss than full-term infants. Neonates with a history of persistent pulmonary hypertension or extracorporeal membrane oxygenation (ECMO) therapy have a 21% incidence of SNHL.[15] Children of any age who develop meningitis must be carefully tested for hearing loss because of both the consequences of the

infections and the ototoxic side effects of many antibiotics used to treat meningitis.[9] Children treated for malignancies with platinum compounds (cisplatin or carboplatin) or who are receiving cranial radiation may develop delayed SNHL and must be followed carefully with audiometry testing.

Mixed Hearing Loss

Hearing loss may also be a combination of conductive hearing deficits and sensorineural hearing deficits. Children with congenital syndromes often have mixed hearing loss.

The management of hearing deficits in children has advanced with new surgical techniques and bone-anchored, bone-conduction hearing aids (Fig. 11.18). Cochlear implantation and advances in hearing aids have improved the treatment of hearing loss dramatically, providing some sound to most children with even severe hearing loss.

EVIDENCE-BASED PRACTICE TIP

An age-appropriate hearing test should be performed for all children with chronic otitis media with effusion, or children with otitis media with effusion who are at risk for hearing loss.[16]

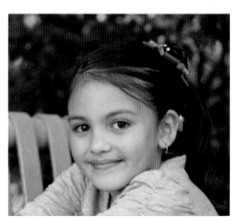

FIGURE 11.18 Child with a bone-anchored hearing aid (BAHA) fitted. (Gan R, et al. Management of hearing loss in children. *Paediatr Child Health.* 2016; 26(1):15–20.)

Acute Otitis Media and Otitis Media with Effusion

AOM is an inflammation within the middle ear that is often acute but can be recurrent or chronic, lasting more than 3 months. AOM is one of the most common conditions seen in pediatric practice in young children between 6 months and 3 years of age.[17] Children exposed to daycare or crowded living situations are prone to upper respiratory infections that may result in inflammation in the middle ear. Exposure to secondhand smoke has also been shown to increase the risk for AOM, whereas breastfeeding has been shown to be protective.[18] There is a genetic component to OM, with a higher incidence of OM in children who have older siblings or parents with a significant history of OM.

Abnormal clearance of middle ear fluid is the cornerstone of AOM and OME. Viruses and bacteria from the nasal pharynx enter the middle ear via the eustachian tube opening in the oropharynx. Young children are more prone to AOM because of their short, horizontal, less mature eustachian tubes and more frequent upper respiratory tract infections. Children with nasal allergy are also more prone to AOM because inflammation of the respiratory tract associated with allergies often causes swelling and obstruction of the eustachian tube, trapping fluid. Viruses or bacteria in the middle ear from respiratory infection cause further inflammation and often obstruction. Children with craniofacial defects or immunodeficiencies are at greatest risk for ear infections, and children with placement of nasogastric tubes also have a higher susceptibility.

The majority of AOM infections are presumed to be of viral etiology. *Streptococcus pneumoniae*, *Haemophilus influenzae*, and *Moraxella catarrhalis* are the most common bacterial pathogens found in AOM. Expanded immunization schedules covering an increased number of phenotypes of *H. influenzae* and pneumococcal strains have resulted in decreased incidence of AOM caused by these organisms.

The presenting symptoms of AOM include rapid onset of ear pain or *otalgia*, fever, irritability, disrupted sleep pattern and occasionally *otorrhea*, or drainage from the ear. Severe conjunctivitis may also be present. Physical assessment should include careful otoscopy and pneumatic otoscopy to determine inflammation in the middle ear. AOM results in moderate to marked bulging of the tympanic membrane, a purulent effusion in the middle ear, and hemorrhagic redness, making bony landmarks difficult to see (Fig. 11.15B).[17] The light reflex becomes diffuse and abnormally positioned on the tympanic membrane or absent. With pneumatic otoscopy the normal fluttering of the membrane is not present because of the increased fluid pressure in the middle ear. The tympanic membrane is usually erythematous, often with increased vascularity; however, these findings can also be present in a child who has been crying, and color should not be used as the primary finding to diagnose AOM in young children. Persistent otitis media is classified as chronic when there is chronic inflammation of the middle ear that does not self-resolve or persists over time. Underlying causes include bacterial colonization of the mucosa, poor local immunocompetence, eustachian tube dysfunction, and other anatomical abnormalities.[4]

OME is a more common finding than AOM and is defined as middle ear effusion without signs or symptoms of AOM.[16] OME presents with opacity of the tympanic membrane caused by a clear or serous transparent effusion in the middle ear or a cloudy nontransparent effusion.[17] OME causes decreased movement of the tympanic membrane on pneumatic otoscopy or tympanogram, a retracted or concave membrane, and visible air bubbles or a fluid line indicating eustachian tube dysfunction. OME may occur after AOM as the acute infection resolves but before air pressure equilibrates, from eustachian tube dysfunction without acute infection, or during an upper respiratory infection. Chronic OME, or an effusion that persists for 3 months or longer, interferes with sound wave transmission into the middle ear and is a common cause of conductive hearing loss. By school age, 90% of children will experience one to four episodes of OME per year.[16] Children with Down syndrome or cleft palate are at higher risk of developing OME. An age-appropriate hearing test should be performed for all children with chronic OME or children with OME who are at risk for hearing loss.

Diagnosing AOM or OME with certainty in infants and young children can be a challenge. Positioning and restraining an irritable child, presence of cerumen in a narrowly curved ear canal, and difficulty obtaining a proper seal of the ear canal for pneumatic otoscopy or tympanostomy all make certainty of diagnosis difficult. Bilateral AOM occurs more frequently in the child who is younger than 24 months than in children with unilateral AOM. Occurrence of bilateral AOM should not be a determining criterion for treatment.[17] Treatment guidelines and algorithms for AOM and OME are well established and take into consideration the child's age, duration of symptoms, and risk factors.[18]

Vestibular Disorders Affecting Children

Vestibular inputs in the inner ear are essential to balance and gait stability.[19] There is a growing recognition of vestibular system dysfunction in children resulting in gaze instability, dizziness, and balance problems. A study in children from 3 to 17 years found an overall prevalence of dizziness and balance problems was 5.3% and increased with age from 4.1% for children aged 3 to 5 years to 7.5% for children aged 15 to 17 years of age.[20] Children should be screened for *Meniere's disease*, a disorder of the inner ear that is associated with episodic vertigo, tinnitus, aural fullness, and hearing loss. Although Meniere's disease is most common in middle-aged adults, it can occur at any age. Dizziness, vertigo, disequilibrium, and unsteadiness can cause life-altering disability and health care burden. Increased risk factors

associated with dizziness and balance problems include children with history of LBW or VLBW, intellectual disability, developmental delay, frequent headaches or migraines, recurrent AOM or hearing loss, or history of seizures. It is important for pediatric health care providers to screen children for vestibular problems and refer children to a pediatric neurologist, otolaryngologist, or early developmental intervention program.[19,20]

TELEHEALTH TIPS

Telehealth, or telemedicine, is a growing field that has seen exponential growth in the last decade.[21] Telehealth facilitates continuity of care for patients with socioeconomic constraints, patients who are immunocompromised and/or homebound, and maintains infectious disease precautions between providers and patients.[22] A successful telehealth experience requires provider training, a cooperative pediatric patient, adequate internet connection, and access to appropriate devices to support the visit. Although telehealth can be conducted by phone or video, video is the preferred method due to visual feedback that is similar to an office visit. The provider and patient/caregiver can make eye contact, pick up on nonverbal communication from the patient, and the provider can visualize some physical findings (if applicable).

During a video telehealth visit, several aspects of the ear exam can be assessed. The auricle can be visually inspected for size, shape, position, pits or skin tags, erythema, swelling, or discharge. The young child may be able to state if they have ear pain, but not the location or quality. The older developmentally appropriate child can verbalize the location, duration, and quality of the ear pain when prompted with probing questions. Visual inspection of the inner ear is possible during a telehealth visit. Synchronous video otoscopy and hearing screening has been successful in several telehealth studies.[23] Internet-based software matched with smartphones are available on the market to aid in the external auditory canal and middle ear exam. This diagnostic information can be forwarded to the provider as a video or still image. However, image quality and cerumen impaction limit visualization during otoscopy. Video otoscopy has been shown to provide better imaging and a more reliable diagnosis compared to still images. Hearing exam data (tele-audiometry) during the visit further support diagnoses.

There are several audiometry applications for smart devices (iPad, tablet, smartphones). Sound quality is of particular importance when conducting a hearing screen remotely. PC-based software has been used to configure video conferencing for synchronous hearing screening when the provider and the patient are in different locations. There are several challenges to internet- and computer-based tele-audiometry. The provider and the parent need to be trained on how to use the applications so that the child can be supported throughout the testing. In addition, ambient noise and undiagnosed cerumen impactions or middle ear effusions during hearing screens negatively impacts measurement and compromises test reliability.[23,24] Sensitivity and specificity of telehealth hearing screen is higher in children 5 years and older.[23] Data is limited in tele-audiometry for young children and children with special health care needs that are difficult to test.

SUMMARY OF EXAMINATION

- Before examining the ear, inspect the head, face, and neck for any asymmetry. The superior portion of the auricle should be equal in height to the outer canthus of the eye.
- Inspect the auricles for size, shape, symmetry, deformity, placement, discharge, and color.
- Inspect the tympanic membrane for contour, intactness, color, translucency, and presence of visible landmarks (umbo, handle of malleus, and light reflex).

- The light reflex is usually found between the 4 o'clock and 6 o'clock position on the right tympanic membrane and 6 o'clock to 8 o'clock on the left tympanic membrane.
- Mobility of the tympanic membrane, an important indication of middle ear pressure, can be assessed with a pneumatic attachment to the otoscope or by use of a tympanometer.
- Ear drainage in the external canal should alert the examiner to otitis externa, a ruptured tympanic membrane, patent tympanostomy tubes, or cholesteatoma.
- Ten percent of childhood hearing loss is acquired after birth. Routinely screen for hearing deficits and begin pure-tone audiometry at 3 years of age.
- Adhere to current guidelines for treatment of AOM and OME in infants and children.
- Vestibular disorders should be considered in children with gaze instability, dizziness, and balance problems.
- A successful telehealth experience requires provider training, a cooperative pediatric patient, adequate internet connection, and access to appropriate devices to support the visit.

DOCUMENTATION

Term Neonate
Ears: Auricle well formed, symmetrical, with normal alignment. External canals patent with small amount of white residue. Tympanic membranes partially visible, gray, opaque, without visible light reflex or bony landmarks.
Adolescent
Ears: Auricles well formed, symmetrical, with two healed piercings on outer border of helix and one healed piercing in center of lobe. No masses, erythema, or tenderness noted. External canals with minimal dark brown cerumen. Tympanic membranes pearly gray, concave, light reflex and bony landmarks visible. + movement with insufflation. Screening audiometry—NL. 1000–4000 frequency (Hz) at 25 decibels (dB).

REFERENCES

1. Saha R, Srimani P, Mazumdar A, Mazumdar S. Morphological variations of middle ear ossicles and its clinical implications. *J Clin Diagn Res*. 2017;11(1):AC01–AC04.

2. Myers RP, Duncan AN, Girotto JA. Deformational plagiocephaly. In: Kleigman R, Stanton B, St. Geme J, Schor N, eds. *Nelson Textbook of Pediatrics*. 20th ed. Elsevier; 2015:2819–2823.

3. Schoem S, Darrow D. *Pediatric Otolaryngology for Primary Care*. 2nd ed. American Academy of Pediatrics; 2020.

4. Luers JC, Hüttenbrink KB. Surgical anatomy and pathology of the middle ear. *J Anat*. 2016;228(1):338–353.

5. Isaacson G. Endoscopic anatomy of the pediatric middle ear. *Otolaryngol Head Neck Surg*. 2014;150(1):6–15.

6. Mozaffari M, Jiang D, Tucker AS. Developmental aspects of the tympanic membrane: shedding light on function and disease. *Genesis*. 2020;58(3-4):e23348.

7. Ryan PJ, Patel NP. Endoscopic management of pediatric cholesteatoma. *J Otol*. 2020;15(1):17–26.

8. Gettelfinger JD, Dahl JP. Syndromic hearing loss: A brief review of common presentations and genetics. *J Pediatr Genet*. 2018;7(1):1–8.

9. Ciorba A, Corazzi V, Negossi L, Tazzari R, Bianchini C, Aimoni C. Moderate-severe hearing loss in children: A diagnostic and rehabilitative challenge. *J Int Adv Otol*. 2017;13(3):407–413.

10. Subbiah K, Mason CA, Gaffney M, Grosse SD. Intervention for deaf and hard of hearing infants: CDC's hearing screening and follow-up survey, United States, 2006–2016. *J Early Hear Detect Interv*. 2018;3(2):1–7.

11. Yoshinaga-Itano C, Manchaiah V, Hunnicutt C. Outcomes of universal newborn screening programs: systematic review. *J Clin Med*. 2021;10(13):2784–2807.

12. Yoshinago-Itano C, Sedey AL, Wiggin M, Chung W. Early hearing detection and vocabulary of children with hearing loss. *Pediatrics*. 2017;140(2):e20162964.

13. Stewart JE, Bentley JE. Hearing loss in pediatrics: What the medical home needs to know. *Pediatr Clin North Am*. 2019;66(2):425–436.

14. Foulon I, De Brucker Y, Buyl R, et al. Hearing loss with congenital cytomegalovirus infection. *Pediatrics*. 2019;144(2):e20183095.

15. Murray MF, Nield T, Larson-Tuttle C, Istvan S, Friedland P. Sensorineural hearing loss at 9-13 years of age in children with a history of neonatal extracorporeal membrane oxygenation. *Arch Dis Child Fetal Neonatal Ed*. 2011;96:F128–132.

16. Rosenfeld RM, Shin JJ, Schwartz SR, et al. Clinical practice guideline: Otitis media with effusion executive summary (update). *Otolaryngol Head Neck Surg*. 2016;154(2):201–214.

17. Uitti JM, Laine MK, Tahtinen PA, Ruuskanen O, Ruohola A. Symptoms and otoscopic signs in bilateral and unilateral acute otitis media. *Pediatrics*. 2013;131(2):e398–405.

18. Liberthal AS, Carroll AE, Chonmaitree T, et al. Diagnosis and management of acute otitis media. *Pediatrics*. 2013;131(3):e964–e999.

19. Young AS, Rosengren SM, Welgampola MS. Disorders of the inner-ear balance organs and their pathways. In: Day BL, Lord SR, eds. *Handbook of Clinical Neurology*. 3rd ed. Elsevier; 2018:385–398.

20. Li CM, Hoffman HJ, Ward BK, Cohen HS, Rine RM. Epidemiology of dizziness and balance problems in children in the United States: A population-based study. *J Pediatr*. 2016;171:240–247.

21. Beule AG. Telemedical methods in otorhinolaryngology. *Laryngorhinootologie*. 2019;98(S01):s152–s172.

22. Fieux M, Duret S, Bawazeer N, et al. Telemedicine for ENT: Effect on quality care during Covid-19 pandemic. *Eur Ann Otorhinolaryngol Head Neck Dis*. 2020;137(4):257–261.

23. Govender SM, Mars M. The use of telehealth services to facilitate audiological management for children: A scoping review and content analysis. *J Telemed Telecare*. 2017;23(3):392–401.

24. Levy DA, Hill DR, Bia FJ, et al. Tablet-based hearing screening in children aged 5 to 17 in rural Dominican Republic. *Otol Neurotol*. 2018;39(7):823–828.

CHAPTER 12

NOSE, MOUTH, AND THROAT

Adebola M. Olarewaju

A thorough assessment of the nose, mouth, and throat is an essential part of the pediatric physical examination. Infants and children have frequent upper respiratory infections, viral infections, and nasal allergies, such as allergic rhinitis, which are common disorders that affect the *nasopharynx*. Viewing the *oropharynx* is particularly important when looking for a focus of infection in a febrile child. The oral health of children is, also, key to overall health, and the pediatric health care provider is an important link in oral health assessment and preventing dental caries.

EMBRYOLOGIC DEVELOPMENT

In general, facial development starts from the lateral edge to the center of the face. The facial structures develop in the embryo during the first few weeks of gestation. The tongue, lips, gums, and tooth enamel all evolve from the ectoderm of the primitive mouth, the *stomodeum*, early in the fourth week. The lips are formed during the fourth to eighth weeks of gestation. The primary teeth (deciduous teeth) and salivary glands are formed between the sixth and eighth weeks of fetal life. By the sixth fetal month, the ducts are hollow and begin producing saliva. Calcification of the *primary teeth* begins in the fourth month of fetal life and is complete by 1 year of age. Any insult during pregnancy to the sensitive process of tooth formation can result in an anomaly in the color, size, or shape of the primary or permanent dentition. Early development of the nose begins during the fifth week of gestation, with development of muscle, bone, and cartilage complete by the 12th week of gestation.

The *palate* evolves from fusion of the maxillary prominences during the seventh and eighth weeks of gestation. It is completely formed by the 12th week of gestation during the fusion of the primary and secondary palates becoming the hard and soft palate. Failure in fusion results in *cleft palate*. Worldwide, cleft palates are a common congenital anomaly. The prevalence of cleft palates varies widely between countries at a rate of 3 to 20 per 10,000. In the United States the prevalence is 7.7 per 10,000.[1] Cleft lip can be an isolated defect or associated with cleft palate or a component of a congenital syndrome (Fig. 12.1A, B). The etiology is multifactorial involving both genetic and environmental risk factors in both syndromic and nonsyndromic clefts. Several risk factors associated with cleft type have been identified and include maternal smoking, alcohol consumption, diabetes, maternal nutrition and folic acid intake, and maternal medications (e.g., anticonvulsants).[1] A *subcutaneous cleft, located in the soft* palate, also can occur during this period with incomplete fusion of the palate; it often goes undetected in the newborn and is associated with persistent abnormal speech patterns.

DEVELOPMENTAL VARIATIONS

Table 12.1 presents the physiological variations to be monitored from infancy to adolescence. Table 12.2 reviews the development of the sinuses from infancy through adolescence.

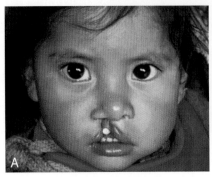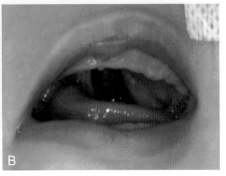

FIGURE 12.1 (A) Cleft lip. (B) Posterior cleft soft palate. ([B] From Farhadieh D, et al, eds. *Plastic Surgery Principles and Practice.* Elsevier; 2022.)

TABLE 12.1	PHYSIOLOGIC VARIATIONS OF THE NOSE, MOUTH, AND THROAT	
Age-group	**Physiologic Variations**
Newborn	Nose cartilage is soft, malleable; deformities in external appearance from intrauterine or birth positioning usually resolve spontaneously; congenital anatomic deformities, obstructive masses, or traumatic obstruction can occlude the nasal passages Natal teeth may be present Epstein pearls, small whitish nodules or cysts, at juncture of hard and soft palates may be visible in first month of life; Bohn nodules, or mucous gland cysts, may be present on gum surface in first 2–3 months Rooting, gag, sucking reflexes are present A short tight lingual frenulum attached to the inferior tip of the tongue may impede movement of the tongue and breastfeeding
Infancy	Anatomically small airway passages Occlusion of nasal pathways can occur with nasal secretions Deciduous teeth appear between 6 and 24 months Rooting, sucking reflexes wane about 4–6 months Drooling increases as salivary gland production increases Anterior permanent teeth begin to calcify at 3–12 months Ethmoid and maxillary sinuses present but undeveloped
Early childhood	Tonsils, adenoids enlarge and may remain 2+ to 3+ Nasal passages enlarge allowing easier airflow Maxillary and ethmoid sinuses present but sphenoid and frontal sinuses limited in size and function Sinuses not normally assessed in children until middle childhood because of their limited development Swallowing coordination improves, drooling decreases Permanent molars begin to calcify at 18 months to 3 years

TABLE 12.1	PHYSIOLOGIC VARIATIONS OF THE NOSE, MOUTH, AND THROAT—CONT'D
Age-group	**Physiologic Variations**
Middle childhood	Tonsils and adenoids usually begin to atrophy returning to size 1+ to 2+ Horizontal creases on anterior nose may develop in children with nasal rhinitis/allergies Deciduous teeth begin to shed; permanent teeth erupt causing change in facial structure, appearance Bridge of nose becomes more prominent Third molar, last permanent tooth, is formed and begins calcifying
Adolescence	All permanent teeth present Bridge of nose formed by bone creating pyramid shape Frontal and sphenoid sinuses completely formed and functioning

TABLE 12.2	DEVELOPMENT OF SINUS CAVITIES
Sinus Cavity	**Development**
Maxillary	Present at birth; first sinuses to develop significantly; can be seen radiologically at 4–5 months of age; open beneath the middle turbinate into the middle meatus; rapid growth occurs between birth and 4 years of age and 6–12 years of age.
Frontal	Last sinuses to develop, beginning around 7 years of age and do not develop fully until late adolescence. Secretions drain into the middle meatus. The walls of the frontal sinus border the orbital and intracranial cavities, which can increase the risk for frontal sinus infections spreading directly into these adjacent structures.
Ethmoid	Present at birth, but not developed, grow rapidly during the first 4 years and are fully developed by 12–14 years of age; first seen radiologically at 1 year of age. Ethmoid sinuses are divided into anterior portion, draining into the middle meatus, and posterior portion, which drains into the superior meatus.
Sphenoid	Undeveloped at birth and do not begin to grow rapidly until 3–5 years of age; development complete between 12 and 15 years of age. Lie anterior to the pituitary fossa. Optic nerve and carotid artery are located on the lateral wall of the sinuses, offering a potential route for spread of infection into the central nervous system.

Data from Schoem SR, Darrow DH. *Pediatric Otolaryngology.* Elk Grove: American Academy of Pediatrics; 2012.

ANATOMY AND PHYSIOLOGY

External Nose

The nose of the newborn and young infant is generally flattened and malleable (Fig. 12.2). In the neonate, the septum is composed of cartilage; ossification occurs during childhood. The nose develops a bony structure by early adolescence. The soft tissue of the nose can

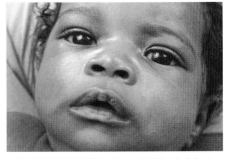

FIGURE 12.2 Flattened nasal bridge in infant.

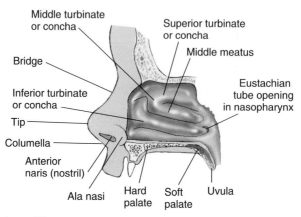

FIGURE 12.3 Anatomy of the nose.

continue to grow and change shape until late adolescence. Typically, adolescents will reach facial maturity by 18 years of age. The nose is divided into four sections: the proximal bony portion, often referred to as the *nasal bridge;* the mid cartilaginous vault; the tip, *columella,* and *nares;* and the interior *vestibule* (Fig. 12.3).

Nasal breathing is the normal breathing pattern, and infants and young children are prone to increased airway resistance, because they have anatomically small airway passages. Nasal congestion in the neonate is a common normal finding, and a nasal bulb syringe is often used to gently remove secretions from the small narrow nasal passages to clear the airway during breastfeeding and bottle-feeding. In the past, it was thought that newborns are obligatory nasal breathers for the first few months of life. However, research has demonstrated newborns can switch from nasal to mouth breathing as needed, so they are actually "preferential" nasal breathers.[2] Respiratory compromise or distress occurs rapidly in young infants when the nasal passages become occluded. The most common reason for occlusion is mucosal congestion or increased secretions, but congenital anatomical deformities, obstructive masses, or traumatic obstruction can also occlude the nasal passages. Nasal resistance is a key factor in total airway resistance, and nasal occlusion may contribute to half of total airway resistance.

Internal Nose

The internal nose, the *vestibule,* is divided by the bony and cartilaginous *nasal septum.* The septum is rarely perfectly straight, and a significant deviation of the septum at birth or resulting from the birth process or trauma must be assessed to determine whether it interferes with nasal breathing. The perpendicular plate of the nasal septum ossifies by 3 years of age. The anterior portion of the vestibule is lined with vascular squamous epithelium that has tiny hair follicles and secretes mucus. Most nose bleeds, or *epistaxis,* result from a network of small blood vessels found in the anterior superficial portion of the septal mucosa known as the *Kiesselbach plexus.* The posterior portion is lined with fragile respiratory epithelium. The lateral walls of the nose are composed of horizontal bony structures known as the *superior, middle,* and *inferior turbinates,* which mature throughout childhood and resemble those of the adult by 12 years of age (Fig. 12.3). They are covered with vascular mucous membranes. Furrows between the bony structures provide recesses to filter and humidify the air and form a nasal passage, or *meatus.*

The posterior *ethmoid sinuses* drain into the superior meatus, and the *paranasal sinuses* drain into the middle meatus. The inferior meatus is mostly nonfunctioning until approximately 6 years of age, except that it drains the *nasolacrimal duct*. Therefore, the nose has increased drainage in children, particularly during periods of crying or eye irritation. In cases of allergic rhinitis, exposure to allergens recognized by immunoglobulin E (IgE) receptors results in inflammation in the nasopharynx. As a result, the nasal mucosa is pale and may appear blueish in color with edematous nasal turbinates. The space between the posterior portion of the turbinates and the posterior wall of the nasopharynx is called the *choana* and is of little significance in children unless blocked or narrowed by a congenital abnormality such as *choanal atresia*, a bony or membranous blockage of one or both *naris* posterior to the nasal turbinates, resulting in blockage of the airway and respiratory distress in the newborn. Approximately 30% of cases of choanal atresia are bilateral and 70% are unilateral.[3] It occurs in 1 in 5000 to 7000 births and occurs more often in infants assigned female at birth. In newborns, choanal atresia is most commonly associated with the CHARGE syndrome (Coloboma, congenital Heart disease, choanal Atresia, growth Retardation and cognitive delays, Genital hypoplasia, and Ear deformities) and may also be found in Crouzon, frontonasal dysplasia, mandibulofacial dystosis, Pfeiffer, and Treacher Collins syndromes.[4]

Cranial nerve I (olfactory) innervates the nasal area. The *olfactory receptor* cells line the upper reaches of the nasal cavity in the olfactory epithelium and innervate the olfactory nerve. Olfactory learning begins in utero and is well developed in the newborn. It assists newborns in recognizing the distinct smell of their mother's breast milk. Nasal congestion or mucus plugging limits airflow up to the receptors and can block the sensation of smell.

Nasopharynx

The *nasopharynx* forms the superior portion of the pharynx. The *eustachian tube* opening is located along the lateral walls of the nasopharynx (Fig. 12.3). Adenoidal tissue is lymphatic tissue found along the superior posterior wall of the oropharynx and is also referred to as the *pharyngeal tonsils*. The inferior border of the nasopharynx is formed by the soft palate. The nasopharynx is surrounded by bone, ensuring patency unless trauma occurs. In allergic rhinitis, postnasal drip is clear rhinorrhea visible in the posterior oropharynx. Symptoms include an itchy throat, sore throat, frequent swallowing, and/or throat clearing.

Sinuses

The paranasal sinuses consist of paired cavities: maxillary, ethmoid, frontal, and sphenoid sinuses. The *maxillary* and *ethmoid* sinuses are present at birth but are small. The *frontal* sinuses begin to develop by 7 years of age, and the *sphenoid* sinuses develop in adolescence. As the sinuses develop, they become air-filled cavities, and when mature, they are lined with ciliated epithelium-containing goblet cells and submucosal glands that produce mucin glycoproteins and immune mediators. The sinuses reach their final maturity between 12 and 14 years of age (Fig. 12.4; Table 12.2).[5]

Mouth and Oropharynx

The *oral cavity* is composed of the lips, cheeks, hard and soft palates, teeth, posterior pharynx, tongue (Fig. 12.5), sensory cells for taste, and the mandible that supports the lower gums and teeth. The cheeks form the lateral walls that are lined with *buccal mucosa*. Cheeks may be particularly prominent in young children because of the buccal fat pad. The cheeks and lips are innervated by *cranial nerves V (trigeminal)* and *VII (facial)*. The central nervous system controls the complex mechanisms of the mouth needed for sucking, swallowing, breathing, and vocalization. The *hard palate* is the anterior two-thirds of the palate and separates the nasal and oral cavities. The posterior third of the palate is the *soft palate*, which is contiguous with the lateral pharyngeal wall. It provides a slightly mobile barrier between the nasopharynx and oropharynx and is essential for normal articulation and speech intonation. Hyperplastic lymphoid tissue may develop

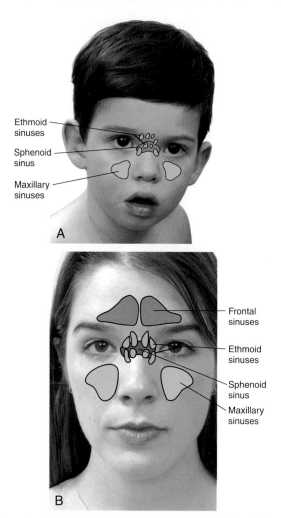

FIGURE 12.4 **(A)** Sinus development in childhood. **(B)** Sinus development in adolescence.

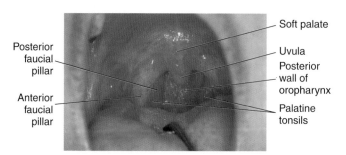

FIGURE 12.5 Anatomy of the posterior oral cavity. (From Fehrenbach M, Herring S. *Illustrated Anatomy of the Head and Neck.* 4th ed. 4, St. Louis: Elsevier; 2012.)

in the posterior oropharynx in children with allergic rhinitis.

Tonsils

The *palatine tonsils* form the anterior and posterior tonsillar pillars. Tonsillar size is graded on a scale of 1+ to 4+ (Table 12.3 and Fig. 12.6). Additional tonsillar tissues surround the posterior pharynx but are not visible on examination. The *uvula* hangs down from the middle of the soft palate in line with the anterior pillar, or *palatoglossus muscle*. A *bifid uvula*, a cleft uvula that is incomplete or completely split into two parts, is an anomaly that results from disruption of the palate development and may indicate a *submucosal cleft palate*. It may also

be associated with nasal polyps. However, nasal polyps are more common in children with cystic fibrosis and nasal allergies.

PEDIATRIC PEARLS

In the infant, the palatine tonsils are not normally visible, but by 2 years of age, they are usually seen extending medially into the oropharynx. They generally are at their peak size between 2 and 6 years of age and then begin to atrophy or decrease in size along with other lymphatic tissue.

Enlarged tonsils and adenoids can partially occlude the posterior pharynx during sleep resulting in sleep-disordered breathing (SDB).

TABLE 12.3	TONSILLAR SIZE
Size	**Description**
1+	Tonsils visible slightly beyond tonsillar pillars
2+	Tonsils visible midway between tonsillar pillars and uvula
3+	Tonsils nearly touching the uvula
4+	Tonsils touching at midline occluding the oropharynx

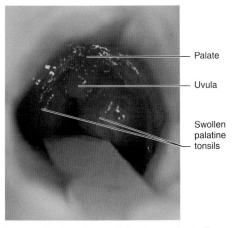

Palate

Uvula

Swollen palatine tonsils

FIGURE 12.6 Enlarged tonsils in child. (From Thibodeau G, Patton K. *The Human Body in Health and Disease*. 5th ed. St. Louis: Mosby; 2010.)

Teeth

The mandibular central incisors are the first to erupt in the majority of infants, followed by the maxillary central incisors, the upper and lower lateral incisors, first molars, cuspids or canine teeth, and then the second molars. Tooth *eruption*, movement of the tooth through alveolar bone and gums, normally occurs between 4 and 12 months of age for the first tooth. *Eruption* occurs once approximately two-thirds of the root for the tooth is developed. The maxillary incisors usually erupt 1 to 2 months after the mandibular incisors. The eruption of the 20 primary teeth should be complete between 24 and 30 months of age (Fig. 12.7A, C). The timing and sequence of tooth eruption depend on genetic, nutritional, environmental, and systemic factors. Delayed eruption of the primary teeth can occur in premature infants, infants who were small for gestational age, infants or children with metabolic or chromosomal abnormalities, or children with severe malnutrition. A familial pattern of delayed tooth eruption can also occur across generations.

The permanent teeth begin developing in the mandible during the first 6 months of life. The period of *eruption* of the *mixed dentition* occurs between 5 and 13 years of age, beginning with the eruption of the first permanent

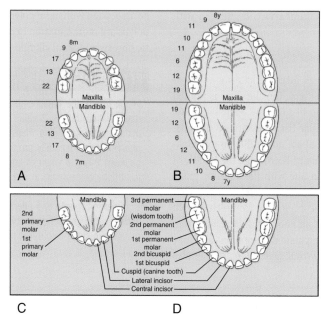

FIGURE 12.7 Ages of tooth eruption. **(A)** Primary dentition of maxilla. **(B)** Permanent dentition. **(C)** Primary dentition of mandible. **(D)** Permanent dentition of mandible. (From Zitelli BJ, McIntire SC, Norwalk AJ, Garrison J. *Zitelli & Davis' Atlas of Pediatric Physical Diagnosis.* 8th ed. Philadelphia: Elsevier; 2023.)

tooth. *Exfoliation*, or loss of the primary dentition, often begins with the central incisors and follows the eruption pattern. There are 32 permanent teeth (Fig. 12.7B, D). Low birth weight, infection, children who do not eat by mouth (due to lack of mastication), and trauma have been associated with delayed eruption of the permanent teeth. Delayed exfoliation of the primary dentition has also been associated with Down syndrome, hypothyroidism, osteogenesis imperfecta, and other congenital endocrine disorders. Dental enamel can be eroded, resulting in structurally weakened teeth in some conditions such as chronic gastroesophageal reflux disease, bulimia, and celiac disease.

Dental caries are the most common chronic health condition in childhood.[6] Nearly a quarter of children aged 2 to 5 years have dental caries in their primary teeth.[6] The infectious process of dental decay begins early in infancy when the cariogenic bacterium *Streptococcus mutans and lactobacilli* can be transmitted from the caregiver to the infant through oral contact in the first few months of life. Ingestion of a high carbohydrate diet and/or frequent dietary sugars in infants and children provides a substrate for the bacteria to flourish and alters the oral bacterial composition, enhancing the development of dental caries.[6] In addition, health inequities that affects access to dental care, fluoride exposure, and oral hygiene practices can negatively impact dental health.

Tongue

The *tongue* is a mobile muscle, with its anterior two-thirds located in the oral cavity and the posterior one-third located in the oropharynx. The anterior dorsal surface of the tongue is composed of a thick mucous membrane lined with *filiform*, or threadlike, papillae, and the posterior dorsal surface is lined with lymphoid tissue that forms the *lingual tonsil*. The ventral surface of the tongue has a thin mucous membrane with visible vessels and is normally anchored to the floor of the mouth by the *lingual frenulum* (Fig. 12.8).

Cranial nerves IX (glossopharyngeal) and X (vagus) innervate the tongue for sensation and taste, and cranial nerve XII (hypoglossal) innervates the tongue for motor function. The sensation of taste is immature at birth and not fully functional until approximately 2 years of age.

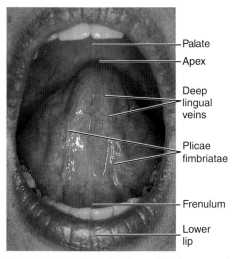

FIGURE 12.8 Ventral surface of the tongue and salivary glands. (From Fehrenbach M, Herring S. *Illustrated Anatomy of the Head and Neck*. 4th ed. St. Louis: Elsevier; 2012.)

Term infants also have a *tongue-thrust reflex* for the first 4 months of life that aids in breast-feeding or bottle-feeding and to protect them from choking, but it is counterproductive when trying to feed solids by spoon. Tongue thrusts with feedings by spoon or while drinking from an open cup can be seen in children with a history of oral aversion and feeding difficulties. At the base of the tongue in the oropharynx lies the *epiglottis*, a glistening pink spoon-shaped appendage that helps direct the passage of food into the esophagus and away from the trachea (Fig. 12.9). *Laryngomalacia*, the most common congenital anomaly of the larynx, is the inappropriate or impaired function of the epiglottis due to redundant or floppy tissue that impairs the infant's ability to breathe or swallow safely. Laryngomalacia accounts for 60% to 70% of cases of stridor, due to turbulent airflow through a stenotic upper airway.[7,8] In the child that is sleeping and growing well, the issue will self-resolve within the first 12 to 24 months of life. In the child with sleep disordered breathing, feeding difficulties, and concern for failure to thrive, surgical intervention with a pediatric otolaryngologist is often required.

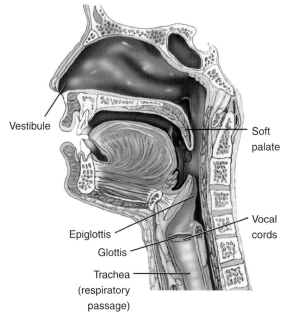

FIGURE 12.9 Sagittal view of mouth and oropharynx.

Salivary Glands

The *salivary glands* are paired exocrine glands that secrete enzymes that aid in initial digestion. The *parotid glands* are the largest salivary glands and are the glands that become inflamed with *mumps*, or *parotitis*. Parotitis, after mumps, is the second most common childhood disease of the salivary glands globally.[9] The *parotid duct*, or *Stensen duct*, empties into the oral cavity opposite the upper second molar. The *submandibular gland* is the second largest gland and is located on the floor of the mouth. The *submandibular ducts*, or *Wharton ducts*, exit into the mouth on either side of the lingual frenulum. The third set of salivary glands is the *sublingual glands*, which release their enzymes through approximately 12 ducts located on the floor of the mouth. The sublingual glands are not visible on examination. Secretions from the salivary glands begin around 6 weeks of age in the term infant, which results in increased drooling by 3 to 4 months of age. As infants mature and become more proficient in swallowing and the lower teeth develop to create a dam, the drooling decreases even though the production of saliva increases. Hundreds of additional salivary glands line the mucous membranes of the mouth and oral pharynx by late adolescence, providing additional serous and mucous secretions.

SYSTEM-SPECIFIC HISTORY

The Information Gathering table presents essential information to gather for different ages and developmental stages when assessing the nose, mouth, and throat.

INFORMATION GATHERING FOR ASSESSING THE NOSE, MOUTH, AND THROAT AT KEY DEVELOPMENTAL STAGES

Age Group	Information to Gather
Preterm and newborn	History of exposure to prenatal infection, including TORCH infections? Exposure to prenatal drug use?
	Perinatal exposure to infection?
	Any difficulty sucking, feeding? Difficulty breathing through nose?
	Is there difficulty with movement of the tongue?
	Any natal teeth or lesions in mouth?
Infancy	Any nasal discharge? Any difficulty sucking, feeding, introducing solid foods?
	Any sores, white patches, or bleeding in mouth?
	Have any teeth erupted? Use of sugar-sweetened beverages in bottle? Is infant on fluoride supplement or is water fluoridated?
	Plans for weaning from breast or bottle?
	Does infant habitually put objects in mouth? Use pacifier or suck thumb or fingers? How frequently?
Early childhood	Does child have difficulty eating solid foods? Does the child have strong food preferences or known food allergies? Does the child use a bottle for milk or juice?
	Does the child put objects in their mouth or nose?
	Are there any concerns about child's speech? Does child's speech have a nasal or congested resonance?
	History of frequent nasal congestion, chronic rhinorrhea, asthma, atopic conditions, itchy throat, sore throat, or tonsillitis? Does the child snore or gasp for breathing during sleep? Have restless sleep patterns? Complain of being tired during the day?

INFORMATION GATHERING FOR ASSESSING THE NOSE, MOUTH, AND THROAT AT KEY DEVELOPMENTAL STAGES—CONT'D

Age Group	Information to Gather
	Has child had nose injuries? Does child put fingers or objects in nose? Recurrent nose bleeds?
	Does child suck a digit or pacifier?
	Does child attend childcare or preschool?
	Age at first dental visit? Recent application of fluoride varnish? Does child brush teeth with parental assistance? Does the child have any missing or injured teeth?
	History of trauma to mouth or gums?
Middle childhood	Any mouth or nose injuries?
	History of frequent nasal congestion, chronic rhinorrhea, asthma, atopic conditions, itchy throat, sore throat, throat clearing, or tonsillitis?
	Any complaints of itchy nose and/or throat? Are symptoms triggered by environmental exposures or changes in season?
	Does child snore or gasp during sleep? Have restless or interrupted sleep pattern? Complain of being tired during the day?
	Has child had nose injuries? Does child put fingers or objects in nose? Recurrent nose bleeds?
	Any known exposure to Group A Streptococcal infection? Has child had a documented GABHS pharyngitis? Other pharyngeal infections?
	Routine dental care? Does child brush and floss? Are teeth aligned properly or is a referral needed for orthodontia?
	Has child had any teeth extracted? Tonsils or adenoids removed?
	Does child participate in competitive contact sports? Wear a mouth guard?
Adolescence	Any injuries to mouth or nose? Recurrent nose bleeds?
	Does adolescent play competitive contact sports? Do they wear a mouth guard?
	History of frequent nasal congestion, chronic rhinorrhea, asthma, atopic conditions, itchy throat, sore throat, throat clearing, or tonsillitis?
	Any complaints of itchy nose and/or throat? Are symptoms triggered by environmental exposures or changes in season?
	Does adolescent snore or gasp during sleep? Have restless sleep? Complain of being tired during the day? Have tonsils or adenoids been removed?
	Has adolescent had previous documented GABHS infections or recently been exposed to Group A Streptococcal infection? Other pharyngeal infections?
	History of oral sex? Are there any oral piercings? Oral lesions/sores?
	Routine dental care, brushing, flossing? Dental braces or orthodontic appliances? Teeth removed or lost due to injury?
	Tobacco or recreational drug use, including vaping, inhalants, or snorted powders?
Environmental risks	Exposure to household tobacco smoke, vaping or recreational drug use? Recreational activities or sports with increased risk of injury to mouth or nose?
	Exposure to potential allergens such as animal hair, pests, mold, pollens, or dust?

GABHS, Group A beta-hemolytic streptococci; *TORCH*, toxoplasmosis, other diseases (syphilis), rubella, cytomegalovirus, herpes simplex virus.

Physical Assessment

Equipment

Equipment needed for examination of the nose, mouth, and throat includes an otoscope with halogen light and speculum, tongue depressor, and gloves for palpation of palate and gums when indicated.

Positioning

Delay the examination of the mouth and nose in the infant and young child until after the "quiet" parts of the exam and the ear examination. If the infant or young child cries, attempt to visualize the mouth and oropharynx with an otoscope halogen light and a tongue depressor. Infants are best positioned on the examination table with the head stabilized to visualize the internal nose and mouth (Fig. 12.10). Examination of the older infant or young child can also occur while the child is sitting in the parent's or caregiver's lap with the head secured by the examiner and the child's arms secured by the parent. The feet may need to be secured between the parent's legs if the child is uncooperative. With the young child on the examination table, the parent may also secure the arms above the head to stabilize the head and visualize the oropharynx.

An alternative position for conducting the inspection of the teeth is to place the child in the "knee-to-knee" position. In this position, the examiner and parent sit face to face with their knees touching to make a comfortable support for the young infant, and the infant or young child's head is placed in the examiners lap to look directly into the child's mouth (Fig. 12.11). This position is best used for examining the teeth and applying fluoride varnish in the older infant and young child.

External Nose

While the child is comfortable, note any flaring or narrowing of the nares with breathing. If an infant is feeding or sleeping, watch carefully for indications of nasal obstruction requiring mouth breathing. Note the shape of the nose, any obvious deviation of the nasal bridge or columella, and the tip of the nose. Older children with chronic nasal drainage such as in allergic rhinitis may present with the *allergic salute* sign—a transverse crease across the nose or nasal bridge caused by repeated upward swipes with the hand. If there is drainage from the nose, note the color, consistency, and quantity and whether it is unilateral or bilateral. Swelling or dark discoloration under the eyes, often called *allergic shiners*, may occur with nasal congestion, *sinusitis*, or nasal allergy. Allergic conditions and upper respiratory infections cause bilateral drainage,

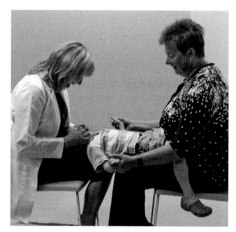

FIGURE   12.11 Knee-to-knee position for dental assessment. (From Clark C. Open mouth, open mind: expanding the role of primary care nurse practitioners. *J Pediatr Health Care.* 2015; 30(5):480–488.)

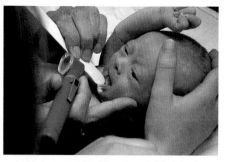

FIGURE   12.10 Position for stabilizing child's head for oral examination. (From iStock)

whereas foreign objects in the nose can cause unilateral, purulent, malodorous discharge. Sinus infections also may cause unilateral drainage. *Epistaxis*—bleeding or hemorrhage from the nose—occurs from irritation of the nasal mucosa, often due to cold, dry environmental conditions, nasal allergy, or as a result of trauma.

Palpate any areas around the nose that appear discolored or inflamed. If there is a history of facial trauma, palpate the bridge of the nose to determine tenderness or pain. If the child has a recent history of head or facial trauma and clear watery nasal discharge, a cerebrospinal fluid leak must be considered and confirmed with imaging. Traumatic fractures of the protective facial bones increase the risk of developing meningitis. Children with obvious deviation of the nose should be referred to a craniofacial specialist for evaluation. Patency of each side of the nose can be determined by placing a tissue in front of one naris at a time while you occlude the other naris. If there is movement of airflow on the nonobstructed side, the tissue will move, confirming patency. In the newborn, this technique assists in diagnosis of choanal atresia; minimal movement may indicate choanal stenosis or blockage in the nasal passage, while absence of movement indicates choanal atresia.

Internal Nose

To inspect the internal nose, use a penlight or otoscope with halogen light and nasal speculum while being careful not to touch the sensitive internal nasal septum (Fig. 12.12). A large ear speculum can be inserted 2 to 3 mm into the nares in older children and adolescents for inspection of the nasal cavity but is not recommended in infants and young children, to avoid trauma. The nares are best visualized in infants and young children who are positioned on the exam table or on the parent's lap.

The vestibule of the nose should be assessed for any blockage by foreign body, polyps, nasal secretions, mucous plugs, or dried blood. The mucosal lining should be assessed for

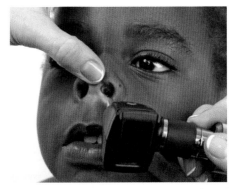

FIGURE 12.12 View of the nasal vestibule and turbinates.

consistency of color, abrasions, lesions, and swelling. The color is normally deep pink, and a thin layer of clear mucus gives it a shiny appearance. The nasal septum should be examined for alignment, perforations, abrasions, bleeding, or crusting. It should be relatively straight and midline in the nose. Significant deviations of the septum may interfere with breathing. The turbinates should be assessed for color and swelling. Pale, swollen mucosa and edema of the turbinates is associated with allergic rhinitis and occlusion of air passage. Inflamed, reddened mucosa and turbinates is associated with respiratory infections. Children with chronic respiratory conditions may develop polyps that appear as shiny sacs extending into the nasal vestibule.

If a foreign body is suspected, attempt to have the child blow out the object while occluding the unaffected side. If this is not successful in dislodging the object, securely position the child on the exam table for removal of the object. In a cooperative child, a gentle probe with a curette or tweezers can be attempted to dislodge the foreign body. If unsuccessful and the object has become adhered to the mucosal wall or nasal septum, refer to a pediatric otolaryngologist for removal.

Sinuses

The maxillary and frontal sinuses can be assessed by physical examination beginning around 7 years of age through inspection and palpation. The facial area over the maxillary and frontal sinuses should be evaluated for swelling, erythema, and tenderness. Percuss with the forefingers or apply mild pressure with the thumbs over the maxillary and frontal sinus area (Fig. 12.13). Evaluate pain, tenderness, and increased sensation in the frontal, ethmoid, or maxillary area, especially if there is a history of prolonged upper respiratory infection. It may be difficult for young school-age children to accurately determine increased pain or tenderness caused by sinus inflammation; therefore, relying on accurate health history and symptom assessment is important in this age group. The diagnosis of sinusitis in children is generally made clinically. Imaging studies are not recommended unless children are unresponsive to medical therapy, develop complications of rhinosinusitis (RS), or who are being considered for surgical intervention.[2]

Mouth

While inspecting the oral cavity, observe for the presence of any unusual odor or lesions. Inspect the lips for color, symmetry, lesions, swelling, dryness, and fissures. The color should be pink at rest and with feeding or crying. Note any asymmetry of movement or drooling that might indicate nerve impairment. Drooling during infancy from 3 to 15 months of age is normal, but drooling later may indicate nerve damage and loss of control of oral secretions. In contrast, poor saliva production in the setting of swelling of one or both parotid glands is concerning for parotitis. Juvenile parotitis usually first presents between 3 to 6 years of age and can become recurrent, and is more common in males.[9] Symptoms include parotid swelling, pain, and fever that last up to 1 week with asymptomatic periods in between episodes. Inspect for skin changes over the gland, facial asymmetry, and facial nerve function. Violaceous skin change may indicate an atypical mycobacterial infection. Perform bimanual palpation of the glands and attempt to express saliva from Stensen's duct. Expressed saliva is typically nonsuppurative but there may be mucous plugs. A painless parotid mass may suggest neoplasm.

Young infants may have a callus or blister on the lip from vigorous sucking (Fig. 12.14). This is particularly common in breastfed infants in the first few months of life. Swelling of the lips may be caused by injury or allergic reaction. Cracked, dry lips can be caused by harsh weather conditions, repeated lip licking or biting, mouth breathing due to nasal allergy, fever, illness, or dehydration. Erythematous papules or erythematous ulcerating vesicles in the mouth or on the lips may indicate a viral infection such as *Coxsackie virus* or *herpes simplex virus* type

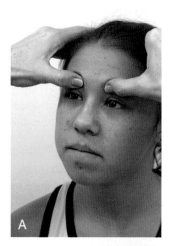
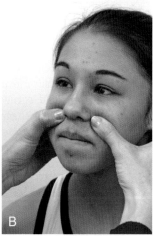

FIGURE 12.13 **(A)** Palpation of ethmoid sinuses. **(B)** Palpation of the maxillary sinuses.

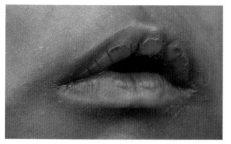

FIGURE 12.14 **Sucking blister.**

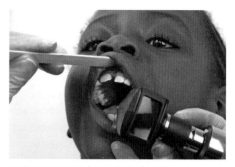

FIGURE 12.15 Inspection of teeth and gums in an older child.

1, respectively. *Halitosis*, mouth odor or bad breath, in children may be caused by poor oral hygiene and dental caries, tonsillitis, or sinusitis. Note the frenulum of the upper lip that connects the upper lip to the gums of the maxilla at the point of the central incisors. It is prominent in the infant and disappears slowly in childhood with growth and development of the maxilla. Trauma to the upper lip and gum in the young child often includes trauma to the frenulum.

Use a tongue blade or tongue depressor to inspect the buccal mucosa and gingivae for color, moisture, symmetry, and lesions (Fig. 12.15). The mucosa is typically shiny, smooth, and moist throughout. The oral mucosa may appear pale in children with darker-pigmented skin and pink in children with lighter-pigmented skin. Use a tongue depressor or a gloved finger to move the tongue and lips to ensure all surfaces of the mucosa are inspected. *Epstein pearls*, white pearly papules at the juncture of the hard and soft palates or on the anterior surface of the buccal mucosa, are common in newborns and resolve spontaneously. With a gloved finger, palpate unusual-looking areas for swelling and tenderness. If the mucosa of the gum in an infant or young child appears inflamed or swollen, palpate for erupting teeth or hematomas. Inspect the maxillary gums for a *cleft alveolus*, incomplete formation or complete absence of the gum, often seen in children with cleft lip and palate. An *eruption cyst or eruption hematoma* is a bluish-purple, blister-like swelling on the gum, which may precede tooth eruption, particularly with the first and second molars. Reddened, swollen, or

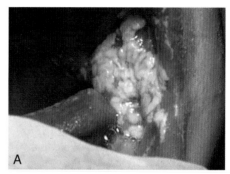

A

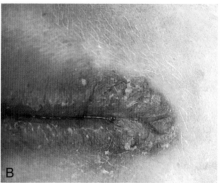

B

FIGURE 12.16 **(A)** Candidiasis of oral mucosa. **(B)** Candidiasis of lip. (From Zitelli BJ, McIntire SC, Norwalk AJ, Garrison J. *Zitelli and Davis' Atlas of Pediatric Physical Diagnosis*. 8th ed. Philadelphia: Elsevier; 2023.)

friable gums can be an indication of poor oral hygiene, infection, or poor nutritional intake. Anticonvulsants may also cause hyperplasia of the gums.

Candidiasis, appearing as bright white superficial lesions on the tongue, gums, and buccal mucosa of the cheeks, is often seen in the young, breastfed infant or in the infant or child after use of oral antibiotics or with chronic infection (Fig. 12.16A, B). The lesions of candidiasis can be differentiated from milk or formula residue by the bright white appearance. *Candidiasis lesions* do not scrape off the oral mucosa with the tongue depressor. *Petechiae*, pinpoint erythematous lesions may be present on the soft palate with streptococcal infections or may be indicative of a bleeding disorder.

Teeth

Inspect and note the number, color, size, and shape of the primary and permanent teeth and the pattern of eruption (Fig. 12.17). *Natal teeth* are prematurely erupted primary teeth that are present at birth. The incidence of natal teeth is approximately 1 in 2000 births and is often seen in infants with cleft palate and other chromosomal deletion syndromes.[10] *Neonatal teeth* erupt in the first month of life, and 90% of neonatal teeth are lower primary teeth, or *mandibular incisors*.[10] Both natal and neonatal teeth are often immature caps of enamel and dentine with poorly formed roots and are unstable in the gum or attached to the gum. Although rare, natal teeth can be a risk of aspiration in the neonatal period. If the teeth are supernumerary, very loose, or cause feeding problems, consultation with a pediatric dentist and extraction may be indicated.[10] Precocious eruption of primary teeth has been associated with precocious puberty.[11]

Inspection of the teeth in infants and young children includes identifying any presence of plaque and caries on the teeth. Check the primary teeth in the infant and young child for *white spot* lesions, or decalcifications, and *brown spot* lesions, or cavitations, indicating the first sign of dental decay (Fig. 12.18A, B). White spot lesions on the anterior tooth surfaces may be a sign of *early childhood caries*. They are caused by early transmission of the bacterium *S. mutans* from parent or caretaker to child and intake of frequent dietary sugars reducing the normal pH of oral secretions, resulting in demineralization of the tooth enamel. The mandibular incisors in infants are protected by the tongue when sucking and therefore are not prone to decay with prolonged bottle-feeding

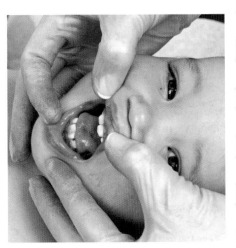

FIGURE 12.17 Inspection of primary teeth.

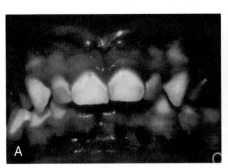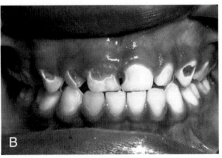

FIGURE 12.18 **(A)** White spot lesions. **(B)** Brown spot lesions. (Courtesy Dr. Francisco Ramos-Gomez, University of California, Los Angeles.)

BOX 12.1   HIGH RISK FOR DENTAL CARIES BETWEEN 6 MONTHS TO 5 YEARS OF AGE

- Primary caregiver has active cavities (family oral health history)
- Decreased or absent oral hygiene practices
- Limited fluoride exposure
- Child has more than three sugary snacks or beverages between meals
- Child is put to bed with bottle containing natural or added sugar
- Child with special health care needs
- Health inequities that affects access to preventive dental care.

Adapted from American Academy of Pediatric Dentistry. Guidelines on caries-risk assessment and management for infants, children, and adolescents. *Pediatr Dent.* 2015/2016; 35(5):E157–E164.

---

or breastfeeding. Dental care should commence as soon as teeth erupt, and daily oral hygiene using a damp cloth or soft infant toothbrush to gently rub the gums and teeth of the infant can prevent plaque development. In older infants and young children, teeth should be brushed at least twice daily with fluoridated toothpaste under parental supervision.

Caries risk assessment is an important component of the assessment of the oral cavity in all children. The US Preventive Task Force recommends establishing a dental home with a comprehensive dental assessment by eruption of the first tooth or 12 months of age.[6] Box 12.1 assists health care providers in assessing children from 6 months to 5 years of age who are at high risk for development of dental decay.[12] Access to a pediatric dental home and application of dental sealants improves oral health outcomes and reduces the incidence of dental caries. Fluoridated drinking water and application of topical fluoride varnish by pediatric health care providers also help to reduce the incidence of early childhood caries.[6,13] Children with special health care needs may be at high risk for dental caries because of oral aversion, oral side effects of medications or special diets, and the child's ability/inability to participate in daily oral hygiene.

Maxillary permanent incisors may erupt widely spaced and protruding outward, and mandibular incisors may erupt behind the primary incisors but align with normal development of the oral cavity unless there is a familial pattern of malocclusion or dental deformities. A slight overlap of the maxillary incisors to the mandibular incisors occurs with normal permanent dentition. Children with significantly misaligned teeth should be referred to a pediatric orthodontist for evaluation and treatment. *Bruxism*, or tooth grinding, which induces moderate wear on the surface of the canines and molars, may be noted on inspection. The peak incidence of bruxism is during the developmental period of mixed dentition. Bruxism rarely damages the dentition in young children but may be significant in older children or children with special health care needs.

EVIDENCE-BASED PRACTICE TIP

Application of fluoride varnish by the pediatric health care provider to the primary teeth beginning in the first year of life are recommended to prevent dental caries. Two or more applications of fluoride varnish per year is effective in preventing caries in infants and children at high-risk for dental disease.[6]

Tongue

Inspect the tongue, noting color, size, and movement. The dorsal surface should appear slightly rough but moist and pink to pale pink. There may be variation in the papillae, giving the dorsal surface a patterned appearance. *Geographic tongue*, a benign inflammation of the dorsal surface of the tongue, causes pink or red

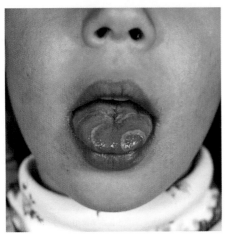

FIGURE 12.19 Geographic tongue. (From Zitelli BJ, McIntire SC, Norwalk AJ, Garrison, J: *Zitelli and Davis' Atlas of Pediatric Physical Diagnosis*, ed 8, Philadelphia, 2023, Elsevier.)

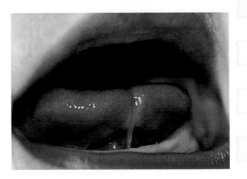

FIGURE 12.20 Ankyloglossia; short lingual frenulum. (Reprinted from Henry L, Hayman R. Ankyloglossia and its impact on breastfeeding. *Nurs Womens Health*. 2014:18(2) with permission from Elsevier.)

areas with absent papillae and a surrounding whitish border (Fig. 12.19).

The ventral surface of the tongue appears thin with prominent vessels without hematomas. Connecting the ventral surface of the tongue to the floor of the mouth is the *lingual frenulum*. The lingual frenulum should allow movement of the tongue past the lips and to the roof of the palate. Movement of the tongue can be assessed through observation while an infant cries or a child vocalizes. Infants who can breastfeed or bottle-feed without difficulty have adequate movement of the tongue, and no further assessment of *cranial nerve XII (hypoglossal)* is needed. Newborns with significant feeding problems should be referred to a pediatric otolaryngologist and a speech or occupational therapist trained and experienced in neonatal feeding problems. A significantly shortened lingual frenulum, *ankyloglossia*, is caused by attachment of the frenulum to the anterior tip of the tongue causing limited tongue mobility (Fig. 12.20). There is no consensus on the definition of posterior ankyloglossia, which is a shortened lingual frenulum that is *near* the tip of the tongue. In some cases,

it may interfere with adequate latch and sucking in the newborn and impair the infant's ability to breastfeed. The diagnosis of ankyloglossia has increased exponentially with an incidence of 2.8% to 10.7% due to the widening definition of ankyloglossia.[14] Surgical intervention may be indicated in some infants and children. A *frenulotomy* or *frenulectomy* is the surgical procedure in which the lingual frenulum is cut. A frenulectomy does not always relieve maternal pain with breastfeeding or improve breastfeeding difficulties.[14] This surgical procedure remains controversial, particularly in relation to later speech development. Data has been insufficient on nonbreastfeeding outcomes.[15] Consultation with a speech pathologist is recommending prior to undergoing the procedure for speech concerns. A frenulectomy is contraindicated in infants with retrognathia, micrognathia, neuromuscular disorders, and coagulopathy.

Macroglossia, an enlarged tongue, can be congenital or acquired and is associated with hypothyroidism, Down syndrome, Beckwith-Wiedemann syndrome, and other congenital anomalies. This is different from *glossoptosis*, the collapse of the tongue base against the posterior pharyngeal wall causing tongue-based obstruction. *Pierre Robin* sequence is associated with glossoptosis, micrognathia, feeding and breathing difficulty, and a high arched or cleft palate. *Micrognathia*, a small jaw or mandible, can be associated with congenital craniofacial anomalies, genetic conditions, or small for gestational age infant and may be associated with feeding and breathing problems.

In the older child and adolescent, ask the child to stick the tongue out past the lips and move the tongue from side to side to test *cranial nerve XII (hypoglossal)*. These maneuvers should be easy to perform without fasciculation of the tongue. The ability to curl the tongue is a hereditary trait in some children. Any lesions, areas of tenderness, or swelling should be palpated to determine the size and depth.

Palate

Inspect the hard palate for openings or lesions in the roof of the mouth. It should appear dome shaped but not deeply indented, lighter in appearance than the skin on the buccal mucosa and soft palate and have transverse firm ridges. In a newborn infant with jaundice, the hard palate appears yellowish. In darker-pigmented infants and children, it is helpful to inspect the hard palate and sclera to assess for jaundice. The hard palate is contiguous with the soft palate and extends to the anterior pillars and the uvula. The soft palate should appear intact and rise symmetrically along with the uvula when the child vocalizes or says "ah." This movement tests for *cranial nerve X (vagus)*. Movement of the soft palate is necessary for the development of normal speech and articulation.

The hard and soft palates should always be palpated in the newborn to determine whether there is any submucosal cleft not visible on inspection or congenital anomalies associated with cleft palate. A gloved finger can be placed on the infant's palate to determine whether the palate is intact. As the infant sucks, evaluate the strength of the suck reflex and the palate surface. After the newborn period, palpation of the palate is not usually performed unless lesions, swelling, or erythema is noted.

Tonsils

Inspect the palatine tonsils for size, color, exudates, pitting or enlarged crypts, or membranous covering. The tonsils are normally the color of the buccal mucosa or slightly lighter, should appear equal in size and position, and should be rated on a scale of 1+ to 4+ during well visits and during periods of illness to evaluate change (Table 12.3). Tonsils that are larger than normal may indicate chronic respiratory allergies, and if reddened indicate infection. White or yellowish exudate in the crypts of the tonsils in the presence of fever or other signs of illness is often associated with bacterial *tonsillitis* or *infectious mononucleosis* and requires further diagnosis and treatment. Unequal size tonsils and color may indicate a *peritonsillar abscess*, requiring further diagnostics, antibacterial therapy, and possible hospitalization. Pitting or enlarged crypts of the tonsils are often seen in children with a history of recurrent throat infections or chronic respiratory allergies (Fig. 12.21). The exact cause and pathogenesis of tonsilloliths, or tonsil stones, is unknown. Tonsil stones are a combination of calcified epithelium, food debris, and bacteria that form in tonsil crypts. Tonsil stones are hard and vary in shape, size, and color. History may include recurrent tonsilitis, sore throat, halitosis, odynophagia, foreign body sensation, or tonsillar hypertrophy.

Some children and adolescents have chronically enlarged tonsils and adenoids that

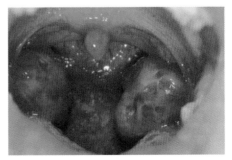

FIGURE 12.21   Large cryptic tonsils. (From Lemmi FO, Lemmi CAE. *Physical Assessment Findings Multiuser CD-ROM*. St. Louis: Saunders; 2000.)

partially block air passage in and out of the oropharynx. During sleep, relaxation of the pharyngeal musculature exacerbates the occlusion of the air passages, resulting in obstruction of airflow and *sleep-disordered breathing (SDB)* and may result in *obstructive sleep apnea (OSA)*. The pediatric health care provider should obtain a health history regarding the child's sleep, sleep pattern, and the occurrence of snoring and apnea. Children with SDB often breathe with their mouth open during sleep to enlarge the air passageway, and dry, cracked lips are a hallmark sign of chronically enlarged tonsils in children.

Sleep-related breathing disorders impact the duration and quality of sleep and have been associated with nasal allergy, craniofacial anomalies, neurologic disorders, laryngomalacia or tracheomalacia, tonsillar hypertrophy, and childhood obesity. In children, the prevalence of OSA is 1.2% to 5.7%.[16] OSA causes comorbid conditions such as growth retardation, enuresis, and chronic morning headaches. Daytime fatigue and inattention related to OSA may impact school performance and have been associated with hyperactivity and behavioral problems[16] Refer the child to a pediatric otolaryngologist if there is a concern for OSA.

The two leading indications for adenotonsillectomy are sleep-disordered breathing and recurrent *throat infections*, a viral or bacterial infection of the pharynx, tonsils, or both.[15] Throat infections are deemed recurrent if they are frequent (seven episodes in the past year, five episodes in the past 2 years, or three episodes per year for the last 3 years), with a documented fever (temperature >38.3°C), cervical lymphadenopathy, tonsillar exudate, or positive group A beta-hemolytic streptococcus test.

Vocalization

Vocalization and speech patterns in infants and children should also be assessed. A high-pitched cry in the newborn or young infant may indicate increased intracranial pressure, stridor may indicate *laryngomalacia*, and a hoarse cry in infants with upper respiratory infection may indicate *croup* or *laryngitis*.

Hoarseness in the neonatal period may be associated with congenital anomalies or a laryngeal hemangioma. In children, prolonged hoarseness should be investigated to determine the etiology that includes acute or chronic infection, benign lesions of the vocal cord folds, gastroesophageal reflux disease, and psychogenic causes. Prolonged unintelligible speech may indicate a speech articulation problem, expressive language delay, cognitive delay, or a hearing problem and should be promptly evaluated and referred for early intervention. Intelligible speech is critical for early success in school and socialization. Evaluation of speech and language delay and initiating speech therapy should not be delayed in hopes that the child will outgrow the problem. See Chapter 3 for further discussion on important developmental milestones for speech and language development and Chapter 11 for hearing assessment.

NOSE, MOUTH, AND THROAT CONDITIONS

Table 12.4 presents abnormal infectious conditions of the mouth and throat in infants, children, and adolescents.

Among children with a viral upper respiratory tract infection, 5% to 13% may progress to acute rhinosinusitis (RS).[17] A portion will develop chronic RS. Symptoms include nasal congestion, nasal discharge that can be clear, mucoid, thick or thin, low-grade fever, irritability, cough, halitosis, and rarely headache, a cardinal sign of sinusitis in adults. Acute bacterial RS should be suspected when symptoms persist beyond 10 days or if there is purulent rhinorrhea for 3 to 4 consecutive days with fever of 39°C or above. RS is defined as chronic if the child has at least two symptoms, purulent rhinorrhea, nasal obstruction, facial pressure/pain, or cough for 90 days consecutively. Since RS usually has a viral origin, no antibiotics should be prescribed, and rarely are nasal decongestants indicated. The consensus on management of acute bacterial RS in children is treatment with antibiotics.[18]

TABLE 12.4	CONDITIONS OF THE MOUTH AND THROAT
Condition	**Descriptions**
Aphthous ulcers	Round to oval lesions with an erythematous halo appearing on buccal mucosa of cheeks, also known as "canker sores." May be painful and associated with fever and pharyngitis. Often resolve spontaneously within 1 week.
Epiglottitis	Edema and inflammation of epiglottis resulting in occlusion of trachea and acute respiratory distress; a medical emergency that may require intubation and radiographs for confirmation of diagnosis; avoid exam of oropharynx; incidence has decreased 80%–90% in children due to vaccine coverage with *Haemophilus influenzae* vaccine.
Gingivostomatitis	Vesicular lesions of lips, tongue, gingivae, oral mucosa resulting in swollen, painful, friable gums; common between 6 months and 3 years of age preceded by fever and irritability. Most often associated with herpes simplex type 1 or post coxsackievirus. Treatment focused on symptom management and prevention of dehydration.
Herpangina (coxsackievirus Groups A and B)	Small vesicles on posterior pharynx, tonsils, soft palate that rupture to form ulcers; occurs in young children with onset of sore throat, fever, malaise. Caused by coxsackievirus Group A. Treatment focused on symptom management and prevention of dehydration.
Mononucleosis	Enlarged tonsils, general malaise, fatigue, lymphadenopathy, splenomegaly usually caused by Epstein-Barr virus (EBV) but can be caused by other organisms such as cytomegalovirus (CMV); confirmed by EBV antibody testing.
Mucoceles	Fluid-filled cavities extending from mucous glands lining the epithelium of oral mucosa. May be associated with mild oral trauma frequently on lower lip. Spontaneous rupture usually occurs with resolution of lesion.
Streptococcal pharyngitis	GABHS pharyngotonsillitis is acute in onset and characterized by high fever, palpable cervical lymphadenopathy, sore throat, headache, and abdominal pain.

GABHS, Group A beta-hemolytic streptococci.

Although the most common etiology for pharyngotonsillitis is viral infection, group A beta-hemolytic streptococci (GABHS) is the most common bacteria associated with pharyngotonsillitis in children and the only indication to treat a "sore throat" with antibiotics. "Strep throat," the common term used for GABHS pharyngitis, peaks in winter and spring, and transmission occurs through spread of droplets. Symptom history may reveal a household contact with similar symptoms or a diagnosed strep throat. Children and adolescents with prior history of GABHS are more susceptible to repeat infection. Signs and symptoms of GABHS pharyngitis are acute in onset and characterized by high fever, palpable cervical lymphadenopathy, sore throat, headache, and abdominal pain, sometimes with nausea and vomiting. Pharyngeal and tonsillar mucosa are typically erythematous with exudate present in 50% to 90% of cases.[2] A rapid antigen detection test (RADT) with confirmative throat culture is necessary to accurately diagnose GABHS.

Although symptoms will resolve within a few days without treatment, early treatment with penicillin (preferred) or amoxicillin, cephalosporins, macrolides, or clindamycin has effectively eradicated the infection and is presumed to prevent sequelae, including rheumatic fever. The incidence of rheumatic carditis is 0.3% in endemic environments. Acute glomerulonephritis is a sequela of a specific nephritogenic strain of GABHS, and 10% to 15% of people infected with this strain of GABHS will develop acute glomerulonephritis regardless of treatment.[2]

TELEHEALTH TIPS

In situations where a telehealth visit is appropriate, it should mirror an office visit in order to guide clinical decision-making.[19,20] Discuss the chief complaint, followed by an assessment and plan. Voice quality is assessed at the start of the visit when there is dialogue between the provider and the child. In infants and young children, voice quality can be assessed with cooing, babbling, or crying. The child should be in a room with an adequate light source so that you can begin with an inspection. Inspect all external anatomy of the face, submandibular area, and neck as you would in an in-person visit. Due to the limitation of current technology, the nasal exam is limited to external inspection. Inspection of the mouth and oropharynx depends on an adequate light source and the child's ability to open their mouth wide. Instruct the caregiver or adolescent to position the light source towards the mouth. Have the caregiver or child use a finger on each side of the mouth to retract the lips and cheek to get a better view of the teeth and gums. Assess cranial nerve function and the ability of the tongue to reach the lower lips and/or roof of the mouth (for ankyloglossia). Examination of the oropharynx in the infant or young child may require a tongue depressor that can be used to depress the tongue.[19] For the older child or adolescent that needs assistance repositioning their tongue, the back of a spoon can be used if a tongue depressor is not available.

In a clinic setting, inspection is followed by palpation. Since the provider is not with the patient, the caregiver and child are encouraged to actively participate in their care. Whether it's an adult caregiver or an adolescent performing a self-exam, the provider needs to ensure that the maneuvers are performed correctly. Instruct the caregiver to palpate over the forehead and cheekbone area for tenderness (sinusitis). Have the caregiver or adolescent patient palpate the submandibular gland for tenderness and swelling (parotitis).

SUMMARY OF EXAMINATION

- In the infant, inspect for patency of nares and note any flaring or narrowing of the nares with breathing.
- An otoscope with halogen light is often used without a speculum to externally visualize the nares in infants and young children.
- Maxillary and ethmoid sinuses are present at birth but are small; the frontal sinuses begin to develop by 7 years of age and the sphenoid sinuses develop in adolescence.
- Percuss with the forefingers or apply mild pressure with the thumbs over the maxillary and frontal sinus area to evaluate tenderness.
- The cheeks and lips are innervated by cranial nerves V (trigeminal) and VII (facial).
- Inspect the lips for color, symmetry, lesions, swelling, dryness, and fissures.
- Delay the examination of the mouth and nose in the infant and young child until after the "quiet" parts of the exam and after the ear examination.
- Inspect the buccal mucosa and gingivae with a tongue depressor for color, moisture, symmetry, and lesions.
- Inspect for tonsillar size and quality. Tonsillar size is graded on a scale of 1+ to 4+.
- Tooth *eruption* normally occurs between 4 and 12 months of age for the first tooth, and eruption of the 20 primary teeth should be complete between 24 and 30 months of age.
- Check the primary teeth in the infant and young child for "white spot" lesions, or decalcifications, and "brown spot" lesions, or cavitations, indicating the first sign of dental decay

- Telehealth via video is the preferred method for assessment of the oropharynx and it supports patient-provider engagement and a similar office visit experience.

DOCUMENTATION

Healthy Newborn
Nose, mouth, and throat: Nares patent bilaterally without flaring, clear nasal discharge. Strong suck. Mucous membranes pink, moist without lesions. Soft and hard palate intact. Uvula and tongue midline, nonprotuberant, gag response intact, without natal teeth.

DOCUMENTATION

Adolescent
Nose, mouth, and throat: No nasal discharge, nasal septum midline, turbinates pink, moist. No facial swelling or tenderness over sinuses. Buccal mucous pink and moist without lesions. Gums pink, firm without bleeding. Thirty-two teeth present in good repair without evidence of active decay. Pharynx pink, tonsils 1+ without exudate or pitting, uvula midline, sensitive gag response.

REFERENCES

1. ElHawary H, Czuzoj-Shulman N, Abenhaim HA, Gilardino MS. Decreasing incidence of palatoplasty in the United States. *J Craniofac Surg.* 2021;32:2710–2712.
2. Schoem SR, Darrow DH. *Pediatric Otolaryngology for Primary Care.* 2nd ed. American Academy of Pediatrics; 2020.
3. Moreddu E, Rizzi M, Adil E, et al. International Pediatric Otolaryngology Group (IPOG) consensus recommendations: Diagnosis, pre-operative, operative and post-operative pediatric choanal atresia care. *Int J Pediatr Otorhinolaryngol.* 2019;123:151–155.
4. Kwong KM. Current updates on choanal atresia. *Front Pediatr.* 2015;3:52–59.
5. Bluestone CD, Simons JP, Healy GB. *Pediatric Otolaryngology.* 5th ed. Elsevier; 2014.
6. US Preventive Services Task Force Davidson KW, Barry MJ, et al. Screening and interventions to prevent dental caries in children younger than 5 years: US preventive services task force recommendation statement. *JAMA.* 2021;326:2172–2178.
7. Clark CM, Kugler K, Carr MM. Common causes of congenital stridor in infants. *JAAPA.* 2018;31:36–40.
8. Hysinger EB. Laryngomalacia, tracheomalacia, and bronchomalacia. *Curr Probl Pediatr Adolesc Health Care.* 2018;48:113–118.
9. Wood J, Toll EC, Hall F, Mahadevan M. Juvenile recurrent parotitis: Review and proposed management algorithm. *Int J Pediatr Otorhinolaryngol.* 2021;142:110617.
10. Zitelli BJ, McIntire SC, Norwalk AJ, Garrison J. *Atlas of Pediatric Physical Diagnosis.* 8th ed. Elsevier; 2021.
11. Bjermer L, Westman M, Holström M, Wickman MC. The complex phathophysiology of allergic rhinits: Scientific rationale for the development of an alternative treatment option. *Allergy Asthma Clin Immul.* 2019;15:24.
12. American Academy of Pediatric Dentistry Caries-risk assessment and management for infants, children, and adolescents. *Pediatr Dent.* 2017;39:197–204.
13. Geissler KH, Dick AW, Goff SL, Whaley C, Kranz AM. Dental fluoride varnish application during medical visits among children who are privately insured. *JAMA Netw Open.* 2021;4:e2122953.
14. Messner AH, Walsh J, Rosenfeld RM, et al. Clinical consensus statement: Ankyloglossia in children. *Otolaryngol Head Neck Surg.* 2020;162:597–611.
15. Chinnadurai S, Francis DO, Epstein RA, Morad A, Kohanim S, McPheeters M. Treatment of ankyloglossia for reasons other than breastfeeding: A systematic review. *Pediatrics.* 2015;135:E1467–E1474.
16. Mitchell RB, Archer SM, Ishman SL, et al. Clinical practice guideline: Tonsillectomy in children (update). *Otolaryngol Head Neck Surg.* 2019;160(1_suppl):S1–S42.
17. Brietzke SE, Shin JJ, Choi S, et al. Clinical consensus statement: Pediatric chronic rhinosinusitis. *Otolaryngol Head Neck Surg.* 2014;151(4):542–553.
18. Leung AK, Hon KL, Chu WC. Acute bacterial sinusitis in children: An updated review. *Drugs Context.* 2020;9:1–11.
19. Singh J, Badr MS, Diebert W, et al. American academy of sleep medicine (AASM) position paper for the use of telemedicine for the diagnosis and treatment of sleep disorders. *J Clin Sleep Med.* 2015;11:1187–1198.
20. McCoul ED. Grasping what we cannot touch: Examining the telemedicine patient. *JAMA Otolaryngol Head Neck Surg.* 2020;146:685–686.

NECK AND LYMPHATIC SYSTEM ASSESSMENT

Bridget Ward Gramkowski

EMBRYOLOGIC DEVELOPMENT

The lymphatic system is established in the mesoderm layer during the third week of embryonic development, and the development of the primary lymphoid organs, the thymus, and bone marrow begins during the fifth to sixth week of fetal development. The secondary lymphoid organs—the spleen, lymph nodes, and lymphoid tissue—develop soon after the primary organs and are well developed at birth. The ectoderm gives rise to the epithelial linings of the glandular cells of the large organs that make up the lymphatic system. Lymph nodes develop over the course of the first year of life.[1,2]

The thyroid gland derives from the endoderm; early in fetal development it descends from the posterior one-third of the tongue down to the anterior upper trachea. Parathyroid glands grow from the dorsal endoderm around the fifth week of intrauterine life and can be seen on a cellular level around 14 weeks of fetal development. These glands are small, usually 5 mm by 3 mm by 1 mm and they weigh less than 50 mg.[3]

DEVELOPMENTAL VARIATIONS

The spleen, lymph nodes, and lymphoid tissue are small at birth and mature rapidly after exposure to antigens or microbes during the postnatal period. The thymus is the largest lymphoid tissue in the body at birth and continues to develop during the first year of life as the immune system develops. At puberty, the thymus begins slowly regressing as the immune system is well established in the lymphoid tissue.[1]

In the newborn, the amount of lymphatic tissue is small. Lymphadenopathy, enlargement of the lymph glands, can often be detected as a result of perinatal infections, particularly in the occipital region. Lymphoid tissue increases throughout the first year of life, and cervical lymph nodes become more pronounced with respiratory infections by 12 to 24 months of age. In the young child, splenomegaly may also occur with episodic viral illness. By school age, tonsillar and adenoidal tissues are approximately the same size as in an adult, and then they increase in volume during pubertal development when tonsillar tissue becomes twice the adult size. During late adolescence the volume of lymphatic tissue begins to decrease and resumes an adult level.[2]

Lymphatic malformation can occur during early embryonic development as a congenital defect of the lymphatic vessels. The lymphatic channels may become blocked, and lymphatic fluid collects in the vessels during embryonic development, forming a mass or cyst that is present at birth but may not be detected until later in the first year of life or in early childhood. A lymphatic cyst or mass generally occurs in the neck, mouth, or tissues around the ear and may be associated with other chromosomal abnormalities.[2]

Worldwide, congenital primary hypothyroidism, primarily due to thyroid dysgenesis, is one of the most common preventable causes of severe neurodevelopmental morbidity and is estimated to occur in 1 in every 2000 births. Prompt treatment is essential to promoting long-term outcomes; the earlier the condition is treated the better the long-term cognitive function of the child.[4] Infants born with abnormal development of the parathyroid gland are associated with a variety of genetic conditions, the most common as 22q11.2 deletion syndrome, or "DiGeorge syndrome."[5] DiGeorge syndrome is the second most common chromosomal disorder after trisomy 21 or "Down syndrome" and is the most common microdeletion disorder, occurring in 1 per 1000 fetuses in every 3000 live births. This syndrome is often associated with immune dysfunction related to athymia (absence of thymus), congenital heart defects, distinctive facial features, neurologic differences, and other systemic alterations.[5]

ANATOMY AND PHYSIOLOGY

Neck

The superficial and deep muscles of the neck support the pivotal rotation of the head. There are nine muscles in the neck and around the thyroid. The sternocleidomastoid or sternomastoid muscle is the largest muscle in the neck, running from the mastoid area at the base of the ear to the clavicle and sternum, and is primarily responsible for turning the head from side to side. The trapezius muscle lies at the back of the neck and is triangular. The origin of the trapezius muscle is in the back at the

12th thoracic vertebra extending to the lateral border of the clavicle and attaches at the posterior edge of the occipital bone. It supports the head movement from side to side and the shoulder movement.[6,7]

The structures in the neck are protected by the deep vertebral muscles, which support the side movements of the head. The trachea is the cartilaginous tube that extends from the larynx to the bronchi in the upper chest beneath the sternum. In infants and children, it is more mobile and more deeply recessed in muscle than in adults. The head and neck region are perfused by the carotid arteries. The external carotid supplies the head, face, and neck, and the internal carotid supplies the cranium. Blood from the cranium is drained through the subclavian and jugular veins.[6,7]

Neck masses typically fall into three categories: developmental, inflammatory, or neoplastic. The most common congenital developmental masses are thyroglossal duct cysts, branchial cleft cysts, dermoid cysts, vascular malformations (see Table 13.1). Reactive lymphadenopathy, infectious lymphadenitis, or Kawasaki disease are the most common inflammatory causes of neck masses. Neoplastic lesions can be benign and include pilomatrixomas, lipomas, fibromas, neurofibromas, and salivary gland tumors.

TABLE 13.1	COMMON CONGENITAL CYSTS AND MASSES OF THE NECK
Condition	Findings
Lymphovascular malformation	Slow flow vascular lesion, formed, benign, usually soft and fluctuant Formed from dilated lymphatic channels of endothelial cells
Branchial cyst	Lateral congenital neck mass, usually anterior to sternocleidomastoid muscle Formed from incomplete obliteration of pharyngeal pouches and clefts during embryologic development
Dermoid cyst	Midline congenital neck mass, nontender, mobile, submental neck mass Formed from epithelium entrapped in tissue during embryologic development
Thyroglossal duct cyst	Midline congenital anterior neck mass Typically presents as a painful, erythematous, and tender mass following an upper respiratory infection

Data adapted from Rajasekaran K, Krakovitz P. Enlarged neck lymph nodes in children. *Pediatr Clin North Am.* 2013;60:923–936.

TABLE 13.2	Neck Conditions
Condition	Description
Congenital hypothyroidism	In symptomatic infants: decreased activity, increased sleep, constipation, jaundice, poor feeding; infant may have dysmorphic facial features myxedematous (puffy face), enlarged tongue, umbilical hernia, hypotonia. One of the most common preventable causes of intellectual disability.
Congenital torticollis	Contracture or fibrosis of sternocleidomastoid muscle on one side, causing homolateral inclination and contralateral rotation of the face and chin (tilting of head to one side); occurs secondary to birth trauma, cervical spine anomalies, or spinal cord congenital deformities, tumors, ocular or neurologic dystonias; may be associated with positional plagiocephaly
Acquired Hypothyroidism	Primary (problem with the thyroid gland itself) and secondary hypothyroidism (problem with function of pituitary or hypothalamus)
Sandifer syndrome	Dystonic movements including spasmodic torsional dystonia (torticollis of the head and neck) and opisthotonos posturing (severe arching of the spine) that occurs up to 10 times a day and last between 1 and 3 minutes. Associated with gastro-esophageal reflux disease (GERD)
Torticollis	Contraction of sternocleidomastoid muscle causing tilting of head toward involved side; can be sequela of upper respiratory infection
DiGeorge syndrome (22q11.2 deletion)	Genetic disorder, varied phenotype including congenital heart disease, absent or missing thymus, parathyroid and/or adenoids (resulting in low immune function and low calcium), cleft palate, scoliosis, hearing loss, kidney abnormalities, growth hormone deficiency, feeding difficulties, minor facial differences, learning and behavioral differences
Turner syndrome	Genetic disorder, a female phenotype; characterized by short stature, webbed neck, pectus excavatum, primary amenorrhea, no development of secondary sexual characteristics

Rarely, malignant neoplasms can occur in the neck such as lymphoma, rhabdomyosarcoma, thyroid carcinoma, and metastatic nasopharyngeal carcinoma.[8] Table 13.2 presents common acute and chronic conditions of the neck in children.

Thyroid

The *thyroid gland* is an endocrine structure located midline on the anterior neck, inferior to the larynx, and has two butterfly-shaped lobes and an isthmus (a narrow strip of tissue) that connects the lobes across the midline of the trachea at the second and third tracheal rings. There are a wide range of morphologic variations to the thyroid including isthmus size and lateral lobe sizing, and the lobes may be asymmetric. It produces the thyroid hormones Triodothyronine (T3) and Tetraiodothyronine (T4) that are manufactured from dietary iodine. The thyroid also produces calcitonin, produced by parafollicular cells (C cells), a hormone that decreases serum calcium concentrations. Together, these hormones contribute to the regulation of metabolism, growth, and serum electrolytes. In children, thyroid hormones are essential for growth of the brain, physical growth, and sexual maturation. In people of all ages, T3 and T4 increase the basal metabolic rate causing increases in body temperature, heart rate, and metabolism.[9]

The thyroid gland is highly vascular, in fact, more than three times more vascular than the brain and six times more vascular than the kidney. Parasympathetic nervous system innervation is by the vagus nerve, which controls hormonal production and secretion, while sympathetic nervous innervation is from ganglia off the sympathetic truck and is primarily responsible for vasculature.[10] The four *parathyroid glands* are small endocrine glands generally located on the posterior side or dorsal surface of the thyroid gland. Like the thyroid gland, they do not contain ducts, and they secrete parathyroid hormone (PTH), which regulates calcium metabolism by increasing serum calcium levels. PTH stimulates release of calcium from the bones and increases calcium absorption from the small intestine.[11]

Lymphatic System

The *lymphatic system* is one of the most sensitive indicators of infection and toxins in children. The lymphatic tissue plays a role in the immune system as a first responder to fight infection through phagocytosis and the production of lymphocytes and antibodies. The lymphatic system forms an extensive network throughout the body and is composed of capillaries, collecting vessels, lymph nodes, and lymphoid organs.[1,2,7]

The bone marrow and thymus, which are the central lymphoid organs, provide the center for the production and maturation of the immune cells.[1] The peripheral lymphoid organs—the spleen, tonsils, appendix, and lymphatic tissue in the respiratory, gastrointestinal, and reproductive systems—concentrate antigens or immunogens and promote the cellular interactions of the immune response throughout the body to seek out and destroy microbes.[1,2]

Lymph is a clear fluid filtered and collected through the lymphatic capillaries from the organs and tissues throughout the body. The fluid consists of white bloods cells and occasionally red blood cells. The collecting vessels or lymphatic vessels are small canals that lie near the blood vessels and carry lymph from the lymphatic capillaries to the lymph glands and back to the bloodstream. Lymph is deposited into the bloodstream through the jugular and subclavian veins in the neck. The lymphatic system also absorbs fat and fat-soluble substances from the intestinal wall. Lymph and fat are transported from the lymph glands to the larger ducts and through venous return to the heart. The lymphatic system plays a major role in the maintenance of fluid balance. This system filters fluid at the lymph nodes and also removes bacteria. Obstruction of lymph flow or removal of lymph nodes causes lymphedema.[1,2]

Lymph glands are small aggregates of lymphoid tissue lying along lymphatic vessels throughout the body and consist of outer cortical layers and an inner medullary layer. The terms lymph gland and *lymph node* are often used interchangeably, and both terms can be applied to the lymphatic system. A gland is an organ that produces a substance or secretion, and a node is a swelling or protuberance. Each lymph node processes lymph from the surrounding anatomic area. People have 500 to 600 lymph nodes scattered throughout the body and clustered into specific regions. Fig. 13.1 illustrates the lymph glands in the head and neck area and gives a view of the lymphatic chains in the body.

The extensive lymphatic system throughout the body provides the pediatric health care provider with a map in times of illness. The patterns of drainage leading to the regional lymph glands are indicative of infections that occur in different areas throughout the body. Regional positioning is correlated with concentration of nodes; for example, the cervical region has roughly 300 lymph nodes. Certain lymph nodes have greater clinical significance. The right supraclavicular lymph gland or "Virchow node" is also termed a "sentinel node." It drains the breast, lung and upper esophagus, and an enlarged lymph node and can be the first sign of malignancy in these regions. In contrast, the left supraclavicular lymph nodes drain more varied and distant regions such as the kidney, cervix, testis, and pancreas.[1,2,12]

Lymph nodes filter lymph using specialized white blood cells that remove a variety of elements including microorganisms,

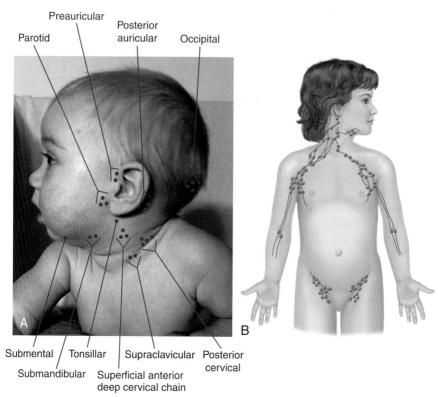

FIGURE 13.1 **(A)** Lymph glands in the head and neck area. **(B)** Lymph glands in the body.

malignant cells, damaged cells, and foreign particles. Lymph node size can double in 24 hours and can be ten times its original size within a week. This dramatic growth is a normative immune reaction to infection but can also signal an autoimmune response. The increased size can be triggered by five mechanisms: 1) cells in the node replicate after detecting an antigen or a malignant cell; 2) neutrophils or malignant cells enter the node; 3) histiocytic cells of the node store foreign material; 4) a cytokine release leads to vascular engorgement and edema; or 5) cellular material results from tissue necrosis.[13]

The head and neck region are the areas of the body with the highest concentration of lymph glands, and even mild infections in children cause swelling in the regional lymph glands. Although lymphadenitis refers to inflamed lymph nodes, the terms lymphadenitis and lymphadenopathy are often used interchangeably. *Lymphadenopathy* in children is generally episodic, benign, and self-limiting and is most often associated with viral infections. In contrast, in people 18 years or older, neck masses should be considered malignant until further evaluation demonstrates the cause.[8,14]

The differential for lymphadenopathy is extensive and can include neoplastic, infectious, inflammatory, reactive, and nondiagnostic causes. Cervical lymphadenitis refers to enlarged, inflamed, and tender lymph node(s) of the neck. Generalized lymphadenopathy indicates a systemic source of infection and is more likely to occur in children than in adults. Accurate assessment and diagnosis may depend on the pediatric health care provider's knowledge of the lymphatic drainage system.[1,2,7] Table 13.3 reviews common conditions presenting with lymphadenopathy.[2,8]

TABLE 13.3	CONDITIONS ASSOCIATED WITH LYMPH NODE FINDINGS
Condition	Lymph Node Findings
Viral infection	Soft to palpation Not fixed to underlying tissue or structures
Bacterial infection	Tender Fluctuant Not fixed to underlying tissue or structures
Abscess formation	Tender, fluctuant lymph node Erythematous Warm to touch
Malignancy	Hard to palpation Often fixed to underlying tissue No signs of acute inflammation

Data adapted from Rajasekaran K, Krakovitz P. Enlarged neck lymph nodes in children. *Pediatr Clin North Am.* 2013;60:923–936.

The tonsils and adenoids are organs of the lymphatic system. The buds of tonsillar tissue are present in the oropharynx at birth but are underdeveloped. As the immune system develops and reacts to respiratory triggers, such as viral, bacterial, and fungal infections and environmental toxins, the tonsils are the first line of defense. The adenoidal tissue is a mass of lymphoid tissue with many crypts that is situated posterior to the nasal cavity. The adenoids are also known as a pharyngeal tonsil or nasopharyngeal tonsil, they have limited blood flow and due to an abundance of folds or crypts can gather bacteria easily. Significant hypertrophy of the adenoidal tissue can partially or completely block airflow through the nasal passages and cause a variety of clinical symptoms including alterations in the quality of the voice, snoring, and mouth breathing. Adenoiditis, the inflammation of the adenoid tissue, often accompanies tonsillitis and occurs mainly in childhood. Since the pharyngeal opening to the auditory tube is at the adenoids, otitis media can be caused by both infection or hypertrophy of the adenoids[15] (see Chapter 12 for more content on the tonsils and adenoids).

The *thymus gland* is embedded beneath the upper sternum above the heart and is a fully developed organ in the term infant (Fig. 13.2).

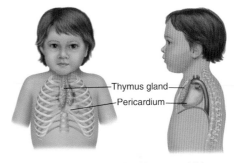

FIGURE 13.2 Thymus gland in young child.

In the infant, the thymus begins to produce mature T lymphocytes and plays an important role in cell-mediated immunity. In puberty, when the immune system is well established, the thymus decreases in size and is gradually mostly replaced by adipose tissue. Thymus tissue persists in the adult but has no demonstrated function. There are genetic disorders that present with thymic alterations or even athymia, such as 22Q11.2 deletion/DiGeorge syndrome,[5,16] as mentioned earlier in the chapter.

The *spleen* lies in the upper left quadrant of the abdomen protected by the rib cage. It is composed of lymphoid tissue and reticuloendothelial cells and is a densely vascular organ.

The spleen filters antigens in the bloodstream and opsonized bacteria (bacteria that is susceptible to phagocytosis). The spleen acts as a part of the immune system and hosts a sequence of activation events similar to the lymph nodes to fight blood-borne infection. In the infant and young child, the spleen stores erythrocytes and filters the blood through the large presence of phagocytes.[17] See Chapter 14 for further discussion of spleen function and assessment.

PHYSIOLOGIC VARIATIONS IN THE LYMPHATIC SYSTEM

Lymph nodes have a characteristic consistency that can be assessed by palpation. Insignificant lymph nodes should be soft and nontender. Tenderness on palpation typically indicates infection. Lymph nodes with a rubbery consistency are associated with lymphomas, and hard, nontender lymph nodes are associated with malignancy and granuloma infections.[2,8,12]

Although the spleen plays an important role in the immune system and the storage of erythrocytes, there are over 1 million people in the United States that have asplenia. Ten percent of these individuals have had a splenectomy due to sickle cell disease. Asplenia can cause clinical complications ranging from fulminant infection to thrombosis to pulmonary hypertension. People at greatest risk for sepsis include children under the age of 5, people 1 to 3 years after surgical splenectomy, or those with immunocompromise. Since these individuals are at greater risk for rapid progression to sepsis, they should seek emergency care if fever or other signs of infection are present.[17]

SYSTEM-SPECIFIC HISTORY

When a child presents with lymphadenopathy or complaints related to the neck, obtaining a complete history is key to an accurate assessment of infection in the pediatric population.

INFORMATION GATHERING FOR THE NECK AND LYMPHATIC SYSTEM AT KEY DEVELOPMENTAL STAGES

Age Group	Questions to Ask
Newborn	Access to prenatal care? Maternal health history of substance use, infections, or autoimmune disease? Prolonged labor with prolonged third stage? Vaginal or cesarean birth? Precipitous delivery? Vacuum-assisted delivery? Shoulder presentation? Preterm birth? Respiratory distress at birth? If neonatal intensive care unit (NICU) stay: length of time, treatments, infections, immunization history? Head tilt? Newborn screening results?
Infancy	Newborn screening results? History of maternal/neonatal infection? History of fever, respiratory infection, exposures? Poor growth or failure to thrive? Any swelling in neck area? Quality of muscle tone and strength, head control? Head tilt?
Early childhood	History of fever/respiratory infection, exposures? International travel? Persistent lymph gland swelling? Head tilt, neck pain/stiffness? Persistent lymph gland swelling?
Middle childhood	Lymphadenopathy? History of fever/respiratory infection? Neck pain/stiffness? Exposures? Fatigue? Loss of appetite? History of anemia? International travel? Family history of infections, tuberculosis?
Adolescence	Lymphadenopathy? Swelling in extremity? History of fever/respiratory infection? Neck pain/stiffness? Fatigue? Weight loss or gain? Neck swelling?
Environmental risks	Contact with common environmental irritants including: chemical cleaning agents, hazardous chemicals, radiation, hazardous waste, pesticides, insecticides, smoke from forest fires, or radiation?

Newborn screening for thyroid disease is required in all states, and results should be confirmed by the pediatric health care provider on the initial postpartum or well-child visit[4,9,18] (see Chapter 6). Newborn screening varies from state to state and country to country, and it is essential for the pediatric provider to be familiar with the conditions screened for in their own region.

The Information Gathering table reviews the areas of assessment that are pertinent for each age group and developmental stage and focuses on exposure to infection.

PHYSICAL ASSESSMENT

Inspection

The neck should be inspected for symmetry, shape, and mobility. In the newborn and very young infant, the neck is shortened, and the musculature is underdeveloped. It is best to inspect the neck with the infant on a firm surface for examination. An unusually short neck may be an indication of a genetic syndrome.[19]

While supporting the neck and shoulders cradled with the thumb and forefingers, use the opposite hand to extend the infant's head back slightly to expose the shortened neck region and conduct a full inspection of posterior, anterior, and lateral regions. This position allows the examiner to determine the symmetry and strength of the musculature of the neck, the alignment of the trachea, and the condition of the skin in the infant and young child. Infants are vulnerable to fungal and bacterial infection of the skin in the anterior neck region. *Torticollis*, or cervical dystonia, has several clinical causes and is defined by a head tilt to one side with limited range of motion of the neck muscles. Importantly, it may be associated with hypotonia or a neurological condition. It is a common finding in infants with plagiocephaly, but can also be caused by viral infection or gastroesophageal reflux disease (GERD) caused by overfeeding.[19]

In the school-aged child, tilting the head back slightly during inspection of the neck will assist the health care provider in evaluating the structures of the neck. The jugular vein is not normally distended in children who are sitting or standing upright. Pulsations in the jugular vein in the neck may be seen when the child is lying supine on the examining table. The jugular vein should appear full but not bulging, and it is normal to observe jugular venous pulsations (JVPs). JVP is normally a gentle undulation visible in good lighting. The pulsations should be of normal rate and amplitude; abnormal pulsations can indicate right-sided heart failure or pericarditis.

Inspect the thyroid gland for size and symmetry and note any swelling or masses. Asking the child to swallow may assist the provider in distinguishing the structure of the neck and movement of the thyroid gland. The thyroid gland should rise as the child swallows. In children who are obese, adipose tissue in the neck region is common and should not be mistaken for an enlarged thyroid gland.[20,21] Visible swelling in the lymph glands on inspection is generally a concerning sign and indicates the need for further diagnostics and prompt consultation and referral.

> ## RED FLAG FINDING IN LYMPHATIC ASSESSMENT
>
> Visible swelling in the lymph glands on inspection is generally a concerning sign in the child or adolescent and indicates the need for further diagnostic workup and treatment if indicated.

Palpation

Neck

Palpation may reveal small neck masses commonly found in children. *Brachial cleft cysts* are smooth, nontender masses on the lateral neck area along the border of the sternocleidomastoid muscle. *Thyroglossal duct cysts* present higher in the neck region. In both cases, surgical removal may be indicated. The most common neck mass in newborns is a *cystic hygroma*, which is a result of sequestered lymph channels. A *cystic hygroma* will transilluminate well and is usually seen laterally or over the clavicle and can be a few to many centimeters in size. Larger *cystic hygromas* may cause feeding difficulties, and in most cases surgical resection is needed.[19]

In the infant and young child, palpate the sternocleidomastoid muscle for masses, strength, and tone, including the clavicular area at the base of the sternocleidomastoid muscle. Any sign of pain or irritability, or resistance to range of motion of the neck or arm in the infant, child, or adolescent, indicates an abnormal finding and requires further evaluation. Resistance to lateral motion of the neck may indicate torticollis, lymph gland swelling, infection, or trauma to the sternocleidomastoid muscle.[7,8,19]

While palpating the neck in the newborn, the examiner should document redundant skin or webbing, which can occur in several conditions including Turner, Noonan, and Down syndromes. The clavicles in newborns should be assessed for birth-related trauma fractures; the examiner may feel crepitus shortly after birth, or the damage may not be evident until a mass is palpated over the clavicle weeks after birth. These newborn fractures typically heal without intervention.[19]

In older children, *carotid pulsations* can be palpated with the finger pads of the second and third fingers in the area between the trachea and the sternocleidomastoid muscle. Evaluate for rate, rhythm, and intensity. Avoid significant pressure to the carotid artery, which may cause a vagal response or hypotension. Auscultation over the vessel may be performed to detect bruits, or blowing sounds but is not routinely performed on children.[7,18]

Infants and young children with unexplained fever, irritability, or a bulging fontanel associated with increased intracranial pressure may indicate pain or neck stiffness during examination of the neck region (See Chapter 19). Meningismus or meningitis, inflammation of the brain and spinal cord, can manifest in the neck. To assess for meningismus, flex the head forward or ventrally with the infant or young child lying on a flat surface or examining table. Pain, irritability, resistance to movement, and range of motion on flexion of the neck is a sign of nuchal rigidity. *Brudzinski sign* or flexion of the lower extremities will occur spontaneously, with flexion of the head forward when meningismus is present to guard or protect the body from pain. *Kernig sign*, pain or resistance to straightening legs or knees from the flexed position, also indicates a positive sign for meningeal irritation. *Opisthotonos*, hyperextension of the neck and spine, indicates severe meningeal irritation.[18,22]

Thyroid

Palpation of the thyroid gland is not usually performed in infants and young children, unless masses or nodular lesions are noted on inspection of the neck. Hypothyroidism or hyperthyroidism can be caused by many disease processes including autoimmune diseases, inflammatory diseases, and cancer. Thyroid disease in infants and young children often presents with systemic symptoms including hypotonia, lethargy, distended abdomen, and enlarged tongue as in congenital hypothyroidism.

In school-aged children and adolescents, palpation of the thyroid gland is most easily approached from the front of the neck in the young child to minimize any fear that may occur during the examination. Continue to include best practices for trauma-informed care including describing your exam before you touch the child or adolescent. Ask the child to tilt their head forward slightly while in a sitting position with the back straight. To guide the examination, the provider may gently support the child's head. Begin by using the forefinger to locate the prominent ring of the tracheal cartilage, the *cricoid cartilage*, which provides a landmark to determine the position of the thyroid gland (Fig. 13.3A). Just lateral to the carotid cartilage, palpate the thyroid gland by placing one hand on one side of the trachea and gently displacing the thyroid tissue to the contralateral side of the neck (see Fig. 13.3B). Repeat this movement to examine both sides

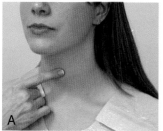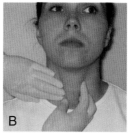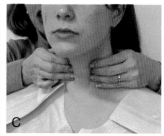

FIGURE 13.3 **(A–C)** Examination of the thyroid gland. **A,** Locate prominent ring of cricoid cartilage. **B,** Palpate thyroid gland with forefingers. **C,** Alternative position for palpation of thyroid gland. ([B], From Fehrenbach M, Herring S. *Illustrated Anatomy of the Head and Neck.* 4th ed. St. Louis, MO: Elsevier; 2012.)

of the thyroid gland. Once positioned, extend the forefingers of both hands, and apply slight pressure for deep palpation along both sides of the trachea and medial to the sternocleidomastoid muscle, and ask the child to swallow. Tilting the head to one side or rotating the neck very gently may help evaluate the size, quality, and firmness of the thyroid gland. With the patient's permission and clear communication from the provider, the thyroid gland can also be examined from behind in adolescents and young adults with the head tilted slightly forward. Using the cricoid cartilage as a landmark, the provider uses the forefingers of both hands to palpate deeply, laterally to the trachea, and medial to the sternocleidomastoid muscle (see Fig. 13.3C). A soft, mushy gland, or any masses or nodules noted on examination of the thyroid gland, are abnormal and require prompt evaluation. A goiter is a firm, nontender, mobile, symmetrical mass in the neck. Enlargement of the thyroid gland may occur with hyperthyroidism, Graves' disease, or Hashimoto thyroiditis.[18,20,21]

Lymphatic System

The provider must be an astute observer when examining the lymphatic system as each region of the body has clusters or chains of lymph glands that can signal infection in adjacent areas.[7,8,12,18] The examination includes palpating lymph glands accessible in four areas: the head and neck, arms, axillae, and inguinal areas of the body. The most effective approach to

TABLE 13.4	SIZING OF LYMPH GLANDS ON EXAMINATION
Size	**Description**
1+	Shotty, firm, nontender, <1 cm to >1–1.5 cm, requires deep palpation
2+	Mobile, detectable on superficial-to-deep palpation, >2–2.5 cm
3+	Palpable superficially, visible on inspection, >3–3.5 cm
4+	Lymph glands are walnut size or larger, nonmobile, tender; skin can be reddened and warm; >4–4.5 cm; visible on inspection

palpation of the lymph nodes is to use the pads of the examiner's second, third, and fourth fingers. The examiner's nails should be short to allow for direct palpation. Superficially massaging an area may not detect nodes, but superficial then deep palpation with the forefingers moving over the neck regions can better determine the size and mobility of a lymph gland.[7,12]

Lymph nodes are generally mobile and nontender and do not feel warm to the touch. Table 13.4 reviews sizing of the lymph nodes commonly used to describe findings on physical exam. Lymph nodes >1 cm in diameter are considered enlarged and defined as lymphadenopathy.[2] Inspect enlarged lymph nodes for erythema or edema. Lymph nodes that

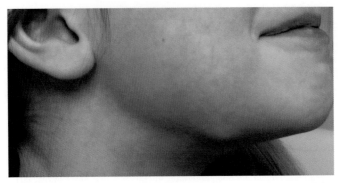

FIGURE 13.4 Enlarged sublingual lymph node. (From Rajasekaran K, Krakovitz P. Enlarged neck lymph nodes in children. *Pediatr Clin North Am.* 2013;60:923–936.)

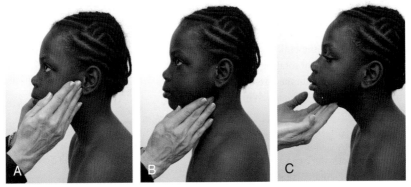

FIGURE 13.5 (A–C) Palpation of the cervical chain in a school-age child.

are immobile, tender, and warm to the touch indicate infection or an abscess and require further diagnostic evaluation and treatment. Symmetry should always be assessed; palpable asymmetry in lymph nodes indicates a clinically significant finding. Typical size of lymph glands varies by region.

The occipital nodes in the infant and young child lie on either side of the occiput just above the base of the skull. In the young infant, the occipital nodes are located well above the hairline, adjacent to the occipital bony prominence, and are commonly palpable with viral respiratory infections.[7] The parotid glands are located anterior to the ear and surround the oral cavity. The submandibular, sublingual, and submental glands are located along the anterior and posterior jaw line and under the anterior jaw.

They are palpable when infection occurs in the tongue, mucous membranes of the mouth, sublingual area extending to the base of the tongue, gums, or when decay or abscess occurs in the teeth (Fig. 13.4).[8,18]

The cervical nodes constitute the largest collection of lymph glands in the body. In children, the cervical glands are often palpable because they experience frequent respiratory infections (Fig. 13.5). The posterior auricular and preauricular nodes are often not palpable in the presence of common viral respiratory infections, but are enlarged and palpable with infection related to the external and internal ear, the pinna, and surrounding skin. The anterior superficial cervical nodes are palpable at the juncture of the mandible and sternocleidomastoid muscle at the neck. This examination

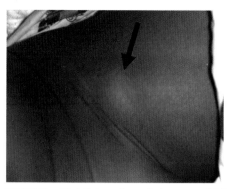

FIGURE 13.6 Enlarged posterior superficial cervical nodes. (From Kelly MN, Tuli SS, Usher S, Tuli SY. A 6-year-old with acute-onset generalized lymphadenopathy. *J Pediatr Health Care.* 2012;26:465–470.)

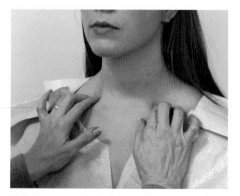

FIGURE 13.7 Palpation of the supraclavicular nodes.

requires both superficial and deep palpation, depending on the age and developmental stage of the child or adolescent. These glands are almost always palpable during throat and respiratory infections, but may be missed due to incorrect positioning of the fingertips during the assessment of the neck. The posterior superficial cervical nodes along the posterior neck area are palpable with systemic infections (Fig. 13.6). Posterior deep cervical nodes are rarely palpable in children and are only identifiable with deep palpation in the older child. In children ages 2 to 12 years old, the examiner will often palpate small, firm, mobile lymph nodes along the cervical chain on physical examination. These are often referred to as "shotty" nodes because of their pellet-like distribution; however, they are clinically insignificant findings due to frequent viral infections.

The supraclavicular nodes, along the clavicle, are rarely palpable and if enlarged may indicate a malignancy (Fig. 13.7). Enlargement of the "Virchow node" at the supraclavicular fossa is considered clinically significant if greater than 1 cm. Abnormal findings in the left supraclavicular node are correlated to abdominal infectious or malignant processes, while right supraclavicular nodes indicate a process in the intrathoracic region. Infraclavicular fossa nodes are associated with breast cancer or malignant lymphoma.

PEDIATRIC PEARLS

Occipital nodes are located high above the hairline in the infant and are often missed by the examiner palpating too low at the nape of the neck. Occipital adenopathy in the newborn may be an indicator of maternal infection during pregnancy, or in the older infant may indicate an acute viral infection. They may be visible on inspection and are often noted by the parent of a young infant.[23]

The axillary, brachial, and subscapular nodes lie anteriorly along the brachial artery and in the axillae along the lateral edge of the pectoralis major muscle. They are generally noted in children only on deep palpation unless enlarged. Examination of the subscapular nodes of the axillary chain is illustrated in Fig. 13.8. The epitrochlear nodes lie along the medial aspect of the arm above the elbow and are palpable over the humerus. The *epitrochlear lymph nodes* can be palpated most easily while moving fingerpads up and down the upper arm. The epitrochlear and *popliteal nodes* are the only peripheral lymph nodes in the lymphatic system and act as collection ducts for the limbs. Infants and children have hyperplastic nodes due to the increased immune activity from birth. Due to continued new exposures to antigens, these nodes stay larger than an adult size until roughly age 12. Palpable nodes in cervical, axillary, and inguinal regions are expected findings throughout this age range (see Table 13.5).[13] In adults, lymph nodes in the axilla and inguinal regions greater than 3 cm are considered clinically significant, while most other lymph nodes are significant if they are greater than 2 cm. In adolescents, pay particular attention to axillae and groin lymph nodes since they

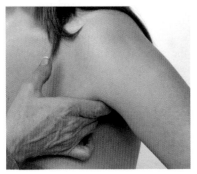

FIGURE 13.8 Palpation of the subscapular nodes of the axillary chain.

drain areas of common sexually transmitted infections and skin infections.[1,2,7,8]

The *inguinal nodes* can be palpated along the juncture of the thigh and abdomen and along the inguinal ligament and the saphenous vein. The horizontal chain of inguinal nodes runs along the inferior groin, and the vertical chain can be palpated on deep palpation along the upper inner thigh. If lymph glands are enlarged in the inguinal area, they are often visible in normal weight children when lying supine on the examining table. Fig. 13.9 shows a young child in the supine position for examination of the inguinal nodes. Inguinal lymphadenopathy often occurs with systemic viral infection in the pediatric patient and is also present in adolescents. Inguinal lymph nodes that are small and hard are similarly insignificant and common; this region can also be described as "shotty."[1,7,12] Table 13.6 reviews some of the causes of regional and systemic lymph node swelling in infants, children, and adolescents.[1,7,12,18]

TABLE 13.5	FREQUENCY AND LOCATION OF PALPABLE LYMPH NODES IN HEALTHY CHILDREN		
Palpable Node	Neonate	Age <2 Years	Age >2 Years
Cervical	+	++	++
Postauricular	-	+	-
Occipital	-	++	+
Submandibular	-	+	++
Supraclavicular	-	-	-
Axillary	+	+++	+++
Epitrochlear	-	-	-
Inguinal	+	+++	+++
Popliteal	-	-	-
None	++	++	++

+++ Normally found in <50% of children, ++ normally found in 25% to 50% of children, +normally found in 5% to 25% of children, -normally found in <5% of children

Data adapted from Jackson, MA, Day, JC. Lymphatic System and Generalized Lymphadenopathy. In Long SS, Prober CG & Fischer M Ed. *Principles and Practice of Pediatric Infectious Diseases.* 5th ed. Elsevier, Philadelphia, PA, 2018. Data sourced from Barnji M, Stone RK, Kaul, A et al. Palpable lymph nodes in healthy newborn infants. *Pediatrics.* 1986;78:573; Herzog LW. Prevalence of lymphadenopathy of the head and neck in infants and children. *Clin Pediatr,* 1983;22:485.

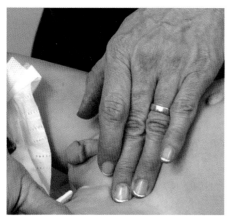

FIGURE 13.9 Palpation of inguinal nodes in a young child.

Palpation of the spleen is an important part of the examination for the lymphatic system, and tenderness and enlargement of the spleen on deep palpation indicates the need for further diagnostic evaluation. The examination of the spleen is reviewed in Chapter 14.

DIAGNOSTICS

Laboratory evaluation of lymphadenopathy in infants and children typically includes: a complete blood count (CBC) with differential, peripheral blood smear, blood culture, erythrocyte sedimentation rate (ESR) and/or C-reactive protein (CRP), lactate dehydrogenase (LDH), and serology for cytomegalovirus (CMV) and Epstein-Barr virus (EBV) or

TABLE 13.6	**REGIONAL AND SYSTEMIC CAUSES OF LYMPHADENOPATHY**
Region	**Related Causes**
Occipital	Scalp infections such as seborrheic dermatitis, tinea capitis, pediculosis/head lice; viral syndromes such as varicella, measles, rubella, roseola; viral respiratory infections (i.e., rhinovirus, RSV, postimmunization)
Preauricular, parotid, postauricular, and superficial cervical	Infection of pinna (ear), otitis externa, middle ear infection; parotitis
Cervical—tonsillar, sublingual, submandibular, deep cervical	Tonsillitis, pharyngitis (group A streptococcal [GAS], mycoplasma pneumonia), stomatitis; tooth decay, dental abscess; ear infection; oral mucosa/mucous membrane infections, tongue; cervical lymphadenitis from systemic infections (Epstein-Barr virus [EBV], cytomegalovirus [CMV]); neoplasm or cancer; postimmunization response
Axillary	Breast infections, thoracic wall inflammation, infections of shoulder and arm, systemic infection, or neoplasm in lymphatic system
Supraclavicular and subclavian	Neoplasm or cancer—metastatic cancers from respiratory, gastrointestinal, or lymphatic system
Epitrochlear and popliteal	Forearm and finger infections, infection secondary to fractures, skin infections, neoplasm, or cyst in lower extremity, venous insufficiency, cardiac or renal disorder
Inguinal	Diaper rash, gluteal and perineal infections; skin infections in lower abdominal area; foot and leg infections, systemic viral infections
Generalized lymphadenopathy	Systemic disease occurring in lymphatic, circulatory, respiratory, gastrointestinal, or genitourinary system; infections such as tuberculosis, HIV

HIV, Human immunodeficiency virus; *RSV*, respiratory syncytial virus.

other viral illnesses as indicated by history or exam. Additional testing may also be indicated for rapid streptococcal antigen test and throat culture, purified protein derivative (PPD) intradermal testing or interferon-gamma release assay QuantiFeron testing, and a chest radiograph.[24] In a child or adolescent with an enlarged thyroid or signs and symptoms of thyroid disease such as rapid weight changes, fatigue, or growth failure, an analysis of thyroxine (T_4), and TSH should be performed.

Ultrasound (US) is used, if indicated, for initial imaging of palpable neck masses in infants and children to avoid radiation exposure with computed tomography (CT).[2] Magnetic resonance imaging (MRI) may be indicated for pediatric neck masses compared with CT as it limits radiation exposure, but requires sedation and is less readily available. CT imaging may be necessary in some cases for differentiation of cysts or solid neck lesions. Biopsy of the lymph nodes may be indicated when the diagnosis is unclear after initial workup, systemic symptoms persist, or an isolated, enlarged lymph node or nonmobile mass persists that does not respond to antibiotic therapy.[24]

ASSESSMENT FOR CHILD MALTREATMENT

It is essential to detect any inflicted injury to a child and report this finding as mandated reporters. When an injured child is returned to the unsafe settings, there is up to a 50% chance the child will be injured again.[25] In a study examining more than 39,000 children admitted for child abuse over a 15-year time period, nonaccidental trauma (NAT) has been found to have some fracture patterns that can assist in clinical diagnosis of maltreatment.[26] Fractures in infancy should be carefully evaluated for cause, since these injuries are often associated with physical abuse. Clavicular fracture is a more common finding in children ages 5 to 8 years old who had been physically abused.[26] Adolescents who have experienced physical abuse often have more facial fractures (43%).[27]

Bruising to the neck is unlikely to occur accidentally, particularly in infancy and early childhood, and should raise concern for abuse.[25] Red flags during history taking include inconsistent history of injury, implausible explanation for the injury, and delay in seeking care.[25]

TELEHEALTH TIPS

Utilizing video telehealth, the neck can be examined for strength to gravity and range of motion. Lymph regions can be inspected with the help of the child and their caregiver. The examiner can request that the caregiver perform some of the physical exam maneuvers described in the physical assessment section above. Caregivers can be instructed to attempt palpation; however, if the clinician has concern based on history or the limitations of telehealth, they should refer the child to an in - person appointment. Full histories can be accessed via phone or video telehealth and based on the child's age and presenting history a triage decision can be made by the tele-examiner for further follow-up and subsequent type of visit (in - person or telehealth).[28]

SUMMARY OF EXAMINATION

- Inspect neck for symmetry, shape, and mobility.
- Palpate neck for any swelling, masses, or nodules.
- Palpation of the thyroid gland is often omitted in infants and young children unless masses or nodular lesions are noted on inspection.
- To examine the thyroid, begin by locating the cricoid cartilage as a landmark for examination of the thyroid gland. Palpate the thyroid gland by placing one hand on one side of the trachea and gently displacing the thyroid tissue to the contralateral side of the neck. Apply slight pressure with the forefingers. Ask the child or adolescent to swallow.

- Any masses or nodules on the neck require diagnostic evaluation and referral when indicated.
- Examination of the lymphatic system includes inspection and palpation of lymph glands regionally (head and neck, arms, axillae, and inguinal areas of the body) during the physical examination.
- Visible swelling in the lymph glands on inspection is a concerning sign in the child or adolescent and indicates the need for further diagnostics and prompt consultation and referral.
- In the young infant, the occipital nodes are located well above the hairline, adjacent to the occipital bony prominence, and are commonly palpable with viral respiratory infections.
- The inguinal nodes can be palpated along the juncture of the thigh and abdomen over the inguinal area along the inguinal ligament.
- Lymph nodes are generally symmetric, mobile, and nontender and are not warm to the touch.

- Lymph nodes that are asymmetric, immobile, tender, and warm indicate infection or an abscess and require further diagnostic evaluation and treatment.

DOCUMENTATION

Term Newborn or Infant
Neck: Supple, full range of motion (ROM), no masses

DOCUMENTATION

9-Year-Old Child
Neck: Supple, full range of motion (ROM), no lymphadenopathy, palpable adipose tissue over anterior neck region, thyroid firm, without nodules or masses.

DOCUMENTATION

Adolescent With Lymphadenopathy
Neck: 3+ tonsillar lymph nodes, mobile, warm, tender to touch; neck supple with full range of motion (ROM), no meningismus noted.

REFERENCES

1. Paessler ME. Lymph nodes. *Color Atlas of Human Fetal and Neonatal Histology*. Cham: Springer International Publishing; 2019:269–273.
2. Breslin JW, Yang Y, Scallan JP, Sweat RS, Adderley SP, Murfee WL. Lymphatic vessel network structure and physiology. *Compr Physiol*. 2018;9:207–299.
3. Guilmette J, Sadow PM. Parathyroid pathology. *Surg Pathol Clin*. 2019;12:1007–1019.
4. Wassner AJ. Congenital hypothyroidism. *Clin Perinatol*. 2018;45:1–18.
5. National Organization for Rare Disorders. 22Q112 deletion syndrome. https://rarediseases.org/rare-diseases/chromosome-22q11-2-deletion-syndrome. Accessed March 1, 2022.
6. Sargent B, Kaplan SL, Coulter C, Baker C. Congenital muscular torticollis: Bridging the gap between research and clinical practice. *Pediatrics*. 2019;144:e20190582.
7. In Brickley LS, Szilagyi PG, Hoffman RM & Soriano RP Ed. *Bates' guide to physical examination and history taking*. 13th ed. Walters Kluwer, Philadelphia, PA. 2021.
8. Meier JD, Grimmer JF. Evaluation and management of neck masses in children. *Am Fam Physician*. 2014;89:353–358.
9. Leung AKC, Leung AAC. Evaluation and management of the child with hypothyroidism. *World J Pediatr*. 2019;15:124–134.
10. Hanley P, Lord K, Bauer AJ. Thyroid disorders in children and adolescents: a review. *JAMA Pediatr*. 2016;170:1008–1019.
11. Felsenfeld AJ, Levine BS. Calcitonin, the forgotten hormone: does it deserve to be forgotten? *Clin Kidney J*. 2015;8:180–187.
12. Stanford Medicine 25: Promoting the Culture of Bedside Medicine. Lymphatic Exam https://stanfordmedicine25.stanford.edu/the25/lymph.html. Accessed March 9, 2022.
13. Jackson, MA, Day, JC. Lymphatic System and Generalized Lymphadenopathy. In Long SS, Prober CG & Fischer M Ed. *Principles and Practice of Pediatric Infectious Diseases*. 5th ed. Elsevier, Philadelphia, PA, 2018.
14. Unsal O, Soytas P, Hascicek SO, Coskun BU. Clinical approach to pediatric neck masses: Retrospective analysis of 98 cases. *North Clin Istanb*. 2017;4:225–232.
15. Wang H. Chronic adenoiditis *J Int Med Res*. 2020;48:300060520971458.
16. McDonald-McGinn DM, Sullivan KE, Marino B, et al. 22q11.2 deletion syndrome. *Nat Rev Dis Primers*. 2015;1:15071.
17. Lee GM. Preventing infections in children and adults with asplenia. *Hematology Am Soc Hematol Educ Program*. 2020;2020:328–335.

18. Szilagyi P. Assessing children: infancy through adolescence. In: Bickley LS, Szilagyi PG, Hoffman RM, Soriano RP, eds. *Bates' Guide to Physical Examination and History Taking*. 13th ed. Philadelphia, PA: Wolters Kluwer; 2021:799–923.

19. Johnson P. Head, eyes, ears, nose, mouth and neck assessment. In: Tappero E, Honeyfield M, eds. *Physical Assessment of the Newborn: A Comprehensive Approach to the Art of Physical Examination*. 6th ed. New York, NY: Springer; 2019:61–78.

20. Stanford Medicine 25: Promoting the Culture of Bedside Medicine. Thyroid Exam https://stanfordmedicine25.stanford.edu/the25/thyroid.html

21. Children's Hospital of Philadelphia: Pediatric Exams. Normal and Abnormal Thyroid. https://www.chop.edu/video/pediatric-exams-normal-and-abnormal-thyroid. Accessed March 6, 2022.

22. Tracy A, Waterfield T. How to use clinical signs of meningitis. *Arch Dis Child Educ Pract Ed*. 2020;105:46–49.

23. Alves Rosa J, Calle-Toro JS, Kidd M, Andronikou S. Normal head and neck lymph nodes in the paediatric population. *Clin Radiol*. 2021;76:315.e1–315.e7.

24. Up to Date: Peripheral Lymphadenopathy in Children: Diagnostic Tests. https://www-uptodate-com.ucsf.idm.oclc.org/contents/peripheral-lymphadenopathy-in-children-evaluation-and-diagnostic-approach. Accessed March 11, 2022.

25. Schilling S, Christian CW. Child physical abuse and neglect. *Child Adolesc Psychiatr Clin N Am*. 2014;23:309–ix.

26. McCarroll JE, Fisher JE, Cozza SJ, Robichaux RJ, Fullerton CS. Characteristics, classification, and prevention of child maltreatment fatalities. *Mil Med*. 2017;182:e1551–e1557.

27. Quiroz HJ, Yoo JJ, Casey LC, et al. Can we increase detection? A nationwide analysis of age-related fractures in child abuse. *J Pediatr Surg*. 2021;56(1):153–158. https://doi.org/10.1016/j.jpedsurg.2020.09.027. Epub 2020 Oct 13. PMID:33153723.

28. American College of Physicians: Telemedicine: A practical Guide for Incorporation into your Practice. https://www.acponline.org/cme-moc/online-learning-center/telemedicine-a-practical-guide-for-incorporation-into-your-practice. Accessed March 14, 2022.

ABDOMEN AND RECTUM

Laura C. Cooke; Michelle Klosterman

Assessment of the abdomen and rectum involves the evaluation of multiple organ systems and functions, including the gastrointestinal, renal, vascular, endocrine, immune, and internal reproductive systems. The health care provider should always maintain a holistic view of the child, adolescent, and family during the assessment, which may help distinguish physical versus psychosomatic origin of symptoms in the pediatric population and help focus the abdominal examination.

EMBRYOLOGIC DEVELOPMENT

The primitive gut forms during the fourth week of gestation from the dorsal section of the yolk sac. It begins as a hollow tube arising from the endoderm, which then forms the *foregut, midgut*, and *hindgut*. The *foregut* develops into the esophagus, stomach, upper portion of the duodenum (bile duct entrance), liver, biliary system, and pancreas. It is perfused by the celiac artery. The *midgut* develops into the distal duodenum and the remainder of the small intestine, cecum, appendix, ascending colon, and most of the proximal portion of the transverse colon; it is perfused by the superior mesenteric artery. The hindgut develops into the remaining transverse colon, descending colon, sigmoid colon, rectum, and superior portion of the anal canal; it is perfused by the inferior mesenteric artery.

By the end of the sixth week of gestation, the gut herniates outside of the abdominal cavity, where it rotates 90 degrees counterclockwise and continues to elongate. By the 10th week of gestation, the gut returns to the abdominal cavity and rotates another 180 degrees counterclockwise.

With the normal intestinal rotation, the stomach and pancreas rotate into the left upper quadrant (LUQ) and are pressed against the dorsal abdominal wall to fuse into position.

The pancreas arises from ectodermal cells from the most caudal part of the foregut and develops into dorsal and ventral buds. The dorsal bud is larger and becomes the major portion of the pancreas. The dorsal and ventral buds fuse to form the main pancreatic duct. Secretion of insulin begins around the 20th week of gestation. Up until the 14th week, the spleen is only a hematopoietic organ. Between weeks 15 and 18, the spleen then loses its hematopoietic function and transforms into an organ of the immune system.

The liver begins as a bud that develops on the distal part of the foregut and grows into the *septum transversum*, where it divides into two parts. The larger part develops into the right and left lobes of the liver, and the second smaller division of the hepatic bud develops into the biliary system. Hematopoiesis begins at the sixth week of gestation and is responsible for the large size of the liver. It is approximately 10% of the total weight of the fetus. Bile begins to form at 16 weeks of gestation, giving meconium its dark green color.

Development of the kidney begins with a primitive, transitory structure called the *pronephros*, or forekidney, which arises near the segments of the spinal cord. These segments appear early in the fourth week of gestation on either side of the nephrogenic cord. The pronephros itself soon degenerates but leaves behind its ducts for the next kidney formation, the *mesonephros*, or midkidney, to utilize. In the fifth week, the *metanephros*, or hindkidney, begins to develop and becomes the permanent kidney. By the eighth week, the hindkidney begins to produce urine and continues to do so throughout the fetal period.

The adrenal glands develop from the medulla, which originates from the neuroectoderm. At the seventh week of gestation, the medulla attaches to the fetal cortex, which develops from the mesoderm, and by the eighth week, the fetal cortex begins to encapsulate the medulla. The fetal adrenal gland is 20 times larger than the adult adrenal and is large compared with the kidneys. However, the adrenals rapidly decrease in size as the fetal cortex regresses and completely disappear by 4 years of age, when they are replaced by the adult cortex.

ANATOMY AND PHYSIOLOGY

The abdomen is the area of the torso from the diaphragm to the pelvic floor and is a three-dimensional space within which many organs overlap one another (Fig. 14.1). It is lined by the *peritoneum*, a serous membrane covering the abdominal viscera. The membrane of the peritoneum creates a smooth, moist surface that allows the abdominal viscera to glide freely within the confines of the abdominal wall and also provides protection.

The *liver* lies immediately below the right diaphragm and is the largest and heaviest organ in the body. It is composed of the right and left hepatic lobes and is an extremely vascular organ. The liver is perfused by the hepatic artery, which arises from the *abdominal aorta*, and by the portal vein, which delivers blood from the spleen, pancreas, and intestines. The liver metabolizes carbohydrates, fats, and proteins. It also breaks down toxic substances and drugs; stores vitamins and iron; produces antibodies, bile, prothrombin, and fibrinogen for coagulation; and excretes waste products. The hepatic veins return blood to the vena cava. Within the inferior surface of the liver lies the *gallbladder*, a sac-like organ. The liver excretes bile into the hepatic duct, which is collected and stored in the gallbladder. Bile is secreted into the duodenum via the cystic duct and the common bile duct to aid in the digestion of fats.

Below the left diaphragm, from posterior to anterior, respectively, lie the spleen, pancreas, and stomach. The *spleen* is a concave organ made mostly of lymphoid tissue that lies around the posterior fundus of the stomach. The spleen filters and breaks down red blood cells and produces white blood cells (lymphocytes and monocytes). It also stores blood, which can be released into the vascular system during an acute blood loss. The *pancreas* is nestled between the spleen and stomach and crosses the midline over the major vessels. The pancreatic head extends to the duodenum and the tail reaches almost to the spleen. It is responsible for producing enzymes needed for the metabolism of proteins, fats, and carbohydrates; these enzymes are excreted into the duodenum via the pancreatic duct and aid digestion. The pancreas also produces insulin and glucagon, which are secreted directly into the bloodstream, helping regulate blood glucose levels and endocrine function. The *stomach* is the most anterior organ in the LUQ of the abdomen. It is connected proximally to the esophagus, which enters through the diaphragm at the *esophageal hiatus*. The stomach receives food from the esophagus through the lower esophageal sphincter. It secretes hydrochloric acid and digestive enzymes, which are used to metabolize proteins and fats. When the stomach is distended, it is stimulated to contract and expel its contents through the pyloric sphincter into the *duodenum*, the first portion of the small intestine.

The *duodenum* is C-shaped and curls around the head of the pancreas. The pancreatic and bile ducts empty into the upper portion of the duodenum. The duodenum transitions to the *jejunum*, which is responsible for much of the absorption of water, proteins, carbohydrates, and vitamins. The *ileum* composes the last and longest part of the small intestine and absorbs bile salts, vitamins C and B_{12}, and chloride. Intestinal contents leave the ileum through the *ileocecal valve* and empty into the *cecum*, located in the right lower quadrant of the abdomen, which is the beginning of the large intestine (Fig. 14.2). The *appendix*, a long, narrow, tubular structure, arises from the base of the cecum. The large intestine lies anteriorly over the small intestine, ascends along the right anterior abdominal wall, and forms the *ascending colon*; it traverses the abdomen to the splenic flexure, forming the *transverse colon*, and descends along the left

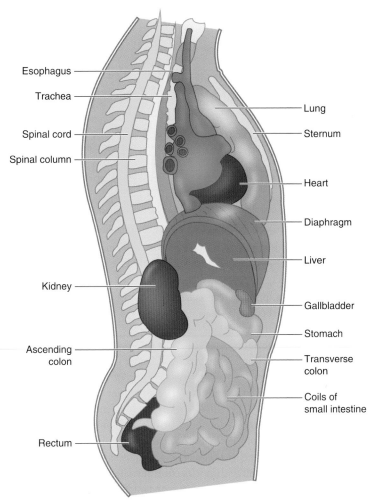

FIGURE 14.1 Side view of the torso and abdomen.

Esophagus
Trachea
Spinal cord
Spinal column
Kidney
Ascending colon
Rectum

Lung
Sternum
Heart
Diaphragm
Liver
Gallbladder
Stomach
Transverse colon
Coils of small intestine

lateral abdomen wall as the *descending colon*. At the level of the iliac crest, the colon becomes the S-shaped *sigmoid* colon. It descends into the pelvic cavity and turns medially to form a loop at the level of the mid-sacrum. The sigmoid colon connects to the *rectum*, which lies behind the bladder in males and the uterus in females. It stores feces until it is expelled through the *anal canal* and out the *anus*, which is located within a ring of nerves and muscle fibers midway between the tip of the *coccyx* and the *scrotum* or *vaginal fourchette*. The anal canal and anus remain closed involuntarily by way of a ring of smooth muscle, the *internal anal sphincter*,

and voluntarily by a ring of skeletal muscle, the *external anal sphincter*.

The *kidneys* lie on either side of the vertebral column in the retroperitoneal space below the liver and spleen. The right kidney tends to be lower than the left because it lies below the right lobe of the liver. Kidneys have a lobulated appearance at birth, which disappears with the development of the glomeruli and tubules in the first year of life. The kidneys are perfused by the renal arteries and filter and reabsorb water, electrolytes, glucose, and some proteins. They regulate blood pressure, electrolytes, and the acid-base composition of blood and other body

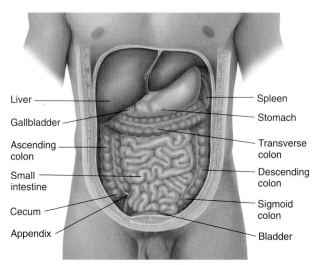

FIGURE 14.2 Anatomic structures of the abdominal cavity in an adolescent male. (From Ball JW, et al. Seidel's Guide to Physical Examination: An Interprofessional Approach. 10th ed. St. Louis: Elsevier; 2023.)

fluids; actively excrete metabolic waste products; and produce urine. The kidneys are capped by the adrenal glands, pyramid-shaped organs that synthesize, store, and secrete epinephrine and norepinephrine in response to stress. The adrenals also produce the corticosteroids, which affect glucose metabolism, electrolyte and fluid balance, and immune system function.

Urine is excreted from the kidney into the *ureters*, long, thin muscular tubules that transport urine to the bladder. The *ureters* connect to the superior pole of the renal pelvis. They descend posteriorly to the peritoneum and slightly medially in front of the psoas major muscle into the pelvic cavity, implanting into the superior posterior wall of the *urinary bladder*. The oblique insertion of the ureters through the bladder wall creates a one-way valvular mechanism that prevents the reflux of urine. The urinary bladder lies anterior to the uterus, or anterior to the rectum in bodies without a uterus. When filled to its capacity, the bladder then contracts and releases urine through the bladder neck and out the *urethra*. The urethra is normally located at the tip of the penis or between the clitoris and vagina. In nonpregnant birthing-capable individuals, the reproductive organs lie within the pelvis between the bladder (anterior pelvis) and the rectum (posterior pelvis). They include the *ovaries, uterine* or *fallopian tubes*,

and *uterus*. These organs descend into the pelvic cavity during normal growth and development and ascend into the abdominal cavity during pregnancy or with ovarian cysts or other abnormalities (see Chapter 17 for further discussion).

Finally, a layer of fascia and then muscle covers the anterior abdomen. The *rectus abdominis* muscle extends the entire length of the front of the abdomen and is separated by the *linea alba* in the midline. The *transverse abdominis* and *internal* and *external oblique muscles* cover the lateral abdomen. The *umbilicus* lies in the midline usually below the midpoint of the abdomen (Fig. 14.3).

PHYSIOLOGIC VARIATIONS

Many aspects of the development of the organs and structures in the abdomen continue into the first few years of life. The muscle tone of the lower esophageal sphincter is not fully developed until 1 month of age and may remain slightly weak for the first year. The stomach is round until approximately 2 years of age and then elongates into its adult shape and position by about 7 years of age. Stomach capacity is also smaller in the infant, whereas emptying time is faster, which results in the pattern of small and frequent feedings. The small bowel grows from approximately 270 cm at birth to up to 550 cm

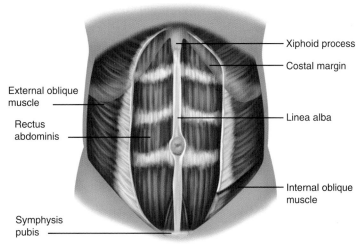

FIGURE 14.3 Abdominal musculature in adolescent.

by 4 years of age. The liver constitutes 5% of the term neonate's body weight, versus 2% in the adult. The kidneys also remain relatively large for the size of the abdomen until adolescence.

SYSTEM-SPECIFIC HISTORY

Information gathering for the assessment of the abdomen should include questions regarding diet, elimination, medications, environmental exposures, and a thorough psychosocial history (see Information Gathering table). Evaluation of abdominal symptoms that may be related to the genitourinary tract are discussed in more depth in Chapters 15 and 17. An assessment of the menstrual cycle and history of sexual activity in adolescents is also essential.

INFORMATION GATHERING AT KEY DEVELOPMENTAL STAGES

Age Group	Topics to Address
Preterm and newborn	Exposure to prenatal drug use, infection Family history of GI conditions Birth weight and gestational age First meconium and stooling/voiding patterns Amount and type of feedings Spitting up or vomiting Jaundice Any abnormal prenatal ultrasound findings, results of amniocentesis, genetic workup (polyhydramnios, gastric bubble, intestine location, hydronephrosis)
Infancy	Weight gain and growth pattern Amount and type of feedings Food allergies or sensitivities Stooling/voiding patterns Blood, mucus, or grease in stool Spitting up or vomiting Persistent unusual discomfort during/after feeds (e.g., back arching, prolonged crying, or refusal to eat) Family history of chronic constipation

Continued

INFORMATION GATHERING AT KEY DEVELOPMENTAL STAGES—CONT'D

Age Group	Topics to Address

Early childhood	Weight gain and growth pattern
	Diet history and fluid intake
	Ingestion of nonnutritive substances (Pica)
	Presence and patterns of abdominal pain
	Stooling/voiding patterns, including
	    Toilet training
	    Constipation or stool withholding
	    Enuresis or encopresis
	    Blood, mucus, or oil/grease in stool
	Symptoms of UTI (abdominal pain, dysuria, enuresis)
	Recent illnesses
	Psychosocial stressors including transition to childcare or preschool and any family dysfunction

Middle childhood	Weight gain and growth pattern Diet history and fluid intake Presence and patterns of abdominal pain Stooling/voiding patterns, including Constipation or stool withholding Enuresis or encopresis Blood, mucus, or grease in stool Symptoms of UTI (frequency, dysuria, urgency) Recent illnesses Psychosocial stressors including bullying, any family dysfunction, or sexual abuse
Adolescence	Weight gain and growth pattern Diet history and fluid intake Body image and risk for disordered eating/purging Laxative use/abuse Presence and patterns of abdominal pain Stooling and voiding patterns Blood, mucus in stool Symptoms or history of UTI Menstrual history (if applicable) Sexual activity and use of contraception and barrier methods Symptoms or history of STI Psychosocial stressors including bullying and intimate partner violence
Environmental risks (all ages)	Home, child-care, or school exposures to infectious disease Family members with chronic abdominal pain or diarrhea Cultural practices for feeding or complementary/alternative healing Recent travel to areas with endemic food- or water-borne illness Recent backpacking or camping Exposure to contaminated foods Environmental lead exposure Food insecurity Exposure to stressors or ACE

ACE, Adverse childhood experiences; *GI,* gastrointestinal; *STI,* sexually transmitted infection; *UTI,* urinary tract infection.

Abdominal Pain

When a complaint of abdominal pain is reported, the examiner must elicit a detailed history of the pain. Information regarding the character and severity of the pain, onset and duration, presence of nocturnal awakening, location or radiation, position of comfort, things that alleviate or worsen the pain, history of trauma, and any associated symptoms of fever, vomiting, anorexia, constipation, diarrhea, or frequent stooling with or without noting blood, are important in narrowing the scope of the differential diagnosis. A complaint of recurrent pain related to meals or after meals should be elicited in the history. A detailed history can help in determining whether the abdominal pain is acute or chronic. Psychosocial and family stressors and bullying should also be considered in evaluating abdominal pain. Remember that abdominal pain can be referred from an extra-abdominal source or can be a condition associated with systemic disease. For example, abdominal pain is common in children with beta-streptococcal pharyngitis, lower lobe pneumonia, sickle cell anemia, cystic fibrosis, Henoch-Schönlein purpura (Immune globulin A Vasculitis), and many other conditions.

EVIDENCE-BASED PRACTICE TIP

When a child presents with chronic abdominal pain, a primary goal is to determine whether the pain has a functional or organic cause, to create an effective management plan. However, confirming the presence or absence of an organic disease is not enough to determine the degree of impairment a child may experience related to chronic abdominal pain. Evidence shows that children with centrally mediated abdominal pain syndrome (formerly known as functional abdominal pain) experience a significant decrease in quality of life and are more prone to impairment in social, psychological, and academic functioning.[1,2] Therefore, it is imperative to include an evaluation of functional impairment for any child with chronic abdominal pain.

RED FLAG IN ABDOMINAL ASSESSMENT

Nocturnal awakening with pain and/or stooling may be a red flag in the school-age child and requires further assessment and diagnostic workup as indicated.

PHYSICAL ASSESSMENT

Equipment

In performing an abdominal exam in an infant or child, good lighting, warm hands, and a stethoscope may be all the equipment necessary. Diagnostic imaging can play an important complementary role in the assessment of some abdominal complaints, but it is essential that the decision to use such resources be warranted and evidence-based.[3] A proper physical examination by the health care provider—whether in person or by telehealth visit—remains essential to determining the best course of action and the level of acuity of the presenting condition. If the assessment reveals abdominal pain accompanied by any red flags (Box 14.1), further evaluation through laboratory analysis and/or diagnostic imaging may be warranted.[4,5]

Preparation and Positioning

Infants and toddlers can initially sit comfortably on the parent's lap directly facing the examiner. Inspection and auscultation of the abdomen can be done with the child sitting upright. For light and deep palpation, the examiner should be seated in a knee-to-knee position with the parent and with the child lying with head and torso in the parent's lap and the hips and legs in the examiner's lap or supported on the parent's lap with the parent leaning back (Fig. 14.4). The initial examination can occur with the child partially dressed and the diaper can be unfastened or pants and underwear pulled below the groin area. For older children and adolescents, the abdomen

BOX 14.1 RED FLAG SYMPTOMS AND SIGNS IN CHILDREN WITH RECURRENT ABDOMINAL PAIN

Symptoms and Key Features in the History
Involuntary weight loss
Chronic diarrhea
Blood in stool or urine
Gynecologic symptoms (e.g., menstrual irregularities, vaginal discharge)
Family or personal history of IBD/celiac disease
Nocturnal waking with abdominal pain or diarrhea
Persistent vomiting (especially if bilious)
Urinary symptoms (e.g., dysuria, enuresis)
Pain radiating through to the back (pancreatitis) or loins (renal pain)
Joint pains, mouth sores, skin rash, unexplained fevers

Signs on Physical Exam
Slowing of linear growth
Clubbing
Mouth ulcers
Abdominal masses
Anorexia/delayed puberty
Hypertension/tachycardia
Perineal changes (tags/fistulas)

Data adapted from Brown LK, Beattie RM, Tighe MP. Practical management of functional abdominal pain in children. *Archiv Dis Child.* 2016;101(7):677–683.

should be assessed on the examination table. It is important for the examiner to consistently place the older child or adolescent in the same position when preparing for the abdominal examination—ideally with the head on the examiner's left and the right side of the child's body in front of the examiner, to more easily palpate the abdominal organs. This will aid in accurate anatomic findings and accurate diagnosis of abdominal symptoms and conditions.

The abdomen is divided into four equal quadrants, with the transverse and midsagittal planes intersecting at the umbilicus (Fig. 14.5A). For a child or adolescent who presents with abdominal pain or for other abdominal presentations, use a mapping technique with nine sections (Fig. 14.5B) to accurately describe findings in the electronic health record. Mentally visualizing the anatomic location of the organs and adopting a mapping technique for abdominal assessment is key to an accurate and informative examination. See Box 14.2 for a list of symptoms or conditions related to different abdominal regions. There may be some variation in the anatomic positions of the organs in children and adolescents depending on the body type, respiratory phase at the time of the exam, the amount of contents within the stomach or bladder, and the amount of palpable stool in the abdomen.

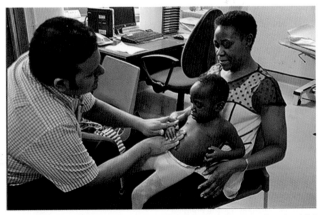

FIGURE 14.4 Knee-to-knee position for examining abdomen in infancy and early childhood. (From Glynn M, Drake, WM, eds. Hutchison's Clinical Methods: An Integrated Approach to Clinical Practice. 25th ed. Elsevier; 2023.)

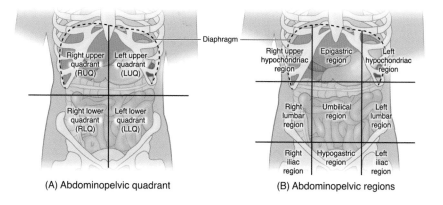

Diaphragm

(A) Abdominopelvic quadrant

Right upper quadrant (RUQ)
Left upper quadrant (LUQ)
Right lower quadrant (RLQ)
Left lower quadrant (LLQ)

(B) Abdominopelvic regions

Right upper hypochondriac region
Epigastric region
Left hypochondriac region
Right lumbar region
Umbilical region
Left lumbar region
Right iliac region
Hypogastric region
Left iliac region

FIGURE 14.5 **(A)** Four abdominopelvic quadrants. **(B)** Nine abdominopelvic regions.

BOX 14.2 ABNORMAL CONDITIONS OF THE ABDOMEN

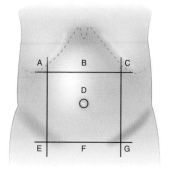

A, Right Upper Quadrant
Hepatitis
Cholecystitis
Liver, renal, or adrenal neoplasm
Hydronephrosis
Pyloric stenosis
Pancreatitis
High fecal impaction
Intussusception

B, Epigastric
Esophagitis:
-chemical (gastroesophageal reflux)
-immunologic (e.g., EoE)
-Infective (e.g., herpes simplex)
-Traumatic
-systemic (e.g., Crohn's)
Cholecystitis
Foreign body ingestion
Disorders of gut-brain interaction)
    (e.g., functional dyspepsia)
Hepatitis
Pancreatitis

C, Left Upper Quadrant
Renal or adrenal neoplasm
Hydronephrosis
Pancreatitis
Splenic mass
Mononucleosis
High fecal impaction

Continued

BOX 14.2 Abnormal Conditions of the Abdomen—Cont'd

D, Periumbilical
Acute gastroenteritis
Constipation
Disorders of gut-brain interac-
    tion (e.g., abdominal migraine;
    centrally mediated abdominal pain
    syndrome)
Appendicitis (referred)
Umbilical hernia
Peptic ulcer disease
Infectious gastritis (e.g., *H. pylori*)
Reactive gastritis (e.g., NSAIDs)

E, Right Lower Quadrant	**F, Suprapubic**	**G, Left Lower Quadrant**
Appendicitis	Bladder distention	Constipation
Intestinal obstruction	Urinary tract infection	Intestinal obstruction
Ovarian torsion or cyst	Bladder neoplasm	Hirschsprung disease
Mittelschmerz	Ovarian torsion or cyst	Ovarian torsion or cyst
Dysmenorrhea	Mittelschmerz	Mittelschmerz
Ectopic pregnancy	Dysmenorrhea	Dysmenorrhea
Mesenteric lymphadenitis	Ectopic pregnancy	Ectopic pregnancy
Incarcerated hernia	Pelvic inflammatory disease	Incarcerated hernia
Lymphoma		Lymphoma
Pyelonephritis		Pyelonephritis
Renal neoplasm		Renal neoplasm

Data from Rakel RE, Rakel DP. *Textbook of Family Medicine*. 9th ed. Elsevier Saunders; 2016.

Inspection

Examination of the abdomen begins with the initial inspection of the child or adolescent's facial expression and color, attitude, activity level, and level of comfort to determine any distress. Observe whether the child has difficulty walking or climbing onto or off the exam table. Children with peritoneal irritation often walk cautiously and resist lying on the exam table. Ask the child to hop or jump and note whether these movements elicit pain. If the child is guarding the abdomen, prefers to keep the legs flexed, or if the abdomen is rigid, this can indicate diffuse peritonitis.

Begin the abdominal assessment by extending each leg and note if pain is elicited and its location. Inspect the abdomen by noting its contour, symmetry, skin texture, color, and integrity. Note any lesions, rashes, pigment variations, piercings, gastrostomy tubes, or scars. Scars can indicate previous abdominal surgery and should always be explored during history taking. View the abdomen from the side and note the shape and anteroposterior dimension. Infants and young children have less developed abdominal musculature, so the abdomen is more protuberant and rounded. Young children to 4 years of age will have a "potbellied" appearance while supine or standing (Fig. 14.6). If the abdomen is scaphoid at any age, it can indicate malnutrition or displaced abdominal organs, as with a diaphragmatic hernia or intestinal atresia in a newborn. If the abdominal contour is distended, it can indicate an intestinal obstruction, a mass, organomegaly, or ascites. Fullness over the symphysis pubis can be seen in a thin child with a full bladder. Asymmetry of the abdomen

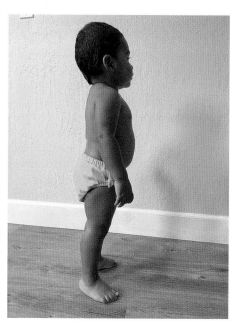

FIGURE   14.6 **Potbelly stance of the toddler.** (Courtesy Tiffany Lambright.)

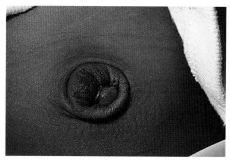

FIGURE   14.7 Umbilical granuloma. (From Eichenfield LF, et al., eds. *Neonatal and Infant Dermatology.* 3rd ed. Elsevier; 2015.)

may indicate a mass, organomegaly, hollow organ distention, or curvature of the spine.

Observe for any pulsations. It is normal to see pulsations in the epigastric area of a young infant or very thin child. Distended veins in the abdominal integument could indicate vascular compression or obstruction, hypertension, or intestinal obstruction. If an intestinal obstruction is suspected, note any obvious loops of bowel, and observe for peristaltic waves on the surface by viewing the abdomen at eye level.

Inspect the umbilicus for any signs of drainage, infection, hernia, or mass. In the initial newborn exam, inspect the cord for the umbilical vessels, two arteries, and a single vein. The arteries are smaller and have a thicker vessel wall. Infants with a two-vessel cord may have congenital anomalies and should be referred for further diagnosis and evaluation. Most umbilical cord remnants detach by the 10th day of life but can take up to 3 weeks to slough. Once the cord has detached, the stump should dry and heal within a few days. Occasionally,

umbilical granulomas or granular tissue at the base of the umbilicus can be present and drain serous or seropurulent fluid or occasionally blood (Fig. 14.7). For persistent umbilical granulomas, cauterization or surgical ligation of the stump may be needed. Any prolonged drainage should be investigated for presence of a *urachal remnant* or *cyst.* If stool is noted coming from the umbilicus, an *omphalomesenteric duct remnant* is present, and the infant should be referred immediately to a pediatric surgeon. Any sign of infection in the umbilicus should be aggressively treated in the neonate. *Neonatal omphalitis* is a rapidly progressing, acute, and potentially fatal infection of the abdominal wall caused by a bacterial pathogen. Any infant with purulent discharge or sign of cellulitis should be treated with systemic antibiotics and referred immediately if the infection progresses.

Note any protrusion or mass in the umbilicus. Observe the midline of the abdomen of the infant or young child while reclining or sitting. A wide bulging superior to the umbilicus is likely *diastasis recti abdominis* (Fig. 14.8), a common finding in children when the rectus abdominis muscle does not meet in the midline. Diastasis recti abdominis does not create any functional problem during infancy and early childhood and usually diminishes or resolves as the child grows and the abdominal muscles strengthen.

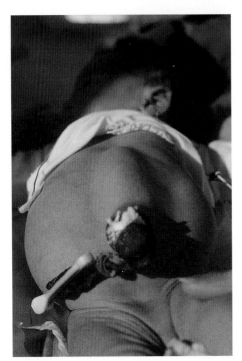

FIGURE 14.8 Diastasis recti. (From Clark DA. *Atlas of Neonatology*. 7th ed. Philadelphia: Saunders; 2000.)

Auscultation

Auscultation of the abdomen should be done before palpation or percussion to prevent any alteration in bowel sounds that may occur from manipulation of the area. Systematically listen to each quadrant or section of the abdomen with a stethoscope. In the infant and young child, auscultate the abdomen during the quiet parts of the physical exam (i.e., the cardiac and respiratory assessment). Bowel sounds can be heard within the first few hours of life and indicate peristalsis and movement of contents through the bowels. Normal bowel sounds are heard every 10 to 20 seconds, and frequency may be approximately 5 to 30 bowel sounds in 1 minute. Hypoactive (more than 30 seconds apart) or absent bowel sounds (none heard within 3 to 5 minutes) may indicate a *paralytic ileus*, or inactivity of the intestines, as in constipation. Hyperactive bowel sounds indicate rapid movement through the intestines, usually associated with diarrhea or a mechanical obstruction. If the child is hypertensive, auscultate for bruits using the bell of the stethoscope to assess for signs of renovascular disease. A newborn with a *scaphoid* abdomen or signs of respiratory distress should be carefully evaluated for bowel sounds or decreased breath sounds in the chest, which may indicate a *diaphragmatic hernia*. During auscultation of the abdomen, the examiner can carefully watch the child's facial expression to identify areas of tenderness while lightly pressing the stethoscope against each section of the abdomen.

Palpation

Palpation is the most important technique in assessing the abdomen and identifies areas of tenderness, masses, organomegaly, ascites, and signs of inflammation or peritonitis. It should not be omitted even with a child who is having difficulty cooperating with the exam. The ideal position for palpation of the abdomen is to have the child lie supine with the knees and hips gently flexed to relax the abdominal wall.

Begin with light palpation using the pads of the forefingers to assess the four quadrants of the abdomen. Use a firm therapeutic touch for palpation. Massaging the abdomen should be avoided. Observe the child's facial expression to note any signs of pain, discomfort, or areas of tenderness. If areas of tenderness are detected with light palpation, examine those areas last when performing deep palpation.

PEDIATRIC PEARLS

Give infants a pacifier to suck or distract the young child in the parent's lap with a toy or favorite stuffed animal, to help relax the abdomen during the abdominal exam. If a child is ticklish during palpation, place his or her hand under your hand with your fingers interlaced and palpate the abdomen together. Distraction with conversation is also effective in eliciting cooperation throughout the exam.

Deep palpation requires a firmer therapeutic touch, and the child may resist palpation because of fear or pain over areas of inflammation. It may be helpful to use two-handed palpation with the nondominant hand to exert pressure over the examining hand when evaluating the abdomen in obese children and adolescents. *McBurney's sign*, tenderness with deep palpation of the right lower quadrant, or referred right lower quadrant pain with deep palpation of the left lower quadrant, *Rovsing's sign*, could be suspicious for *appendicitis* and should be further evaluated and referred. With deep palpation, pain can also be assessed with *rebound tenderness*. To produce *rebound tenderness*, place fingertips at a 90-degree angle against the abdomen and gently but firmly press into the abdomen. Quickly lift the hand off the abdomen and note if any pain is elicited. The child with *rebound tenderness* will have more pain when the examiner's hand is lifted from the abdomen than with deep palpation. Pain with rebound of the abdomen may be a sign of inflammation or *peritonitis*. *Rigidity* of the abdomen is the involuntary tightening of the abdominal musculature that occurs in response to underlying inflammation in the abdomen. *Peritonitis* may be indicated if pain is worse when the examiner lifts the hand off the abdomen when testing for *rebound tenderness*. *Guarding* is the voluntary contraction of the abdominal wall musculature to prevent pain and may subside if the child relaxes.

To palpate the liver, place the fingertips at the right midclavicular line below the right rib cage parallel to the umbilicus. While moving the fingers slightly up and inward towards the right costal margin, feel for a firm nudge by the liver tip on inspiration. Note the distance between the location of the costal margin and liver tip. The liver may be palpable in an infant or toddler 1 to 2 cm below the right costal margin. Hepatomegaly is suspected in any child whose liver is palpable more than 3 cm below the costal margin. In the obese child or adolescent, hepatomegaly is highly suspect for nonalcoholic fatty liver disease (NAFLD) and should prompt further evaluation through laboratory and imaging studies.[6] Other causes of an enlarged liver include systemic infection, tumors, hepatic storage disorders, biliary masses, intrahepatic vascular disease, and cardiac disease.

To palpate the spleen, position the fingertips in the left midclavicular line below the costal margin and feel for firmness on inspiration (Fig. 14.9A and B). An alternative technique in infants is to palpate the spleen between the thumb and forefinger of the right hand. The spleen can be felt in about 5% to 10% of children and should be slightly mobile. If splenomegaly is suspected, ultrasound examination can differentiate spleen enlargement from other masses that may arise in the LUQ. Splenomegaly can be caused by infection, inflammation, blood dyscrasias, a mass, or vascular and oncologic conditions. The spleen is a very vascular organ and should be *gently* palpated if injury/trauma is suspected. If blunt trauma to the abdomen is suspected, avoid

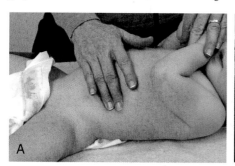
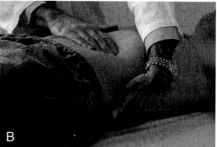

FIGURE 14.9 **(A)** Palpating the spleen in the toddler. **(B)** Two-handed palpation of the spleen in an adolescent. ([B] From Talley N. *Clinical Examination: A Systematic Guide to Physical Diagnosis.* 6th ed. Sydney: Churchill Livingstone; 2010.)

deep palpation of the spleen or liver. If the liver or spleen is lacerated, a clot *tamponading* the laceration could be dislodged, causing further bleeding with deep palpation.

The kidneys can sometimes be palpated in infants. Place the left hand behind the right flank of the infant and, using the fingertips of the right hand, palpate deeply in the right upper quadrant (RUQ) to the right of the midline. The right kidney may be "trapped" between the hands. Repeat the technique, placing the right hand behind the infant's left flank, and use the left fingertips to palpate the left kidney in the LUQ. The kidneys should be round, smooth, and firm. A distended bladder may be palpated in the midline above the symphysis pubis, which may indicate a vesicoureteral or bladder neck obstruction, acute bladder retention, or neurogenic bladder.

Palpate the umbilicus for masses or herniation. The most common umbilical disorder is an *umbilical hernia* in which the intestine protrudes through the abdominal fascia, or *linea alba* (Fig. 14.10). The umbilicus appears to protrude especially when the child is crying, stooling, or coughing, but generally it can be easily reduced when the examiner applies light pressure with the fingertips to the umbilicus. Palpate the fascia below the umbilicus with the fingertips to determine the size of the defect. If the opening is larger than the width of two fingers or the child is older than 3 years of age,

surgical closure may be necessary. Incarceration of an umbilical hernia is very rare. Most will spontaneously close by the time the child is 3 or 4 years of age. The most common umbilical mass is a *dermoid cyst*. It appears as a firm, skin-covered, nonreducible mass within the umbilicus that may have a slight discoloration and can be lobulated. Other cysts or an *umbilical polyp* should be referred to a pediatric surgeon for evaluation. *Diastasis recti abdominis* (Fig. 14.8) can be noted with light palpation over the midquadrant. An infant between the ages of 3 and 8 weeks of age with projectile, nonbilious vomiting may have *pyloric stenosis*. Examine the infant while the abdomen is relaxed and palpate in the upper abdomen, slightly right of the midline for a firm, olive-shaped mass, which is highly suspicious for a hypertrophic pylorus. If a child presents with constipation, a sausage-shaped mass of stool may be palpated in the left lower quadrant (LLQ) or in the midline below the umbilicus or *rectosigmoid* colon. The palpation of stool throughout the abdomen may indicate fecal impaction.

Palpate the groin bilaterally for femoral arterial pulses and the presence of lymph nodes (Fig. 14.11). Check the groin area for a mass or *inguinal hernia*. Note any persistent bulging in the groin. Palpate to determine size and reducibility. If the inguinal bulge or *hernia* can be reduced, referral is indicated for elective surgery and repair. An irreducible or incarcerated hernia is a surgical emergency. Scars from

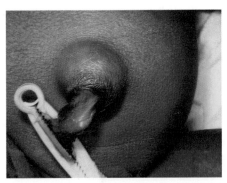

FIGURE 14.10 Umbilical hernia. (From Clark DA. *Atlas of Neonatology*. 7th ed. Philadelphia: Saunders; 2000.)

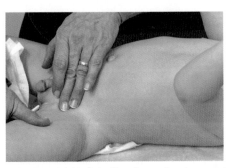

FIGURE 14.11 Palpating femoral pulses and lymph nodes.

previous surgical hernia repairs should also be evaluated. An incisional hernia may be present, should be evaluated, and referred.

Percussion

Percussion of the abdomen can help to identify whether distention of the abdomen is caused by air, a mass, or fluid (Fig. 14.12). When percussing, place your nondominant hand firmly against the abdominal wall so that only your middle finger is resting on the skin. With a relaxed wrist, tap on the distal interphalangeal joint of your middle finger two or three times with the tip of the middle finger of your dominant hand. Air or gas in the abdominal cavity creates a hollow, drum-like sound, or *tympany*, in tapping firmly over the area. Tympany is common in infants and young children because they swallow air while feeding or crying. Percussion can also delineate rough dimensions of solid masses and organs, although in most settings diagnostic imaging is used to confirm the accuracy of any abdominal findings. To measure liver size, percuss superiorly between the ribs until no dullness is noted. The upper edge of the liver should be detected at the right midclavicular line near the fifth intercostal space. Mark this point and measure its distance from the lower edge of the liver. The lower edge of the liver should not extend more than 1 to 2 cm below the costal margin. This technique identifies only the anterior surface of the liver and not the anteroposterior dimension. Fluid in the abdomen creates a dull sound when percussing over the area and may indicate the presence of *ascites* in the abdominal cavity.

Rectal Examination

A rectal exam should be performed if there is concern regarding anal or rectal patency, anal discomfort, constipation or sphincter tone, fissures, hemorrhoids, or rectal polyps.[9] Abdominal pain may be an indication for a rectal exam depending on the child's or adolescent's health history.

If the abdominal exam and health history are unclear, or the information obtained from a rectal exam would assist in the diagnosis, it should be approached carefully with informed consent of child and parent. Explain clearly to the parent and child or adolescent the need for the rectal exam. Keep in mind that a rectal exam is physically invasive, and many children will no longer cooperate with a physical exam after a rectal exam has been performed. If it is necessary to perform a rectal exam, do so at the very end of the physical examination, using the talk-through approach as presented in Chapter 1 and Chapter 17.

Position the child on the side with knees flexed (fetal position). An infant or toddler can lie supine with the hips and knees flexed. Assess the sacrum for dimples, sinuses, or tufts of hair. Note the location of the anus; if displaced anteriorly, it could predispose a child to issues such as constipation. Inspect the anus for rashes, fissures, skin tags, or discoloration.

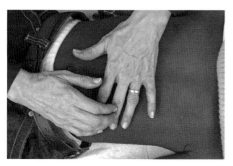

FIGURE 14.12 Percussion of the abdomen.

Contraction of the external anal sphincter (anal wink reflex) is a normal response to stroking of the skin in the perineum. Gently insert a gloved, lubricated finger (usually the smallest finger for infants; the index finger for an older child) into the rectal vault and feel for any narrowing (Fig. 14.13). Assess sphincter tone. Feel for any masses or polyps or pressure compressing the lumen of the rectum. Note whether there is stool in the rectum and whether it is hard or soft. If an explosive stool is elicited with the rectal exam, it may be a sign of a rectal obstruction, such as *Hirschsprung disease*. Gently press toward the right lower quadrant and observe whether this elicits a pain response, which can support a diagnosis of appendicitis. Alternately press in all directions and note any pain. If any stool is retrieved from the exam, perform a guaiac test on the specimen if there is concern for occult blood in the stool, keeping in mind that trauma during a rectal exam may affect the result.

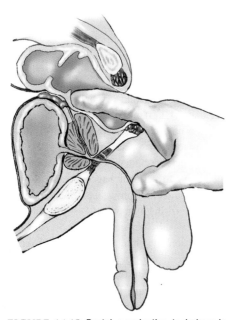

FIGURE 14.13 Rectal examination technique in an older child.

EVIDENCE-BASED PRACTICE TIP

If trauma or sexual abuse is suspected, physical signs during the rectal exam that may be concerning—but not diagnostic—include decreased anal muscle tone, anal dilation and/or perianal venous congestion.[10]

DIAGNOSTIC PROCEDURES

Several diagnostic procedures may be useful to aid in the assessment of abdominal and rectal complaints.[11] Guaiac stool testing or a urine dipstick may be easily performed in the clinic setting or office. Laboratory analyses that could be useful include analysis of urine or stool, serum evaluation of liver, kidney, and pancreas function, monitoring of electrolytes, or checking for antibody markers, including for inflammatory bowel disease (IBD) or celiac disease. When indicated, abdominal ultrasound is often the first step in diagnostic imaging, depending on the child's health history and physical examination findings. Proceed with radiographic procedures such as a kidneys-ureters-bladder (KUB) x-ray or magnetic resonance imaging (MRI), if needed, to locate and measure organs or masses or detect intestinal inflammation, obstruction, or perforation. A computed tomography (CT) scan should be performed with caution, in consultation with pediatric surgery or gastroenterology, when indicated. Endoscopy of the upper or lower gastrointestinal (GI) tract may be useful to visualize anatomy, lesions, and obtain biopsies; for example, to evaluate for inflammation of the esophagus due to gastroesophageal reflux disease.

ABDOMINAL CONDITIONS

Box 14.2 presents conditions of the abdomen according to where the signs or symptoms may occur. Keep in mind that many conditions involve diffuse abdominal pain, and children often have a difficult time localizing pain to a specific region.

TELEHEALTH TIPS

Telehealth is a reliable resource for health care providers and their patients. In the telehealth visit, the examiner must perform the assessment without hands-on medical equipment. The use of observation, thorough history taking, and adapting techniques to guide your patient in front of the camera can yield helpful details.[12,13] Although there may be limitations, a clinician can obtain useful information when objective data is collected properly. A little creativity with tools in the home, such as a scale for weight, measuring tape for height, thermometer for temperature, and even a watch to count pulse, can provide helpful data for assessment.[12] However, there are barriers to a virtual visit where the abdomen and rectum need evaluation.[14] The rectal exam cannot be performed via telehealth due to privacy requirements. In situations that a rectal exam is needed emergently, an in-person visit should be scheduled.[13] See Box 14.3 for abdominal exam techniques via telehealth.

BOX 14.3 TELEHEALTH ABDOMINAL EXAM

Observation:
If possible, have the patient stand and turn to the side to observe the shape of the abdomen
Assess the abdomen visually for scars, rash, distention, ostomy, gastrostomy tube
If unable to see these areas clearly, you can request the patient or caregiver to send you a photo via secured electronic record
Palpation: Assessing abdomen for pain or mass when a caregiver is available to assist
Ask patient to lie flat on couch or bed
Ask caregiver to palpate the abdomen in all four quadrants with your direction
Ask caregiver to describe if abdomen is soft, firm, distended, fluid wave, mass
Ask patient to describe what they are feeling is tenderness, pressure, pain

Ask patient to describe if any pain is present and where it is located
Ask caregiver to palpate lower and mid back for referred pain

Alternate ways to assess the abdomen if the patient is alone:
Ask patient to face the screen and palpate the abdomen in all four quadrants
With patient facing the screen, ask them to point with one finger where the pain is located
Show the patient a photo of an abdomen's four quadrants and ask them to point out the pain region
Ask patient to stand and hop on one foot or step on a stool and jump off, if able (assesses acute surgical abdomen such as appendicitis)

Data from Benziger CP, Huffman MD, Sweis RN, Stone NJ. The Telehealth Ten: A guide for a patient-assisted virtual physical examination. *American J Med*. 2021;134(1):48–51.
James-Stevenson T. The virtual gastroenterology clinic. *Clinic Gastroenterol Hepatol*. 2020;18(12):2679–2682.

SUMMARY OF EXAMINATION

- A thorough and detailed history is an essential part of the abdominal assessment and should include the medical and family health history, nutrition and elimination habits, a psychosocial evaluation, and a review of pain or other presenting symptoms.
- Infants and young children may be more comfortably assessed in the lap of the parent or caregiver.
- Abdominal assessment should be performed using a mapping technique by mentally dividing the abdomen into four quadrants or nine regions.
- Begin inspection of the abdomen by observing the child or adolescent's posture, behavior, and activity level; then inspect the abdomen for size, shape, and pulsations.
- Auscultate each quadrant of the abdomen before palpation and note the quality and frequency of bowel sounds.
- Use light palpation to identify areas of tenderness before deep palpation.

- During palpation, note size of organs if palpable, presence of tenderness or pain on palpation, any guarding or rigidity in the abdomen, and the size and quality of any masses.
- Perform percussion to identify the presence of air or gas and to estimate the size of solid organs or masses.
- A rectal examination should be performed only when applicable and, if so, should be done at the end of the physical exam.
- Adapting the virtual abdominal exam during telehealth visits, the clinician can collect essential, objective data for the assessment and diagnosis of patients outside the clinical environment.

DOCUMENTATION

1-Month-Old Term Infant
Abdomen: Abdomen symmetrical, soft, round, nontender without masses or organomegaly. Liver palpated 2 cm below right costal margin. Normal bowel sounds over all quadrants. Umbilicus clean, dry without hernia, mass, inflammation, or discharge. Epigastric pulsations noted. Percussion tones tympanic.

12-Year-Old With Abdominal Pain
Abdomen: Abdomen symmetrical, flat, tender with guarding throughout, and rebound tenderness noted in RLQ. Bowel sounds hypoactive, especially in the lower quadrants. No masses or hepatomegaly, spleen tip nonpalpable.

REFERENCES

1. Ayonrinde OT, Ayonrinde OA, Adams LA, et al. The relationship between abdominal pain and emotional wellbeing in children and adolescents in the Raine Study. *Sci Rep*. 2020;10(1):1646.
2. Reed-Knight B, Maddux MH, Deacy AD, et al. Brain–gut interactions and maintenance factors in pediatric gastroenterological disorders: recommendations for clinical care. *Clin Pract Pediatr Psychol*. 2017;5(1):93–105.
3. Malinak R. Evaluation & management of functional abdominal pain in children. *Osteopath Fam Physician*. 2017;9(5):32–36.
4. Sanchez TR, Corwin MT, Davoodian BS, Stein-Wexler R. Sonography of abdominal pain in children: appendicitis and its common mimics. *J Med Ultrasound*. 2016;35(3):627–635.
5. Conion TW, Nishisaki A, Singh Y. Moving beyond the stethoscope: diagnostic point-of-care ultrasound in pediatric practice. *Pediatrics*. 2017;144(4):e20191402.
6. Vos MB, Abrams SH, Barlow E, et al. NASPGHAN Clinical practice guideline for the diagnosis and treatment of nonalcoholic fatty liver disease in children: recommendations from the Expert Committee on NAFLD (ECON) and the North American Society of Pediatric Gastroenterology,
Hepatology and Nutrition (NASPGHAN). *J Pediatr Gastroenterol Nutr*. 2017;64(2):319–334.
7. Rothrock SG, Greene SM, Morgan R. Abdominal trauma in infants and children: prompt identification and early management of serious and life-threatening injuries. Part I: injury patterns and initial assessment. *Pediatr Emerg Care*. 2000;16(2):106–115.
8. Henry MK, Bennett CE, Wood JN, Servaes S. Evaluation of the abdomen in the setting of suspected child abuse. *Pediatr Radiol*. 2021;51(6):1044–1050.
9. Orenstein SR, Wald A. Pediatric rectal exam: why, when, and how. *Curr Gastroenterol Rep*. 2016;18(4):1–7.
10. Hobbs CJ, Wright CM. Anal signs of child sexual abuse: a case–control study. *BMC Pediatr*. 2014;14:128.
11. Marcdante KJ, Kliegman RM. *Nelson Essentials of Pediatrics*. 8th ed. Elsevier; 2018.
12. Benziger CP, Huffman MD, Sweis RN, Stone NJ. The Telehealth Ten: a guide for a patient-assisted virtual physical examination. *American J Med*. 2021;134(1):48–51.
13. James-Stevenson T. The virtual gastroenterology clinic. *Clinc Gastroenterol Hepatol*. 2020;18(12):2679–2682.
14. Gajarawala SN, Pelkowski JN. *Telehealth benefits and barriers*. 2021;17(2):218–221.

PENIS, TESTICLES, AND SCROTUM

Angel C. Kuo

The pediatric physical examination is not complete without a thorough evaluation of the developing genitalia. Routine surveillance of the genitourinary system is equally important in all patient encounters; when assessment of the genitalia is performed routinely, abnormalities can be identified and promptly treated. Many parents, children, and adolescents are concerned and anxious about the genitalia, yet they may not feel comfortable expressing those concerns initially. A review of systems in the health history and the routine genital exam offers an opportunity for the parent, child, and/ or adolescent to voice concerns and for the provider to offer reassurance and education on typical development. The provider has a role in fostering dialogue between the parent and child regarding sexual and reproductive health. Establishing this dialogue with families early forms the basis for discussions on sexual and reproductive health during puberty and in the developing adolescent.

EMBRYOLOGIC DEVELOPMENT

The differentiation of the sexual organs begins as early as the third week of embryonic development, dictated by the sex chromosomes at the time of fertilization.[1] The mesoderm is the embryonic layer that becomes smooth and striated muscle tissue, connective tissue, blood vessels, bone marrow, skeletal tissue, and the reproductive and excretory organs. As proliferation of the embryonic layers continues, maturation of the external genitalia in the fetus is established by the 12th week.[1] The sex-determining region of the Y chromosome (SRY gene) activates the differentiation of the embryonic gonad into a testis, without which the gonad would become an ovary. The antimüllerian hormone (AMH) prevents development of the uterus and fallopian tubes, whereas testosterone stimulates the Wolffian ducts to develop into the male reproductive structures, including the epididymis, vas deferens, and seminal vesicles. Testosterone is also the precursor to dihydrotestosterone (DHT), which stimulates the formation of the male urethra, prostate, and external genitalia.[1]

Urine production begins between the 9th and 12th weeks and is excreted into the amniotic cavity through the urethral meatus. During development, the fetus continues the production and excretion of urine, which forms the amniotic fluid. Between the 17th and 20th weeks, the testes, which develop in the abdominal cavity, begin to descend along the inguinal canal into the scrotum, bringing the arteries, veins, lymphatics, and nerves that are encased within the cremaster muscle and spermatic cord.[1] The inguinal canal closes after testicular descent. Incomplete or abnormal embryonic development of the inguinal canal predisposes the newborn to the formation of hydroceles or hernias. Preterm infants are at increased risk for these conditions. At birth, the infant's genitourinary system is functionally immature with limited bladder capacity, an inability to concentrate urine sufficiently, and frequent voiding.

Growth of the fetus and differentiation of the sexual organs can be affected by placental function, the hormonal environment during

275

pregnancy, maternal nutrition, maternal infection, and genetic factors or chromosomal abnormalities. A fetal insult from intrinsic or extrinsic factors during the eighth or ninth week of gestation may lead to major abnormalities of the developing external genitalia. The data on impact from chemical exposure is mixed and inconclusive[2]; however, endocrine-disrupting chemicals do play a role in the development of the endocrine and genitourinary system (see Chapter 5 for further discussion).

ANATOMY AND PHYSIOLOGY

Penis

The penis consists of the shaft, glans, corona, meatus, and prepuce. The shaft is composed of erectile tissue called corpora cavernosa (two lateral columns) and corpus spongiosum (ventral column). The anterior portion of the corpus spongiosum forms the glans penis, the border or edge of which is called the corona. The urethra is within the corpus spongiosum, and the orifice, or urethral meatus, is the slitlike opening just ventral to the tip of the penis (Fig. 15.1).

The prepuce, or foreskin, is the fold of skin at the tip of the penis that covers the glans penis in the uncircumcised male and forms the secondary fold of skin from the urethral meatus to the coronal region of the penis called the frenulum. The skin of the penis is thin, does not contain subcutaneous fat, and is loosely tied to the deeper layer of the dermis and fascia. Often, the skin of the shaft is more darkly pigmented, particularly in children or adolescents with darker pigmentation or darker skin. The skin of the glans penis does not contain hair follicles but does have small glands and papillae that form in the epithelial cells to produce smegma, the white oily material made up of desquamated epithelial cells trapped under the foreskin, which is normal and often mistaken as pathologic (Fig. 15.2). The foreskin is generally nonretractable at birth because of adherence of the inner epithelial lining of the foreskin and glans.[3] Desquamation of the tissue layers continues until the separation of the prepuce and glans penis is complete secondary to intermittent erections and keratinization of the inner epithelium, generally by 6 years of age. Partial adhesions of the foreskin to the prepuce may produce smegma along the coronal region, which often persists throughout

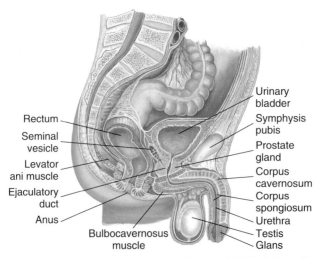

Labels (left): Rectum, Seminal vesicle, Levator ani muscle, Ejaculatory duct, Anus, Bulbocavernosus muscle

Labels (right): Urinary bladder, Symphysis pubis, Prostate gland, Corpus cavernosum, Corpus spongiosum, Urethra, Testis, Glans

FIGURE 15.1 Internal and external genitalia. (From Ball JW et al. *Seidel's Guide to Physical Examination: An Interprofessional Approach.* 10th ed. St. Louis: Elsevier; 2023.)

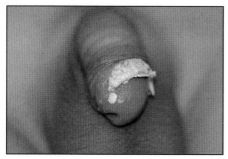

FIGURE 15.2 Smegma. (From Lissauer T, Carrol W. *Illustrated Textbook of Paediatrics.* 6th ed. Elsevier; 2022.)

childhood. In consultation with the health care provider, caregivers may choose for their newborn to undergo circumcision, the excision of the foreskin. If the child has been *circumcised*, then the *glans penis* will be visible without the need to retract any skin.

Scrotum and Testes

The scrotum is made up of a thin layer of skin that forms rugae (folds) and contains the testes. The epididymis is the thin palpable structure along the lateral edge of the posterior side of the testes. Sperm production occurs within the seminiferous tubules in the testes, which connect to the epididymis. The vas deferens is the cordlike structure that is continuous with the base of the epididymis and stores sperm. The spermatic cord extends from the testes to the inguinal ring and is felt only on deep palpation of the testicular sac. The right spermatic cord is shorter in some males, which causes the right testis to hang higher than the left.

Accessory organs include the seminal vesicles, which lay deep in the abdominal cavity alongside the vas deferens and secrete liquid into the semen as it passes from the testes. The opening of the seminal vesicles joins the vas deferens to form ejaculatory ducts and drains to the posterior urethra. The Cowper glands, or bulbourethral glands, lie along the urethra in the male genitalia. These are exocrine glands that produce a viscous secretion that lubricates the urethra for the passage of sperm. It also neutralizes the acidic urethral secretions that could otherwise damage the spermatozoa in the semen. The prostate gland is the small, firm mass that lies within the pelvic cavity. It first becomes palpable on manual examination in the adolescent. The prostate gland surrounds the posterior urethra and secretes an alkaline secretion during ejaculation to promote fertilization. The smooth muscle within the prostate gland assists with urinary elimination. An enlarged prostate gland may cause urinary obstruction.

TABLE 15.1	PHYSIOLOGIC VARIATIONS OF THE PENIS, TESTES AND/OR SCROTUM	
Age Group	**Variation**
Preterm infant	Rugae absent on scrotum in low-birth-weight infant Testes undescended in 20% of infants weighing <2500 g[a]
Newborn	Rugae present from 37 weeks' gestation Note and evaluate any discoloration of scrotum at birth Testis: volume 1–2 mL Length of penis in term infant: 2.5–3.5 cm; size should be palpated during exam Shaft may appear short or retracted in infants with significant suprapubic fat pad
Infancy/early childhood	Foreskin partially retractable over glans penis Testes present in scrotal sac Initial sexual arousal and erection occur with normal sexual exploration or exposure of genitalia

[a]Data from Cavaliere TA. Genitourinary assessment. In: Tappero EP, Honeyfield ME, eds. *Physical Assessment of the Newborn*, 5th ed. Petaluma: NICU INK; 2015, pp. 121–137.

PHYSIOLOGIC VARIATIONS

Table 15.1 presents physiologic variations of the genitalia from infancy to early childhood.

Physiologic Changes in Puberty

Puberty has a gradual onset, and although it is marked by a growth spurt, it may be difficult to ascertain when the first changes in the child begin in the transition to secondary sexual characteristics. Sexual development, or true gonadal activation, begins with an increase in size of the testicles, which is often difficult to determine. Testicular volume should be evaluated and is the most accurate measurement of the progression of puberty in the developing child. In some children, this begins around 10 years of age and is complete in about 3 years, with the normal range extending to 5 years.[4] The sexual maturity rating (SMR) scale, also known as "Tanner stages," helps to classify physical pubertal maturation (Fig. 15.3 and Table 15.2).[4] Genital development and pubic hair may develop at different rates. Ejaculation usually occurs at SMR 3 during the midpoint of sexual development. Fertility is established by SMR 4, although sperm are present in some quantity with ejaculation during SMR 3.

In adolescents, the tempo of growth and maturation is distinctly different between sexes. Most of the rapid linear growth occurs at mid-puberty for those with an XY genotype, due to rising testosterone concentrations. Recent studies have provided evidence that patterns of puberty onset can vary by genetic background.[5]

PREPARATION FOR GENITOURINARY ASSESSMENT

Understanding and respecting cultural differences is an important part of the role of the health care provider, particularly in relation to the assessment of the genitourinary system. Identifying which family members may be a part of the discussion and/or be present during the examination of the genitalia and how to

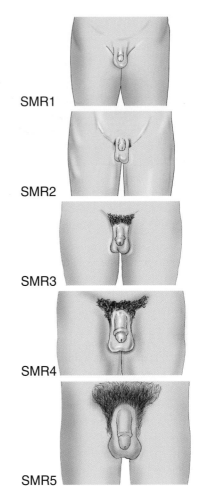

SMR1

SMR2

SMR3

SMR4

SMR5

FIGURE 15.3 Sexual maturity rating or Tanner staging.

approach the exam are the first steps in developing a trusting relationship with the family. Caregiver and family attitudes about sexuality vary widely both within cultures and among cultures. Sexual awakening first occurs in the young child with the discovery of the genitalia as a sensual organ. This initial experience and the caregiver attitude toward developmentally appropriate fondling and exploration may set the stage for either healthy sexual development or a feeling of shame in the child that impacts functioning throughout life. Cultural attitudes concerning sexuality and reproduction may

TABLE 15.2 DEVELOPMENTAL CHANGES IN PUBERTY

Tanner Stage/ Sexual Maturity Rating (SMR)	DEVELOPMENTAL CHANGES			
	Pubic Hair	Penis	Scrotum	Testicular Volume
Tanner stage 1 SMR 1	None	Unchanged from early childhood	Unchanged from early childhood	<1.5 mL
Tanner stage 2 SMR 2	Small amount of light, downy hair along base of penis	Unchanged or slightly enlarged	Enlarged and reddened pigmentation; skin taut and thinner; increased rugation	1.6–6 mL
Tanner stage 3 SMR 3	Moderate amount of curly, pigmented coarse pubic hair extending laterally over symphysis pubis	↑ Length and circumference	Further enlargement	6–12 mL
Tanner stage 4 SMR 4	Abundant adult-like quality	Glans penis broader and larger; penis ↑ length and circumference	Further enlargement and darker pigmentation	12–20 mL
Tanner stage 5 SMR 5	Extends to medial surface of the thighs	Adult size	Adult size	>20 mL

Data from Neinstein LS, Katzman DK, Callahan ST, Gordon CM, Joffe A, Rickert VI. *Neinstein's Adolescent and Young Adult Health Care: A Practical Guide.* 6th ed. Philadelphia: Wolters Kluwer; 2016.

form the basis of conflict between the caregiver and young child or maturing adolescent. Mediating this difference between the adolescent and the caregiver may be the most important and challenging role for the health care provider. In addition, documentation in the health care record provides opportunity to communicate these attitudes to the next provider to ensure consistent delivery of care.

CARE FOR TRANSGENDER AND GENDER-DIVERSE YOUTH

Some youth may identify as *transgender*, where their experienced or expressed gender is different from their assigned or designated sex at birth.[6,7] Gender-diverse individuals may not conform to a gender binary but rather may identify anywhere within or outside of the gender spectrum or may identify as genderless. Transgender and gender-diverse youth may experience symptoms of gender dysphoria, or a discomfort from the misalignment of their identified gender and assigned sex.[7]

Providers should ask for and use the patient's preferred pronoun and chosen name and avoid making assumptions of gender identity based on appearance.[6] While providers are encouraged to use medical terms for the genitalia, for some transgender or gender-diverse youth, such terms may make them uncomfortable; thus, providers should use terminology that the patient uses, or gender-neutral terms such as "genitals" when possible.[8] Unless the youth undergo gender-affirming hormone treatment, their anatomy is still that of the assigned sex at birth and warrant a thorough exam as they feel comfortable.[6]

SYSTEM-SPECIFIC HISTORY

Important information for the assessment of the genitalia at key developmental stages and ages is presented in the Information Gathering table as follows.

INFORMATION GATHERING FOR GENITALIA ASSESSMENT AT KEY DEVELOPMENTAL STAGES

Age Group	Questions to Ask
For all age groups	Gestational and birth history
	History of prenatal exposure to hormone ingestion
	Prenatal exposure to alcohol and/or drug use
	Prenatal exposure to hazardous chemicals and/or pesticides
	Family history of GU abnormalities
	Current medication, including any gender-affirming hormone therapy
	Circumcision status
	Scrotal or inguinal mass; ± pain
	Voiding history (include voiding frequency, voiding stream, ballooning of foreskin [if applicable])
	Elimination history (frequency and consistency)
Preterm, newborn, and infant	History of prenatal infection
	History of significant neonatal infections
	Presence of testes in scrotum at birth
Early childhood, middle childhood	Toilet training process
	Additional voiding history (history of urinary frequency, postponing behavior, daytime and/or nighttime wetting, difficulty, or pain on urination)
	History of balanitis and/or (documented) urinary tract infections
	Physiologic phimosis
Adolescence	Family history of delayed puberty
	Onset of growth spurt and puberty
	Painful erection
	History of balanitis and/or (documented) urinary tract infections
	Testicular pain/swelling
	Penile discharge
	Sexual identity and gender expression; gender-affirming treatment if applicable
	Sexual debut:
	With males, females, or both
	Number of partners
	Types of sexual activity (vaginal, oral, and/or anal intercourse)

Continued

INFORMATION GATHERING FOR GENITALIA ASSESSMENT AT KEY DEVELOPMENTAL STAGES—CONT'D

Age Group	Questions to Ask
	Condom use
	STI exposure/testing/results
	History of coerced or forced sexual contact
	Inability to achieve erection and/or to ejaculate

GU, Genitourinary; *STI*, sexually transmitted infection.

PHYSICAL ASSESSMENT

Preparation

Although there is a tendency toward skipping assessment of the genitalia while performing a physical examination, the provider should be mindful that it is a critical part of evaluating a growing and developing body. If performed regularly by the provider during pediatric well visits, the genital examination then simply becomes an expected part of the routine physical assessment at all ages, including through adolescence. Reticence on the part of the child, adolescent, caregiver, or even the provider is not a reason for omitting the examination of the genitalia, but rather offers an opportunity for a more in-depth approach to the informed consent discussion. As with the rest of the physical examination, the provider should maintain a matter-of-fact approach and use a purposeful technique that is not traumatic for the child or adolescent. For the transgender or gender-diverse youth, additional reassurance can be provided.

Before the start of the genitourinary exam, the provider should discuss the rationale for performing this exam as well as what to expect during the exam. Anticipatory guidance is of utmost importance for all age groups beyond the infant and young child. Parents of adolescents should be asked to leave the exam room after bringing up their own concerns during the health history, and the adolescent should be given the opportunity to share any further information privately. This gives the provider an opportunity to discuss with the adolescent the consent to confidential reproductive health services and the limits to confidentiality, which differ from state to state (see Chapter 4). After a confidential history has been obtained, the adolescent should still be given the option of having the parent or another adult chaperone present during the genital portion of the exam. The presence of a chaperone protects both patients and health care providers and supports ethical practice during sensitive examinations.[9] This practice is recommended regardless of the sex or gender of the patient or provider. Providers should document in the medical record that a chaperone was offered and who was present during the exam, or that the patient declined.[9]

PEDIATRIC PEARLS

In early childhood, the provider should emphasize that the genital exam is only to be done when a parent or guardian is present but not with strangers or other adolescents or adults. In middle childhood, the genital exam is a chance to reinforce typical development, and the exam prepares the child for what to expect as an adolescent. In adolescence, the exam is a chance to be alone with the provider to discuss questions and/or concerns about their genitalia and sexual development, although a chaperone should be offered and provided if desired.

As with all parts of the physical examination in pediatrics, it is important to talk through the assessment of the genitalia and reassure the adolescent of expected findings as well as discuss any concerns when completing the examination. This is also an opportunity to discuss typical growth and development, hygiene issues, and anticipatory guidance. With adolescents, the talk-through exam provides the opportunity to establish rapport and validates feelings and concerns during and after the examination. Adolescents may have underlying questions around issues of "normalcy" or sexual and reproductive health. The pediatric health care provider must be ready to discuss any issues involving sexual and reproductive health in a supportive and professional manner.

Positioning

During the first 4 to 6 months of life, infants are best positioned on the examination table for assessment of the genitalia. Beyond early infancy, the child may be lying on the parent's lap in a knee-to-knee position with the provider or continue to be examined on the exam table. The young child may be lying down or sitting in the tailor position (cross-legged) on the exam table (Fig. 15.4). The middle-age child may be examined lying supine on the

exam table or sitting or standing to enhance gravity of the testicles, as in the adolescent and young adult.[4,10] It is important to have draping available and only expose the child as long as needed for inspection, palpation, and/or education. Lengthy discussions can be done once the child is dressed. Respecting the need for privacy, particularly in the young child and the developing adolescent, establishes a good patient-provider relationship.

Inspection and Palpation

Assessment of the genitalia includes inspection and palpation of the penis, foreskin, urethral meatus, scrotum, testes, rectal sphincter, and perineal skin status. Always inform the child or adolescent before beginning inspection and palpation. Physiologic phimosis, when the foreskin cannot be retracted over the glans penis, is an expected finding until about 6 years of age (Fig. 15.5). Forcible retraction of the foreskin may cause trauma, with increased risk for infection and/or scarring, leading to pathologic phimosis. Good hygiene of the penis and foreskin can decrease the risk of developing infection or adhesions of the foreskin to the glans penis and should be reviewed regularly at well-child visits during childhood.

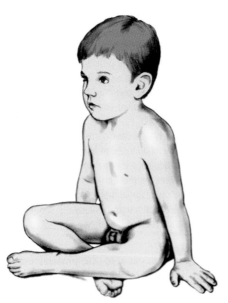

FIGURE 15.4 Young child sitting tailor style (cross-legged) in preparation for testicular exam.

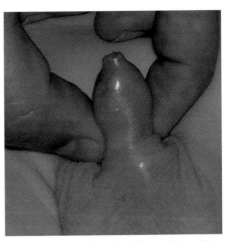

FIGURE 15.5 Physiologic phimosis. (From Abbas T, McCarthy, L. Foreskin and penile problems in childhood. *Surgery*. 2022;40(5):326–331.)

In the newborn, the urethral meatus is normally on the tip of the glans penis. In middle childhood and adolescence, the urethral meatus is a slitlike opening on the ventral side of the glans penis. Examination of the adolescent urethral meatus includes an inspection for erythema or discharge (Fig. 15.6).

Children or adolescents with a penis who do not identify with the male gender may choose to hide their penis through *tucking*, where the penis is pulled backward to the perineum, and testes are pushed into the inguinal canal with use of special undergarments or tape.[12] With the patient's permission, careful inspection of the groin and perineum should include evaluation for issues of skin irritation or other concerns due to tucking.

Inspection of the scrotum includes assessing the fullness, color, median raphe, and rugae, as well as determining SMR. Before palpation of the scrotum in the infant and prepubertal child, the provider should place a hand firmly above the inguinal canal, near the superior anterior iliac crest, milk down the testis along the inguinal canal, and trap the testis in the scrotum with the thumb and index finger of the opposite hand to prevent retraction of the testes (Fig. 15.7). Isolate the testis between the thumb and forefinger and roll within the pads of the fingers to assess for testicular size, shape, consistency, and any point tenderness (Fig. 15.8). The cremasteric reflex causes retraction of the testes into the inguinal canal/abdominal cavity and can be activated by cold, touch, or emotion, particularly in infancy and early childhood. Retractile testis is a testis that may retract on exam but is well-positioned in the scrotum. This may confuse the findings of the exam, prompting unnecessary referral in a typically developing child.

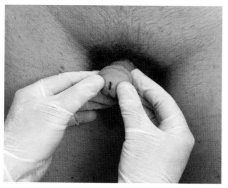

FIGURE 15.6 Examination of urethral meatus in adolescent. (From Swartz MH. *Textbook of Physical Diagnosis.* 8th ed. Philadelphia: Elsevier; 2021.)

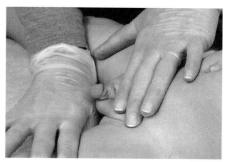

FIGURE 15.7 Trapping of testis in scrotum for examination.

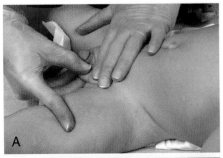

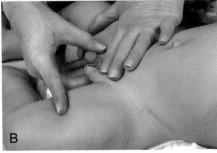

FIGURE 15.8 Palpation of scrotal sac. **(A)** Left testicle. **(B)** Right testicle.

Compare the testes bilaterally for any significant difference in size. Testicular size discrepancy of greater than 15% should be noted for further evaluation.[10] An orchidometer may be used to screen testicular size in the growing and developing child, or to measure atypical testicular size (Fig. 15.9), although

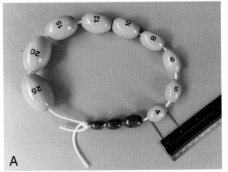

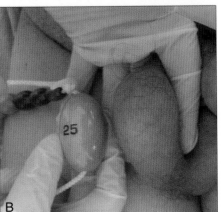

FIGURE 15.9 Orchidometer to evaluate testicular size. ([A] from Zitelli BJ, et al. *Zitelli and Davis' Atlas of Pediatric Physical Diagnosis*. 8th ed. Philadelphia: Elsevier; 2023; [B] from Mana DL, et al. FSH-producing pituitary macroadenoma: Report of 2 cases with clinical manifestations of hormone excess. *AACE Clin Case Rep*. 2016;2(1):e7–e11.)

EVIDENCE-BASED PRACTICE TIP

Cryptorchidism, or undescended testicle, is best evaluated by history and physical examinations initially. Radiologic imaging with ultrasound offers little diagnostic value and increases the cost of health care. Rather than imaging, the optimal next step is referral to a specialist in pediatric urology for evaluation and management.[14] Generally, if testes were detected in the normally formed scrotum in the first 6 months of life but are now present as undescended, they are most likely *retractile* in nature. Acquired cryptorchidism, or ascent of a previously descended testis, may occur in 1%–7% of children assigned male at birth and peaks at 8 years of age.[14] Acquired cryptorchidism also requires further evaluation by a specialist in pediatric urology.

scrotal ultrasound provides a more accurate measurement of testicular volume.[13] If the testis is not palpable in the scrotum of the young child, often a positional change to sitting with legs crossed (tailor style) will facilitate relaxation of the cremasteric muscle and allow for the testes to descend to the scrotal sac (see Fig. 15.4). Careful inspection and palpation of the inguinal, suprapubic, scrotal, and perineal region may reveal an ectopic testis, located outside of the typical path of descent (Fig. 15.10).[14]

In the adolescent, the examiner should palpate for the epididymis on the posterior surface of the testes. It can be felt on the lateral

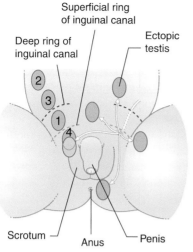

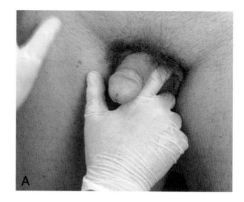

FIGURE 15.10 Ectopic testis. (From de Bruyn R. *Pediatric Ultrasound: How, Why, and When*. 2nd ed. Philadelphia: Churchill Livingstone; 2011.)

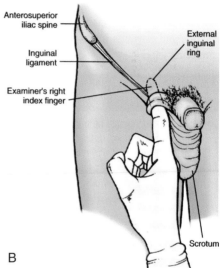

FIGURE 15.11 Examination for inguinal hernia. ([A] from Swartz MH. *Textbook of Physical Diagnosis*. 8th ed. Philadelphia: Elsevier; 2021; [B] from Ball JW, et al. *Seidel's Guide to Physical Examination: An Interprofessional Approach*. 10th ed. St. Louis: Elsevier; 2023.)

surface of the testes as smooth, discreet, and slightly irregular in shape. The vas deferens can be palpated from the testes to the inguinal ring. Palpation of any testicular nodules is an indication for further evaluation to rule out malignancy. The adolescent should be educated about testicular self-examination (TSE) along with a return demonstration.[15] Although there is controversy among some national clinical practice organizations regarding the effectiveness of routine TSE for testicular cancer screening,[15-17] TSE may still be a valuable way for adolescents to detect urogenital health concerns or abnormalities that may lead to testicular cancer or infertility.[15,16]

EVIDENCE-BASED PRACTICE TIP

Some helpful testicular self-examination resources for teens include the following:
Kids Health: http://kidshealth.org/teen/sexual_health/guys/tse.html
MedlinePlus: http://www.nlm.nih.gov/medlineplus/ency/article/003909.htm
American Cancer Society: http://www.cancer.org/cancer/testicularcancer/moreinformation/doihavetesticularcancer/do-i-have-testicular-cancer-self-exam

For young adolescents with SMR or Tanner stage 3 and above, another essential part of the genitourinary exam is the inguinal hernia exam. This is also a routine part of the preparticipation sports physical assessment (see Chapter 18). To determine whether an inguinal hernia may be present, invaginate the skin from the scrotal sac with index finger and advance into the slitlike opening of the inguinal ring (Fig. 15.11). Ask the adolescent to bear down or cough so the protrusion of a mass may be noted as a light "tap" against the examiner's finger. If an inguinal mass is noted, auscultation may occasionally be used to ascertain whether bowel sounds are present, although this technique has been replaced by using ultrasound in most instances. A *reducible* hernia will retract back through the inguinal canal when the child is no longer bearing down and is an indication for a nonurgent referral to a general surgeon for further evaluation and management. An *incarcerated* hernia will not retract and may feel firm, hard, or tender on palpation. This finding requires urgent attention due to the potential for impaired circulation and tissue necrosis and warrants immediate referral for emergency care.

RED FLAG FINDING

An *incarcerated* inguinal hernia is nonreducible and may feel firm, hard, or tender on palpation. This is a medical emergency due to the potential for impaired circulation and tissue necrosis.

SEXUAL ABUSE

A complete physical examination, including thorough evaluation of the genitourinary system, is warranted with any indication or revelation of sexual misconduct on history taken either from parent, caregiver, child, or adolescent. Although in most sexual assault cases there is no apparent visible physical evidence, children and adolescents who are known or suspected victims of sexual assault require careful evaluation for any injuries or biologic material that may be present.[18] If the collection of evidence is anticipated, providers should consult with local experts in forensic evaluation, such as Child Protective Services (CPS), before conducting an exam. The history must be obtained in a safe and private environment, while using open-ended and developmentally appropriate questions. Examination of the oral cavity as well as the genitals and anus require careful inspection. The penis and scrotum should be evaluated for bruising or signs of external trauma, redness, swelling, or discharge. The anus and rectum should be inspected for hemorrhoids, warts, rectal dilatation, rectal fissures, or fistulas that would indicate trauma incurred as a result of intercourse. A digital exam should be performed with a gloved, lubricated finger to evaluate the sphincter tone and the rectal vault (see Chapter 14 for more information about assessment of the rectum). Referral to CPS, consultation with child abuse experts, referral to additional resources, and follow-up visits are recommended.

DIFFERENCE OF SEX DEVELOPMENT

Research continues to define new and multigenetic factors involved in the development of differences of sex development (also known as disorders of sex development; DSD), with newly developed practice guidelines to guide providers.[19] Examples of DSD include disorders of chromosomal sex, disorders of gonadal sex, or disorders of phenotypic sex including ambiguous genitalia. The first step in diagnosing the infant or child with DSD starts with an interprofessional team-based approach.[19] Thorough diagnostic evaluation includes a full body and genital exam and biochemical, genetic, and imaging studies to generate a diagnosis at the molecular genetic level.[19] Family history of a previous spontaneous abortion, stillbirth, or any neonatal death of a sibling should be noted. Family history of excess androgen, congenital adrenal hyperplasia, or an autosomal recessive genotype should also be carefully reviewed.

Perform a careful inspection of any dysmorphic features and examination of the abdominal and genital area. Providers must be mindful to avoid repeated exams and/or excessive photography. There should also be limited number of health care professionals present for the exams, to protect the integrity and privacy of the patient.[19] The key finding of the genital exam is the presence or absence of gonadal or testicular tissue palpable in the scrotum, labioscrotal folds, or inguinal canal (Fig. 15.12).

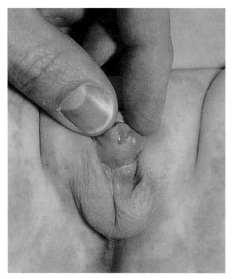

FIGURE 15.12 Ambiguous genitalia. (From Zitelli BJ, et al. *Zitelli and Davis' Atlas of Pediatric Physical Diagnosis.* 8th ed. Philadelphia: Elsevier; 2023.)

Palpable gonads lead to the high probability that the infant has an XY genotype, because ovaries do not descend. Document the size of the penis, location of meatus, and any hyperpigmentation of the labioscrotal folds.

Acute conditions warrant immediate management. Newborns with bilaterally impalpable testes yet a formed phallus should be referred to pediatric urology and pediatric endocrinology for an immediate consult to determine a possible diagnosis of DSD. This can be the consequence of a condition such as congenital adrenal hyperplasia, which could be life threatening if not diagnosed and treated.[10,14] Genetic karyotyping and additional laboratory tests are required to make a sex determination, and immediate referral to a multidisciplinary team, including a neonatologist, primary care provider, pediatric endocrinologist, pediatric urologist, geneticist, psychologist, social worker, and ethicist, is indicated.[19,20]

CONDITIONS OF THE PENIS, TESTES, AND/OR SCROTUM

Table 15.3 summarizes findings that require a referral to a pediatric urologist, and Table 15.4 presents abnormal conditions of the penis,

TABLE 15.3	ABNORMAL FINDINGS OF PENIS, SCROTUM, AND/OR INGUINAL REGION
Area	**Abnormal Findings and Referral Criteria**
Penis	Abnormal position of urethral meatus, ventral or dorsal to tip of penis
	Abnormal curvature of penis
	Micropenis: associated with syndromes and organ abnormalities
	Abnormal discharge, erythema (redness), swelling
	Thickened/scarred foreskin
	Foreskin unable to be retracted (>6 years of age)
	Foreskin unable to return to cover glans (see paraphimosis) **(urologic emergency)**
Scrotum	Painful or red/swollen testicle/scrotum **(urologic emergency)**
	Undescended or absent testes
	Communicative hydrocele (changes in size)
	Hydroceles that prevent assessment of testes (via manual exam or transillumination)
	Hernia
	Onset of puberty before 8 years of age
	Delayed or absent pubertal development
	Presence of skin lesions, vesicles, chancre, or lice
	Testicular size discrepancy of >15%
	Isolated right-sided varicocele
Inguinal region	Inguinal mass or hernia
	Tender lymph nodes

TABLE 15.4 CONDITIONS OF THE PENIS, TESTES, AND/OR SCROTUM

Condition	Image	Description
Adhesions (penile)[a]		Fused layer between glans and prepuce. May have smegma trapped underneath. If physiologic, resolves by adolescent years.
Balanoposthitis/ balanitis		Superficial infection of the penis/foreskin. Redness, swelling, and extreme tenderness of prepuce and glans penis; yellowish discharge may be present. Reoccurrences may cause scarring and/or pathologic phimosis.
Buried penis[b]		Penis partially concealed beneath the scrotum due to post-circumcision healing, or due to excessive skin or an excessive fat pad in pubic region. May lead to urinary obstruction. Generally, the penile size is as expected for age/development.
Chordee[c]		Ventral (downward) curvature of penis due to fibrotic tissue; occurs as an isolated condition or often with hypospadias.
Epididymitis[b]	Inflammation of the epididymis	Inflammation and swelling of epididymis from infection or trauma, often preceded by urethritis, generally associated with sexual activity; accompanied by gradual pain in scrotum, inguinal area, or abdomen; generally, occurs unilaterally. Exam shows point tenderness on epididymis, (+) cremasteric reflex, and (+) Prehn sign (pain relief with elevation of scrotum).
Epispadias[d]	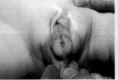	Abnormal placement of the urethral meatus on dorsal surface of penis.

Continued

TABLE 15.4 CONDITIONS OF THE PENIS, TESTES, AND/OR SCROTUM—CONT'D

Condition	Image	Description
Hernia[a]	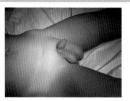	Inguinal mass or protrusion of tissue or bowel through muscle wall due to patent processus vaginalis and intensifies with straining or crying. The mass may be firm and reducible with gentle pressure, or hard and immobile, which requires immediate referral because of the potential for *incarcerated hernia*.
Hydrocele[c]	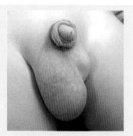	Enlargement of the scrotum due to peritoneal fluid between parietal and visceral layers of tunica vaginalis, which surrounds testis. Scrotum may be taut or firm but nontender on palpation. Transillumination will be clear and may reveal testes in the scrotal sac. Noncommunicating: no connection to the perineum; fluid is nonreducible. Resolves spontaneously. Communicating: patent processus vaginalis (similar to hernia) and thus fluid is reducible with gentle pressure.
Hypospadias[b]	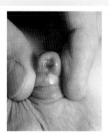	Congenital defect in incomplete development of anterior urethra, corpora cavernosa, and foreskin, which results in abnormal placement of the urethral meatus on the ventral surface of the penis; meatus may be on glans, penile shaft, or penoscrotal junction/perineum. Generally, lack of foreskin on ventral side, and excessive foreskin on dorsal side of glans penis.
Meatal stenosis[e]	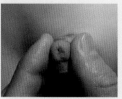	Recurrent inflammation of meatus from prolonged exposure to moist environment; prolonged urethral catheterization or trauma. May also result from friction with diaper or underwear.
Paraphimosis[c]	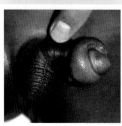	***Urologic emergency!*** Foreskin trapped behind glans penis due to prolonged retraction and swelling/edema from restricted blood flow.

Continued

TABLE 15.4   CONDITIONS OF THE PENIS, TESTES, AND/OR SCROTUM

Condition	Image	Description
Penile torsion[f]	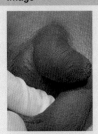	Congenital condition with counterclockwise rotation of the penile shaft, involving glans penis with or without corporal bodies. Often associated with other penile abnormalities (penile chordee or hypospadias).
Phimosis (pathologic)[g]	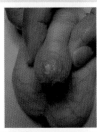	Delayed separation of the prepuce, or foreskin, from the glans penis; may be the result of an incomplete retraction of the foreskin persisting after 6 years of age (see Fig. 15.5) or the result of chronic inflammation causing a secondary phimosis.
Testicular torsion[c]	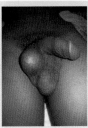	**Urologic emergency!** Twisting of testicle on its spermatic cord; causes **sudden onset of unilateral scrotal/testicular pain**, swelling and tenderness of the scrotal sac, venous obstruction, edema, and organ compromise, which leads to **testicular infarction**. May be associated with nausea and vomiting. Exam shows (–) cremasteric reflex and (–) Prehn sign (pain relief with elevation of the scrotum). Testicular lie is horizontal and potentially high riding. Occurs in 12- to 18-year-olds; peak at 15–16 years. May occur in the newborn period and present as an ecchymotic, nontender testis caused by necrosis of the testis in utero.
Testicular tumor[h]	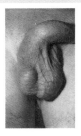	Exam shows firm, circumscribed, painless area of induration or lump within the testis; does not transilluminate. Generally malignant with germ cell origin. The risk of testicular tumor is 10–40 times more in teens with history of cryptorchidism.

TABLE 15.4   CONDITIONS OF THE PENIS, TESTES, AND/OR SCROTUM—CONT'D

Condition	Image	Description
Undescended testis/ cryptorchidism[i]	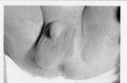	Testis is palpable but cannot be milked into the scrotal sac; may be found along the normal descending pathway, along inguinal ring, upper scrotum, or be *retractile* (normal), or *ectopic (perineum, contralateral scrotum, or femoral);* referral for evaluation by 9 months of age. *Impalpable testis* is generally found intraabdominally. Bilateral *impalpable testes* in a term male raises concerns about disorder of sexual differentiation/virilizing adrenal hyperplasia. *Acquired cryptorchidism* is when a testicle that was previously palpated in the scrotum ascends upwards and is unable to be brought back into the scrotum.
Varicocele[j]	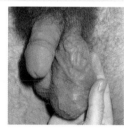	Dilation of internal spermatic vein at venous plexus within spermatic cord; presents as soft mass on spermatic cord ("bag of worms") with or without associated pain; most common on left side and more prominent with straining/standing. Most common inguinoscrotal pathology in male adolescents.
Webbed penis[b]	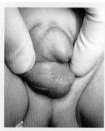	Congenital condition involving a web of skin obscuring the penoscrotal angle in an otherwise normal sized penis. The penis may be concealed by a pubic fat pad or scrotum, or trapped due to phimosis.

[a]From Baldinger L, et al. Abnormalities of the external genitalia. *Clin Perinatol.* 2014;41(3):709–724.

[b]From Zitelli BJ, et al. *Zitelli and Davis' Atlas of Pediatric Physical Diagnosis.* 8th ed. Philadelphia: Elsevier; 2023.

[c]From Kliegman R, St. Geme JW, et al. *Nelson Textbook of Pediatrics.* 21st ed. Philadelphia: Elsevier; 2020.

[d]From Frimberger D. Diagnosis and management of epispadias. *Semin Pediatr Surg.* 2011;20:85–90.

[e]From Acimi S, et al. Prevalence and causes of meatal stenosis in circumcised boys. *J Pediatr Urol.* 2022;18(1):89.e1–89.e6.

[f]From Bhat A, et al. Correction of penile torsion and chordee by mobilization of urethra with spongiosum in chordee without hypospadias. *J Pediatr Urol.* 2014;10(6):1238–1243.

[g]From Abbas T, McCarthy L. Foreskin and penile problems in childhood. *Surgery.* 2022;40(5):326–331.

[h]From Ball JW, et al. *Seidel's Guide to Physical Examination: An Interprofessional Approach.* 10th ed. St. Louis: Elsevier; 2023.

[i]From Godbole PP. Testicular problems in children. *Paediatr Child Health.* 2016;26(6):246–225.

[j]From Swartz MH. *Textbook of Physical Diagnosis.* 8th ed. Philadelphia: Elsevier; 2021.

testes, and/or scrotum in the infant, child, and adolescent.

TELEHEALTH TIPS

As the health care delivery system expands to increased use of telehealth services, providers need to be mindful of the benefits and limitations of using virtual visits for genitourinary assessments.[22,23] Telehealth has increased patients' access to care, as well as increased patient and family satisfaction.[22,24] While history gathering can be done virtually, providers need to be mindful of who else is in the room with the patient and issues of maintaining confidentiality. At the same time, virtual inspection of the genitalia is feasible to the degree that the patient is comfortable in sharing in front of the camera, while palpation by the provider is not feasible through a virtual visit.[23,24] Therefore, telehealth is ideal for some conditions versus others (i.e., inspection of the foreskin feasible but not for palpation of the testes) and may be better served in conjunction with an in-person visit whether as an initial triage visit or as a follow-up to the initial in-person visit and exam.[23,25]

SUMMARY OF EXAMINATION

- Routine examination of the genitourinary system is expected at all routine well visits. It is an opportunity to discuss age-appropriate growth and development, provide anticipatory guidance, and identify any abnormality or pathology early in development. Be familiar with the wide variations of typical development.
- Be mindful and respectful of cultural variations in discussion of genitourinary development and examination. Ask permission to discuss and examine.
- Prepare the child/adolescent by discussing what the exam will entail and provide proper draping as appropriate; be mindful of exposing child/adolescent longer than necessary. Talk through the exam and provide reassurance of normal development.
- Adolescents should be given the opportunity to have the history performed without parents in the room, and an informed consent/confidentiality policy should be discussed.
- Adolescents should be offered a chaperone, either the caregiver or other adult, to be present during the genitourinary exam, and the use or declination of chaperone presence should be documented in the visit note.
- Obtain a thorough history including gestational history, birth history, family history, and voiding/elimination history.
- Assess penis and note foreskin status, penile size, curvature, and meatal location.
- Physiologic phimosis is expected until about 6 years of age. Avoid forceful retraction of foreskin. Discuss care of the uncircumcised penis with the family.
- Assess scrotum and testes at every routine well visit. Determine if palpable testes are descended, retractile, undescended, ascending, or ectopic. Assess testicular size, shape, and consistency and note the presence of any masses or pain. Refer to pediatric urology if testes are undescended by 9 months of age or impalpable at any age.
- Perform a detailed scrotal and testicular examination for any scrotal mass or pain.
- Report and follow up on any suspicion of sexual abuse from history or physical exam.
- Telehealth is feasible for history gathering and for some inspection of genitalia.

DOCUMENTATION

Term Infant at 1 Month of Age
External genitalia: uncircumcised penis, foreskin partially retractable revealing meatus at tip of penis, Ø discharge noted, typical urinary stream, testes ↓↓×2 of age-appropriate size/shape/consistency, Ø hernia/hydrocele.

↓↓, descended.

DOCUMENTATION

Healthy 12-Year-Old
External genitalia: Tanner stage 3, circumcised penis, urethral meatus at tip, Ø discharge noted, scrotum with testes ↓↓×2 with typical shape/consistency, Ø masses palpated, (–) inguinal hernia exam.

↓↓, descended.

REFERENCES

1. Grossman S. *Porth's Pathophysiology: Concepts of Altered Health States.* 9th ed. Wolters Kluwer Health; 2013.
2. Wu Y, Wang J, Wei Y, et al. Contribution of prenatal endocrine-disrupting chemical exposure to genital anomalies in males: The pooled results from current evidence. *Chemosphere.* 2022;286:131844.
3. Dave S, Afshar K, Braga LH, Anderson P. Canadian Urological Association guideline on the care of the normal foreskin and neonatal circumcision in Canadian infants (abridged version). *Can Urol Assoc J.* 2018;12:18–28.
4. Neinstein LS, Katzman DK, Callahan T, Joffe A. *Neinstein's Adolescent and Young Adult Health Care: A Practical Guide.* Wolters Kluwer Health; 2016.
5. Zhu J, Kusa TO, Chan YM. Genetics of pubertal timing. *Current opinion in pediatrics.* 2018;30:532–540.
6. Klein DA, Paradise SL, Goodwin ET. Caring for transgender and gender-diverse persons: What clinicians should know. *Am Fam Physician.* 2018;98:645–653.
7. Safer JD, Tangpricha V. Care of the transgender patient *Ann Intern Med.* 1712019Itc1–itc16.
8. Bosse JD, Nesteby JA, Randall CE. Integrating sexual minority health issues into a health assessment class. *J Prof Nurs.* 2015;31:498–507.
9. Association of Women's Health OaNN The use of chaperones during sensitive examinations and treatments. *Nurs Womens Health.* 2022;26:e7–e8.
10. Butler C, Ellsworth P. Contemporary approach to diagnosis, management, and treatment of varicocele in the adolescent. *Urol Nurs.* 2014;34:271–280.
11. Moreno G, Corbalán J, Peñaloza B, Pantoja T. Topical corticosteroids for treating phimosis in boys. *Cochrane Database Syst Rev.* 2014:Cd008973.
12. Deutsch MB. Binding, packing, and tucking. University of California, San Francisco. Accessed August 18, 2022. https://transcare.ucsf.edu/guidelines/binding-packing-and-tucking
13. Sintim-Damoa A, Cohen HL. Pearls and pitfalls of pediatric scrotal imaging. *Semin Ultrasound CT MR.* 2022;43:115–129.
14. Kolon TF, Herndon CD, Baker LA, et al. Evaluation and treatment of cryptorchidism: AUA guideline. *J Urol.* 2014;192:337–345.
15. Thornton CP. Best practice in teaching male adolescents and young men to perform testicular self-examinations: A review. *J Pediatr Health Care.* 2016;30:518–527.
16. Rovito MJ, Leone JE, Cavayero CT. "Off-label" usage of testicular self-examination (TSE): Benefits beyond cancer detection. *Am J Mens Health.* 2018;12:505–513.
17. U.S. Preventive Services Task Force Screening for testicular cancer: U.S. Preventive Services Task Force reaffirmation recommendation statement. *Ann Intern Med.* 2011;154:483–486.
18. Adams JA, Kellogg ND, Farst KJ, et al. Updated guidelines for the medical assessment and care of children who may have been sexually abused. *J Pediatr Adolesc Gynecol.* 2016;29:81–87.
19. Cools M, Nordenström A, Robeva R, et al. Caring for individuals with a difference of sex development (DSD): A consensus statement. *Nat Rev Endocrinol.* 2018;14:415–429.
20. Tishelman AC, Shumer DE, Nahata L. Disorders of sex development: Pediatric psychology and the genital exam. *J Pediatr Psychol.* 2017;42:530–543.
21. Langan RC, Puente MEE. Scrotal masses. *Am Fam Physician.* 2022;106:184–189.
22. Pettit S, Young E, Jung I. Systematic review of telemedicine in pediatric urology. *J Pediatr Urol.* 2022;18:17–22.
23. Winkelman AJ, Beller HL, Morgan KE, et al. Benefits and barriers to pediatric tele-urology during the COVID-19 pandemic. *J Pediatr Urol.* 2020;16:840.e1–840.e6.
24. Ansary AM, Martinez JN, Scott JD. The virtual physical exam in the 21st century. *J Telemed Telecare.* 2021;27:382–392.
25. Kuo AC, Geleris B, Arnhym A. TeleBBD: Telehealth management of bladder bowel dysfunction—A provider survey of benefits and limitations. *J Pediatr Urol.* 2021;17:792.e1–792.e7.

CHAPTER 16

BREAST

Angela R. B. Todd

Current evidence and recommendations related to the efficacy of breast examination focus on the detection of breast cancer, which is an exceedingly rare diagnosis in children and adolescents; therefore, child and adolescent breast exam recommendations are based on expert practice.[1] The primary intention of the breast exam in children and adolescents is to recognize normal variants, monitor development, and identify nonmalignant pathology. Making assessment of the breast part of the routine physical examination in preadolescents gives the parent or caregiver and child an opportunity to voice any concerns and fosters a dialogue about reproductive health and puberty. It is important to respect privacy and discuss consent when performing the examination of the breast in all children and adolescents.

EMBRYOLOGIC DEVELOPMENT

A mammary ridge forms from the ectodermal layer on day 20 of embryonic development and extends from the forelimb to the hind limb. In the sixth week of fetal development, the nipple and areola form over a bud of breast tissue that is composed of the primary mammary ducts and a loose fibrous tissue or stroma. Fifteen to twenty-five secondary buds then develop and bifurcate into tubules, forming the basis of the duct system.[2] Each duct, as it develops, opens separately into the nipple.

PREPUBERTAL PHYSIOLOGIC VARIATIONS

Breast tissue remains similar in genetically XY (hereafter referred to as "male") and genetically XX (hereafter referred to as "female") children until the onset of puberty. In neonates, breast tissue may be swollen or nodular due to the effects of maternal estrogen crossing the placenta (Fig. 16.1). In general, the nipple and areola are not developed or pigmented with such an enlargement, and no associated signs of puberty are present. This condition usually regresses spontaneously within weeks to months, and in the absence of other secondary sexual characteristics, a biopsy is not indicated.[2] If other signs of puberty appear, then these changes could be the first sign of *precocious puberty*, in which case referral and further diagnostic workup are indicated. Neonatal galactorrhea (witch's milk) is an unusual but normal finding that should resolve within 2 weeks (Fig. 16.2).[3]

Supernumerary nipples may arise from the mammary ridge and be present at birth (Fig. 16.3A). They are often raised, generally require no treatment, and may become imperceptible over time. In most patients, supernumerary nipples are a variation of expected physiology and not associated with pathology. In females, supernumerary nipples will on rare occasion develop a small amount of breast tissue during puberty (see *polymastia* in Table 16.2; Fig. 16.3B). The adolescent may

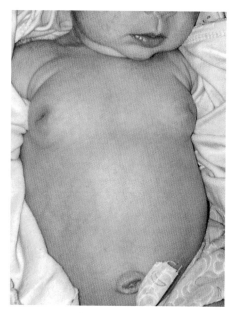

FIGURE 16.1 Estrogen effect in an infant. (From Meshram GG, Kaur N, Hura KS. Breast enlargement in newborns: a folkloric-medical dilemma. *Trop Doct.* 2018;48(2):150–151.)

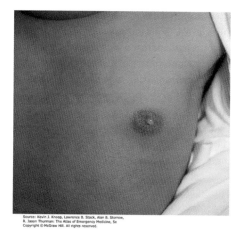

FIGURE 16.2 Witch's milk. (From Basu, R. Galactorrhea of the newborn (witch's milk). Consultant for Pediatricians, Nov 2010; Vol 9, No 11.)

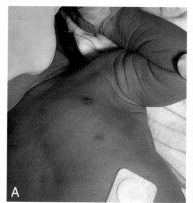
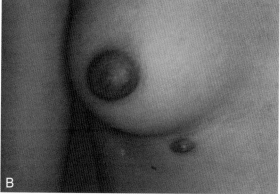

FIGURE 16.3 **A**, Supernumerary nipple. **B**, Supernumerary nipple located in the inframammary fold of the right breast of an adolescent female. ([A] From Eichenfield L, et al. *Neonatal and Infant Dermatology.* 3rd ed. Philadelphia: Elsevier; 2015; [B] From Kliegman RM, et al. *Nelson Textbook of Pediatrics.* 21 st ed. Philadelphia: Elsevier Inc.; 2020: Fig. 566.2)

elect to have cosmetic surgery for removal of the supernumerary breast tissue. Widespread nipples are defined as a nipple spread of greater than 25% of the chest circumference and may be associated with congenital disorders such as Turner syndrome.[3]

PHYSIOLOGIC VARIATIONS

Gynecomastia in Males

At puberty the ductal and periductal mesenchymal breast tissue in male children proliferates under the influence of estrogens, with later involution as testicular androgens rise to adult levels.[2] Male estradiol levels triple during puberty, and androgens ultimately increase 30 times. At one time it was believed that *physiologic gynecomastia*, a benign increase in glandular and stromal breast tissue in pubertal males, was the result of peak estrogen levels occurring prior to peak androgen levels (Fig. 16.4). However, the current understanding identifies leptin, a hormone made by adipose cells to regulate energy balance, as the hormone most likely responsible for pubertal gynecomastia.[2] Most circulating estrogens are produced outside of the testes, and an increase in fatty tissue, as in obesity, may lead to a higher incidence of *gynecomastia* (Box 16.1).

At 14 years of age, up to 64% of adolescent males have some degree of gynecomastia, with only 4% of adolescent males having severe gynecomastia that persists into adulthood.[2] Approximately 50% of males experience the onset of gynecomastia at sexual maturity

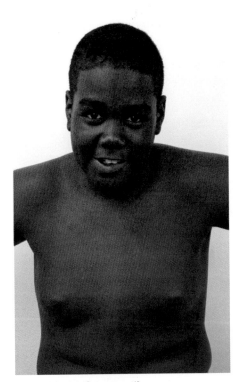

FIGURE 16.4 **Gynecomastia.**

> ### BOX 16.1   Classifications of Gynecomastia
>
> **Grade I:** Small enlargement of the breast in the subareolar area without excess skin
> **Grade IIa:** Moderate enlargement of the breast without excess skin or ptosis
> **Grade IIb:** Moderate enlargement of the breast with some excess skin
> **Grade III:** Significant enlargement of the breast with excess skin and ptosis resembling SMR stage 3 in females (see Table 16.1)

Data from Soliman AT, De Sanctis V, Yassin M. Management of adolescent gynecomastia: an update, *Acta Biomed.* 2017; 88(2):204–213.

rating (SMR; also referred to as "Tanner staging") stage 2 of male genital development, another 20% at SMR stage 1, 20% at SMR stage 3 of male genital development, and 10% beginning at SMR stage 4 (see Chapter 15). In general, adolescent males can be reassured that most cases of *physiologic gynecomastia* will resolve spontaneously within 12 to 18 months, although it can rarely persist after sexual maturity.[3]

Treatment alternatives for persistent *gynecomastia*, including pharmacologic and surgical options, may be appropriate to discuss with youth and families when this condition does not resolve or is particularly distressing. Use of pharmacologic intervention with anti-estrogen drugs could be a reasonable approach if used early in patients with mild to moderate gynecomastia. However, due to lack of data on risks and benefits of anti-estrogen drugs for patients with gynecomastia or for patients with large amounts of breast tissue development, a surgical approach may be needed.[4]

Gynecomastia, although a normal variant, is also present in relation to hormone imbalances due to thyrotoxicosis, cirrhosis, adrenal and testicular neoplasm, primary hypogonadism, chromosome abnormalities such as Klinefelter syndrome, and severe malnutrition.[2] In addition, prescription drugs such as ranitidine, omeprazole, ketoconazole, metronidazole, antiretrovirals, digoxin, spironolactone,

TABLE 16.1	FEMALE BREAST DEVELOPMENT SEXUAL MATURITY RATING (TANNER STAGES)	
Sexual Maturity Rating (SMR)	**Breast Findings**	**Areola and Nipple Findings**
SMR stage 1	Prepubertal; no glandular tissue	Conforms to general chest line; papillae elevated
SMR stage 2	Breast buds present	Areola widens
SMR stage 3	Larger and more elevation; extends beyond areolar parameter	Areola continues to enlarge but remains in contour with breast
SMR stage 4	Larger and more elevation	Areola and papillae begin form a mound projecting from breast contour
SMR stage 5	Adult size (variable); pubertal breast development complete	Areola part of breast contour, nipple projecting above areola

Data from Sass AE, Richards MJ. Adolescence. In: Bunik M, Hay WW, Levin MJ, Abzug MJ, eds. Current Diagnosis & Treatment: Pediatrics, 26th ed. McGraw Hill; 2022.

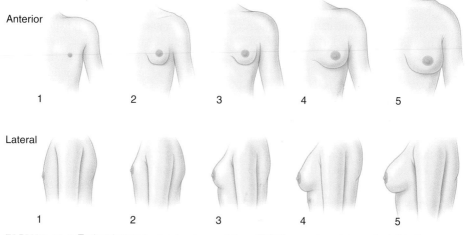

FIGURE 16.5 Typical female breast development, from SMR Tanner stage 1 (prepubertal) to Tanner stage 5 (adult breast). (From Herring J. *Tachdjian's Pediatric Orthopaedics.* 6th ed. Philadelphia: Elsevier; 2022.)

phenothiazines, and some recreational or illicit drugs (e.g., marijuana, anabolic steroids, amphetamines, and alcohol) can cause gynecomastia.[3]

Thelarche in Females

Breast development during puberty involves both multiple hormones and the binding of hormones to breast tissue. Estrogen, especially estradiol, influences ductal development, whereas progesterone influences additional lobular alveolar development.[2] Thyroxine and corticosteroids are also involved in breast development. *Thelarche*, or the beginning of female breast development, is usually the first sign of puberty in females and occurs between 8 and 13 years of age, on average at the age of 11.2 years (Table 16.1; Fig. 16.5).[1]

Full breast development at SMR 5 signals the end of puberty in females. Variations in age at *thelarche* may be affected by factors such as BMI or ancestral background.[5] A longitudinal study of breast development that followed more than 1200 females from childhood to early adolescence found that breast development was influenced significantly by BMI, with those above the 50th percentile reaching SMR 2 at an earlier age. A BMI at or above the 85th percentile was associated with earlier breast development in all groups and was found to be the strongest predictor of earlier age of thelarche.[5]

Premature thelarche is defined as breast development without other signs of puberty, occurring before 7.5 years. Occasionally, a prepubertal child develops an enlargement of one or both breasts, which involves a soft, mobile, subareolar nodule of uniform consistency.[2] Although isolated *premature thelarche* is usually benign and self-limited, the examiner should be sure to evaluate for other signs of precocious puberty.[2]

ANATOMY AND PHYSIOLOGY

Mature female breast tissue at SMR stage 5 extends from the second or third rib to the sixth or seventh rib, and from the sternal margin to the midaxillary area with the nipple located centrally, surrounded by the areola. The breast is composed of glandular and fibrous tissue and subcutaneous and retromammary fat (Fig. 16.6). Fifteen to twenty lobes radiate around the nipple, and each lobe is divided into 20 to 40 lobules of milk-producing acini cells that empty into lactiferous ducts.[2] These cells are small and inconspicuous in the nonpregnant, nonlactating woman. A layer of subcutaneous fibrous tissue provides support for the breast, as do the suspensory ligaments. The muscles forming the floor of the breast are pectoralis major, pectoralis minor, serratus anterior, latissimus dorsi, subscapularis, external oblique, and rectus abdominis. Vascular supply comes from the internal mammary artery and the lateral thoracic artery. The lymph system

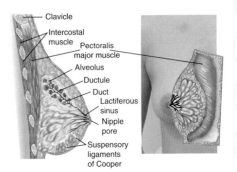

FIGURE 16.6 **Anatomy of the breast.**

drains to the anterior axillary, subscapular, and supraclavicular nodes.

SPECIAL CONSIDERATIONS DURING BREAST DEVELOPMENT

Breast development, an initial sign of secondary sexual development in adolescents, is readily apparent to family members and peers, often eliciting unwanted comments as to presence or absence and size of breast tissue. Breast development is a common issue for teasing, bullying, and sexual harassment in middle school and high school for children of all genders. The health care provider should be mindful that sexual harassment is a major issue for teens, often jeopardizing a teen's mental health and school performance. Adolescents who are victims of appearance-related teasing or bullying are more likely to develop negative self-image and psychological issues such as eating disorders.[6] If the preteen or young adolescent seems particularly concerned or uncomfortable with the health history about breast development or the breast examination, gentle exploration of the issue by the provider, including queries as to teasing or bullying, or unwanted attention from peers, adults, and/or family members should be explored, and the adolescent should be referred for counseling if indicated.

Teens of all genders may desire or attempt to purposefully increase or decrease breast size. Special consideration should be taken with transgender, nonbinary, and gender nonconforming adolescents who may have complex and intense feelings about their changing bodies during puberty. *Gender dysphoria* refers to significant distress or impairment caused by a marked dissonance between the experienced or expressed gender and sex assigned at birth.[7] Recent data has found an increase in adolescents who identify as transgender, with one study showing 1.3% of 16- to 19-year-olds describing clinically significant gender dysphoria in a school survey.[8] Adolescents experiencing *gender dysphoria* may desire to use a *breast binder*, which is a device intended to flatten breast tissue against the chest wall to diminish the appearance of breasts. The health care provider should counsel patients on safety and comfort of breast binders and discuss correct use of such devices.

Transgender, nonbinary, and gender nonconforming children and their families may also present with inquiries about *puberty blockers*, or medications to suppress outward signs of puberty for their sex assigned at birth, such as growth of the Adam's apple, deepening of the voice, or in the case of a child whose sex assigned at birth was female, breast development. Limited evidence on use of *puberty blockers* in children and adolescents with *gender dysphoria* supports general clinical safety as well as psychological benefits to the child.[9] More evidence is needed to form a complete clinical picture of the risks and benefits of *puberty blockers*, and the conversation should be ongoing and multidisciplinary, involving the primary pediatric care provider, psychiatrist, other specialists including endocrinologists, and the parents or caregivers of the child.

Aside from breast development, preadolescent and adolescent patients may present with other breast findings that clinicians should be aware and mindful of. These include body modifications such as nipple piercings. Health care providers should counsel adolescents with nipple piercings on needle safety including not sharing needles, and how to care for piercings. Teens should be given information on signs of infection and when and how to seek care if problems are suspected.

SYSTEM-SPECIFIC HISTORY

The Information Gathering table reviews the important information to be gathered for breast assessment at key developmental stages and for adolescents presenting with breast symptoms or concerns.

PHYSICAL ASSESSMENT

Inspection and Palpation

Prepubertal Breast

Prepubertal breasts are easily inspected and palpated while examining the chest to assess cardiovascular and respiratory status. The health care provider should note any masses or pain, nipple discharge, or signs of premature thelarche, or breast development.

INFORMATION GATHERING FOR BREAST ASSESSMENT AT KEY DEVELOPMENTAL STAGES

Age Group	Questions to Ask
Preadolescents	Breast tenderness or breast buds noted? At what age did breast development begin? Any pain in breast? Other signs of puberty noted? Axillary or pubic hair? Concern about breast development?
Adolescents	Any concerns about breast health, breast development, or breast size? Last menstrual period? Contraceptive use? Breast tenderness or pain noted? Relationship of breast discomfort or pain to menstrual cycle? Previous pregnancy? Any discharge from nipple? Any lump noted in breast or axilla? Redness or irritation on skin? Nipple changes? For adolescents with large breasts: any back or shoulder pain?

Adolescent Male

Pubertal breasts are inspected with the male adolescent supine with his hands behind the head. Place the pads of the three middle fingers at the margins of the breast. Palpate the breast bilaterally for the presence of adipose tissue or breast buds if evaluating for gynecomastia. Note any nodular tissue or firm rubbery masses. In conditions such as a *lipoma* or *dermoid cyst*, the mass is usually noted to one side of the areola.

Adolescent Female

Discussion about breast development in early to middle adolescence provides an opportunity for reassurance and education about expected variations in breast findings. Most adolescent breast complaints are related to normal developmental changes and can be evaluated through an adequate history and physical exam. There is some controversy about the age at which health care providers should perform routine screening for breast malignancies in females, or whether they should be performed as part of a preventative visit at all. The American Cancer Society (ACS), the American Congress of Obstetricians and Gynecologists (ACOG), and the United States Preventive Services Task Force (USPSTF) do not advise performing a clinical breast examination (CBE) as part of a routine visit for children and adolescents.[10–12] Therefore, in the absence of presenting concerns, the provider will have to weigh the benefits of full breast inspection in adolescents who are at low risk for breast cancer against the discomfort they may have to being undressed in front of a provider.

Clinical Breast Examination in the Postpubertal Adolescent

Although malignancies in adolescents are rare and more often due to metastatic disease than to a primary breast malignancy, adolescents and young adults may present with breast concerns that indicate the need for a CBE and further evaluation through ultrasound.

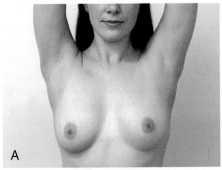

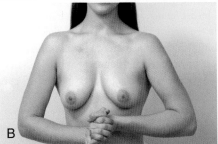

FIGURE 16.7 Inspection of the breast. **A,** Arms extended overhead. **B,** Hands pressed together.

In a full adolescent or young adult breast exam, the breasts are initially inspected with the patient sitting, disrobed to the waist, in the following positions: arms extended overhead, hands pressed against hips or against each other, and leaning forward from the waist (Fig. 16.7). These three positions are most helpful if examining for visual changes in the breast tissue caused by a mass.[3] Palpation of the supraclavicular, infraclavicular, and axillary lymph nodes should follow inspection of the breast and is easiest with the patient sitting and the examiner supporting the patient's arm.

Although the breasts can be palpated sitting and supine, the preferred position for the adolescent is supine. The patient may wear a gown open to the front or a paper drape to provide optimal comfort and privacy. Discuss with the patient that one breast will be undraped at a time to be assessed and, if possible, re-draped when examining the other side. Have the patient place both arms behind their head prior to examination. When both breasts are being evaluated, an adolescent patient may find it most comfortable to place both arms behind the head at the beginning of the exam "as if relaxing on a bed." This position also allows for the provider to visualize both breasts simultaneously if need be and minimizes position changes for the patient.

For purposes of examination, the breast is divided into four quadrants and the "tail of Spence" that extends into the axilla (Fig. 16.8). The breasts should be palpated with the pads (not tips) of the middle three fingers with the

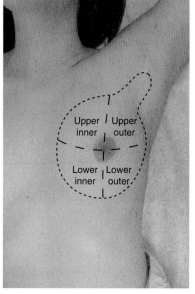

FIGURE 16.8 Quadrants of the left breast, tail of Spence.

fingers palpating over the breast tissue from the sternal margin to the midaxillary area and from the second or third rib to the sixth or seventh rib at the base of the breast. Palpation proceeds stepwise with the fingers to ensure a thorough assessment of the breast tissue. The preferred methods for palpation of the breast are illustrated in Fig. 16.9. When palpating the breast, the examiner should use the dominant hand and stabilize the breast, if necessary, with the nondominant hand. Place the pads of the middle fingers at the margins of the breast to begin palpation, and note any masses, pain, nipple discharge, or signs of premature breast development. If firm, rubbery tissue or a nodular mass is noted, fine palpation is required for accurate sizing and to distinguish among fatty tissue, cysts, and other nodular masses.

It is important to incorporate patient education into the breast examination for the adolescent or adult. During the examination, ask permission to guide the adolescent's hand onto their breast, pointing out landmarks and normal findings in the developing breast, such as the thicker ridge of breast tissue often found in the inferior aspect of the breast and the nodularity of normal adolescent breast tissue especially in the upper outer quadrant. Have the adolescent also feel the ribs underneath the medial border of the breast because this normal finding is often mistaken by adolescents for a breast lump.

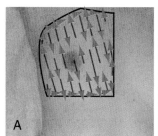
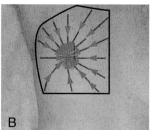
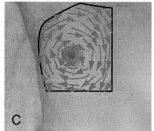

FIGURE 16.9 Methods of breast palpation. **A,** Palpation strip method. **B,** Palpation wedge method. **C,** Palpation circle method.

Asymmetrical breasts are common early in pubertal development in both adolescent males and females (Fig. 16.10).

Breast Self-Awareness

Previously it was recommended to perform and teach how to do a *breast self-exam (BSE)* as a way of increasing young women's investment in their own health care.[3] BSE focused on a routine and repeated inspection and evaluation of the breasts for the purpose of early breast pathology detection.[9] Some adolescent providers believe there is value in teaching adolescents about the texture of glandular breast tissue and normal findings around and under breast tissue, such as ribs and ligaments, which may increase comfort with their own developing bodies. However, there is limited evidence about the effectiveness of BSE in addressing true breast pathology and possible harm from unnecessary imaging or biopsy to rule out cancer in average-risk individuals.[9] The USPSTF and ACOG recommend *against* teaching BSE for adolescents or patients of any age.[9,10]

Teaching *BSE* has been replaced by the concept of teaching breast self-awareness (BSA).[9] BSA may assist the adolescent in accepting their body, increase comfort with the breast examination, and provide an opportunity to reinforce or correct information the adolescent may have received from health classes, media, or relatives about breast health. Both the ACS and ACOG recommend teaching *breast self-awareness* to females aged 20 years and older.[8,9] This includes assisting patients to become familiar with their breasts' normal feel and appearance, focusing on the importance of self-detection and early assessment of abnormal symptoms. BSA can be discussed as part of patient education during a routine well-person or physical exam, during a problem-focused visit involving the breasts, or during a young adolescent or well-child visit in which breast development is being discussed or noted upon exam.

DIAGNOSTIC PROCEDURES

When imaging is indicated, ultrasound is the primary modality due to lower radiation risk and increased sensitivity, since the density of adolescent breast tissue limits the accuracy of mammography. Adolescents with a family

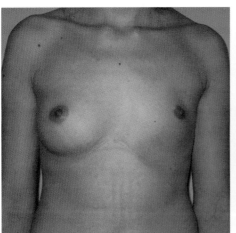 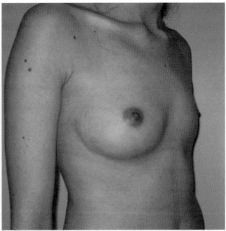

FIGURE 16.10 Asymmetrical breasts. (From Khouri R, Del Vecchio D. Breast reconstruction and augmentation using pre-expansion and autologous fat transplantation. *Clin Plast Surg.* 2009; 36(2):269–280, viii.)

history consistent with hereditary breast cancer, who are BRCA mutation carriers, or who have a history of irradiation to the chest (e.g., treatment of Hodgkin disease), are at a higher risk than the average population of developing breast cancer. These patients will need specialized screening that utilizes imaging to detect malignancy before clinical signs are present. Although recommendations for imaging-based screening vary slightly across different clinical settings, generally, high-risk patients as described above should receive annual mammography with MRI starting at 25 years of age (or 8 years after completion of radiation therapy—whichever comes later).[13]

Breast Conditions

The following are variations of normal that occur with stages of breast development:

- **Physiologic swelling and tenderness**: Breast lobules undergo proliferative changes due to the normal menstrual cycle, leading to pain and discomfort, swelling, and distinct masses that recede after menses.
- **Asymmetry**: In most females, one breast is slightly larger than the other, and this difference may be accentuated by asymmetrical breast development during puberty, which usually corrects by adulthood.
- **Proliferative breast changes**: Formerly called *fibrocystic disease*, increased nodularity is now considered a variation of normal, occurring in more than 50% of women of reproductive age. Adolescents often have painless lumps, which may become tender 1 week before menses. Areas of nodularity may be a few millimeters to 1 cm in diameter.
- **Cysts**: Usually associated with few symptoms, cysts are well circumscribed, small, and freely movable masses, commonly less than 1 cm in adolescents.
- **Montgomery tubercles**: These tubercles arise from sebaceous glands associated with a lactiferous duct. They present as small, soft papules around the areola, with occasional thin, clear to brown discharge and possibly

---

RED FLAGS IN BREAST ASSESSMENT

Concerns requiring a CBE with or without imaging include complaints of breast masses, breast pain, nipple changes (such as a new onset of nipple inversion), skin changes on the breast such as redness or dimpling, and/or nipple discharge.

---

a small lump under the areola. The condition usually resolves without intervention.

Breast cancer in adolescents is extremely rare. Malignant lesions comprise only 0.9% of all surgically excised lesions in the adolescent and young adult age group. Breast variations and benign tumors are presented in Table 16.2.

TELEHEALTH TIPS

Use of telehealth services may be beneficial to patients with certain pediatric breast concerns. A telehealth visit may be a preferable first step to triage certain breast symptoms in pediatric patients who may not otherwise present for care or may not want to undergo a breast exam unless a provider feels it is necessary. Reasons for a telehealth visit may include mild to moderate cyclical breast pain, expected development of breast buds, or assessment of a visual finding such as spontaneous nipple discharge or skin changes. Use of encryption for photos or video visits should always be used, and both the provider and patient should be in a private space during the visit. Assessment of a palpable mass or further workup of a continuing or worsening complaint after a telehealth visit should always be followed by a clinic or office visit and referral as indicated.

SUMMARY OF EXAMINATION

- Prepubertal breast examination in all children is focused on the identification of normal variants, nonmalignant pathology, and monitoring development.

TABLE 16.2	Conditions of the Breast
Condition	**Description**
Breast structure and growth abnormalities	*Amastia* or absence of breast tissue; *Athelia*, absence of nipple, often connected to a chest wall defect or more extensive congenital anomalies; *Polythelia*, the presence of supernumerary nipples; *Polymastia* or breast tissue that develops around supernumerary nipples; *Macromastia*, exceptionally large breasts that may develop as a response to normal hormone changes in adolescence and can cause neck, back, and breast pain
Fibroadenoma	Most common benign breast tumor; firm, rubbery, mobile, nontender; generally 1–5 cm in size. May be excised if large, otherwise observation is recommended
Fat necrosis	A benign condition that is usually the result of trauma to the breast (>50% of cases). May present as a palpable mass with skin changes and/or nipple retraction
Fibrocystic changes	Common benign breast condition affecting >50% of females; characterized by mild swelling, tenderness, and palpable nodularity from dense glandular tissue; commonly associated with hormonal/cyclical mastalgia
Breast abscess/mastitis	Most common in lactating/breastfeeding patients, may occur in nonlactating patients. Presents as a painful area of erythema with local and, later, systemic signs of infection. If a palpable mass is present, or purulent discharge from the nipple, an abscess is suspected, and incision and drainage may be needed. Treatment is antibiotics and other conservative measures
Nipple discharge (spontaneous or nonspontaneous)	Generally, unilateral, single-duct, and spontaneous discharge is most concerning for breast pathology, as is bloody discharge. Bloody or watery/serous discharge may indicate a malignancy or intraductal lesion; purulent discharge may accompany an abscess. Milky discharge (galactorrhea) is more common and may be the result of hormonal imbalance, current or recent pregnancy, various medications including some SSRIs and oral contraceptives, head trauma, or pituitary tumor. Nonspontaneous discharge (only occurring when the breast/nipple is expressed) that is not clear, bloody, or black/green in appearance may be the result of excessive stimulation of the breasts/nipples

Data from Karam A. The breast. In: DeCherney AH, Nathan L, Laufer N, Roman AS, eds. *CURRENT Diagnosis & Treatment: Obstetrics & Gynecology. 12th ed.* McGraw Hill; 2019.

- Focus on the developing breast may be embarrassing and uncomfortable for pubertal children and early adolescents.
- Pubertal gynecomastia is common in approximately 50% of developing male adolescents and may be a source of concern for youth and families.
- Thelarche is the first sign of puberty in developing female adolescents.
- Breast development is often a common issue for teasing, bullying, and sexual harassment in middle school and high school.
- Children and adolescents who are transgender, nonbinary, or gender nonconforming

may experience *gender dysphoria* and inquire about ways to decrease the appearance of breast tissue.
- There is insufficient evidence recommending CBE for screening in adolescents and young adults.

- SBE is no longer recommended, but SBA can be a useful tool in patient education about changing bodies and variations in normal developing breasts, focusing on the importance of self-detection and early assessment of symptoms.

DOCUMENTATION

9-Year-Old
Chest: Symmetrical, lungs clear to auscultation bilaterally, no lymphadenopathy, breasts SMR 2, breast bud noted under R areola, warm and tender to touch, nonerythematous, L breast without swelling or tenderness.

DOCUMENTATION

16-Year-Old
Chest: Symmetrical, lungs clear to auscultation bilaterally, no lymphadenopathy, breasts SMR 4, symmetrical, no discreet masses, no nipple retractions or dimpling, no discharge, no skin changes.

REFERENCES

1. DiVasta A, Weldon C, Labow B. The breast: examination and lesions. In: *Emans SJ, Laufer MR, DiVasta AD, eds. Emans, Laufer, Goldstein's Pediatric and Adolescent Gynecology.* 7th ed. Philadelphia: Lippincott Williams & Wilkins; 2019.
2. Kaneda HJ, Mack J, Kasales CJ, Schetter S. Pediatric and adolescent breast masses: a review of pathophysiology, imaging, diagnosis, and treatment. *AJR Am J Roentgenol.* 2013;200:W204–W212.
3. Gooding H, DiVasta A. Breast disorders and gynecomastia. In: Neinstein L, Katzman D, eds. *Adolescent and Young Adult Health Care: A Practical Guide.* 6th ed. Philadelphia: Walters Kluwer; 2016.
4. Soliman AT, De Sanctis V, Yassin M. Management of adolescent gynecomastia: an update. *Acta Biomed.* 2017;88:204–213.
5. Biro FM, Greenspan LC, Galvez MP, et al. Onset of breast development in a longitudinal cohort. *Pediatrics.* 2013;132:1019–1027.
6. Day S, Bussey K, Trompeter N, Mitchison D. The impact of teasing and bullying victimization on disordered eating and body image disturbance among adolescents: a systematic review. *Trauma Violence Abuse.* 2022;23:985–1006.
7. Ristori J, Steensma TD. Gender dysphoria in childhood. *Int Rev Psychiatry.* 2016;28:13–20.

8. Kaltiala-Heino R, Bergman H, Työläjärvi M, Frisén L. Gender dysphoria in adolescence: current perspectives. *Adolesc Health Med Ther.* 2018;9:31–41.
9. Mahfouda S, Moore JK, Siafarikas A, Zepf FD, Lin A. Puberty suppression in transgender children and adolescents. *Lancet Diabetes Endocrinol.* 2017;5(10):816–826.
10. American Cancer Society. *American Cancer Society recommendations for early breast cancer detection in women without breast symptoms: American Cancer Society.* 2021 [updated 4/22/21; cited 12/23/21]. Available from: http://www.cancer.org/cancer/breastcancer/moreinformation/breastcancerearlydetection/breast-cancer-early-detection-acs-recs.
11. American College of Obstetricians and Gynecologists Breast cancer risk assessment and screening in average-risk women. Practice Bulletin No. 179. American College of Obstetricians and Gynecologists. *Obstet Gynecol.* 2017;130:e1–16.
12. Siu AL, USPST Force. Screening for breast cancer: U.S. Preventive Services Task Force Recommendation Statement. *Ann Intern Med.* 2016;164:279–296.
13. Monticciolo DL, Newell MS, Moy L, Niell B, Monsees B, Sickles EA. Breast cancer screening in women at higher-than-average risk: Recommendations From the ACR. *J Am Coll Radiol.* 2018;15:408–414.

CHAPTER 17

VULVA, VAGINA, AND INTERNAL PELVIC ASSESSMENT

Angela R. B. Todd

The genital examination is a recommended yet underperformed part of the routine physical for children and adolescents. Routine performance of the genital exam allows the health care provider to build skills and familiarity with normal variants in the genitourinary system and establish a baseline from which to monitor individual development and provide information and reassurance to children, youth, and parents or caregivers. However, health care providers may be underprepared to recognize normal genital findings in the prepubescent vulva and vagina and may be unfamiliar with common variations.[1]

With knowledge of normal development of the reproductive anatomy, the health care provider can incorporate the routine examination of the genitalia into well-child care. The review of systems and genital exam offer an opportunity to foster a three-way conversation between the child, provider, and caregiver about anatomy, consent, and body autonomy. For religious and cultural reasons or personal preference, caregivers, children, and adolescents may be more likely to request providers of the same gender for the breast and genital exam. In nonemergent situations, it is important to honor this request, either within the practice setting or by referral, and to respect privacy and confidentiality in performing the examination and discussing findings.

EMBRYOLOGIC DEVELOPMENT

At 5 to 6 weeks of gestation, fetal gonads are bipotential, capable of differentiating into either a testis or an ovary. Both genetically XY (hereafter referred to as "male") and genetically XX (hereafter referred to as "female") embryos have one pair of primary sex organs, or gonads, and two pairs of ducts, *wolffian* ducts and *müllerian* ducts. During the sixth week, the primordial germ cells migrate into the primary sex cords and begin to differentiate. Leydig and Sertoli cells appear in male embryos, producing testosterone and anti-müllerian hormone. In female embryos the gonads do not produce testosterone, and the gonads develop into ovaries. The wolffian ducts deteriorate, and the müllerian ducts develop into the uterus, upper vaginal tract, and fallopian tubes. The external genitalia differentiate at between 8 and 12 weeks of gestation (Fig. 17.1). Active mitosis continues and thousands of germ cells, *oocytes*, are produced. A newborn female may have 2 million primary oocytes at birth. However, after birth, no further oogonia occurs.[2]

DEVELOPMENTAL AND PHYSIOLOGIC VARIATIONS

In preterm neonates, the *labia majora* may not cover the *labia minora*, and the *clitoris* will be prominent. Term newborns will have enlarged labia majora, which usually cover other external structures, a relatively large clitoris, and labia minora with dull pink epithelium, because of maternal estrogen effects (Fig. 17.2). A creamy white or slightly blood-tinged discharge is normal for up to 10 days after birth. The *hymen* is relatively thicker, pink-white, and redundant, and may remain so up until 2 to 4 years of age (Fig. 17.3).[3]

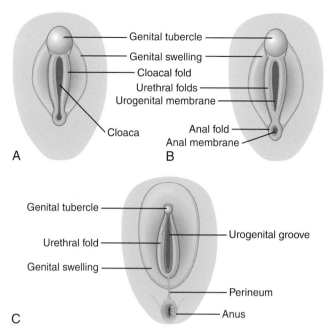

FIGURE 17.1 Development of the external genitalia. **(A)** Early development before completion of the urorectal septum. **(B)** Separation of the anus from the urogenital sinus lined by the urethral folds. **(C)** Development of the genital swelling. (From Crum C, et al.: *Diagnostic Gynecologic and Obstetric Pathology*, ed 3, Philadelphia, 2018, Elsevier.)

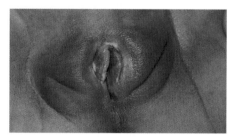

FIGURE 17.2 Newborn with estrogen effect. (From Zitelli BJ, et al.: *Atlas of Pediatric Physical Diagnosis*, ed 8, Philadelphia, 2023, Elsevier. Courtesy Ian Holzman, MD, Mt. Sinai Medical Center, New York, NY.)

Disorders of sexual differentiation (DSD) have their genesis in early fetal development and result from developmental variations in one or more of the three components of sex determination and differentiation: chromosomal sex, gonadal sex, and/or phenotypic sex. Manifestations of some types of DSD are evident at birth in the newborn with ambiguous genitalia, and infants with ambiguous genitalia should

be referred in the neonatal period to a tertiary center with a comprehensive multidisciplinary team with an ethicist.[4] Other types of DSD may become evident only in early adolescence with variations in secondary sexual development (see Chapter 15 for further discussion).

In the absence of congenital anomalies, all female infants are born with a hymen, which can present in a variety of configurations. Commonly, the hymen is *fimbriated, redundant, annular,* or *crescentic* (Fig. 17.4). Annular hymens are more common at birth, whereas crescentic hymens are more common in children older than 3 years. Fig. 17.5 illustrates hymen types that are rare—*septate, cribriform,* and *imperforate.* Table 17.1 presents congenital anomalies in development of the female genitalia.

ANATOMY AND PHYSIOLOGY

After the newborn period and before menarche, the clitoris is approximately 3 mm in length and 3 mm in transverse diameter. In

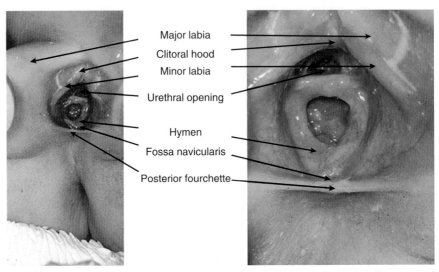

Major labia

Clitoral hood

Minor labia

Urethral opening

Hymen

Fossa navicularis

Posterior fourchette

FIGURE 17.3 External genitalia of the prepubertal child. (From Baren J, Rothrock S, Brennan J, et al.: *Pediatric Emergency Medicine*, Philadelphia, 2008, Saunders.)

TABLE 17.1	CONGENITAL ANOMALIES IN THE DEVELOPMENT OF THE VULVA AND VAGINA
Condition	**Description**
Ambiguous genitalia	Partially fused labia, enlarged clitoris; hypospadias, or bilateral cryptorchidism in an infant with an apparent penis and testes are signs of a possible intersex condition (see Chapter 15)
Hydrocolpos	Vaginal secretions collecting behind an imperforate hymen at birth may appear as small cystic mass between labia
Müllerian agenesis (class 1)	Congenital absence of or hypoplasia of fallopian tubes, uterine corpus, uterine cervix, and proximal portion or entirety of the vaginal canal. Commonly diagnosed when an adolescent presents with primary amenorrhea or for first pelvic exam; however, can be recognized at birth if vaginal obstruction is pronounced

Data from Manipalviratn S, Trivax B, Huang A, Rosen AM, Zalles L. Genetic disorders & sex chromosome abnormalities. In: DeCherney AH, Nathan L, Laufer N, Roman AS, eds. CURRENT Diagnosis & Treatment: Obstetrics & Gynecology, 12e. McGraw Hill; 2019. Congenital Genitourinary Abnormalities. In: Cunningham F, Leveno KJ, Dashe JS, Hoffman BL, Spong CY, Casey BM, eds. Williams Obstetrics, 26e. McGraw Hill; 2022.

prepubertal preschool- and school-age children, hymens are thinner, generally redder (with genital color varying depending on skin color and ancestry), and more sensitive to touch. The prepubertal *vagina* is rigid, nonelastic, and thin-walled. The prepubertal vaginal wall is lined by columnar epithelium, which normally appears redder than the squamous epithelium lining the vagina of pubertal adolescents and adults. During early puberty, the effects of increased circulating estrogens are seen on the vulva, as labia minora develop more fully and the hymen thickens, lightens in color, and is more redundant.[3] Table 17.2 presents pubertal changes of the vagina.

During puberty, *adrenarche*, an increase in androgen secretion that initiates the development of pubic and axillary hair, occurs shortly after *thelarche*, the development of the breast (Fig. 17.6). The mean age of pubic hair growth inception in females is 9 to 10 years of age but may occur as early as 7 to 8 years of age in some

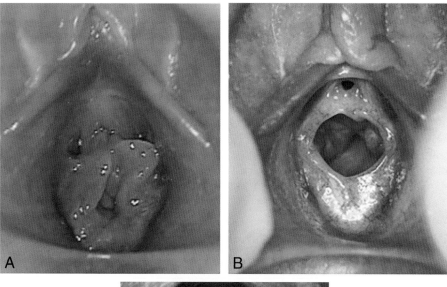

FIGURE 17.4 Variations in normal hymens. **(A)** Redundant. **(B)** Annular. **(C)** Crescentic. (From Zitelli BJ, et al.: *Atlas of Pediatric Physical Diagnosis*, ed 8, Philadelphia, 2023, Elsevier.)

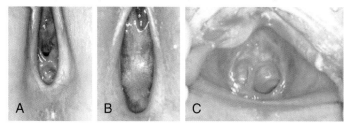

FIGURE 17.5 Abnormal hymens. **(A)** Cribriform. **(B)** Imperforate. **(C)** Septate. (**[A** and **B]** From McCann JJ, Kerns DL. *The Anatomy of Child and Adolescent Sexual Abuse: A CD-ROM Atlas/Reference*, St. Louis, 1999, Intercorp Inc.; **[C]** From Lahoti SL, McClain N, Girardet R, et al. Evaluating the child for sexual abuse. *Am Fam Physician* 63[5]:883–892, 2001.)

TABLE 17.2   PUBERTAL CHANGES OF THE VAGINA

Vaginal Changes	Prepubertal	Pubertal
Vaginal pH	6.5–7.5 (alkaline)	<4.5
Vaginal mucosa	Columnar epithelium (red)	Stratified squamous epithelium (pink); presence of columnar epithelium on ectocervix, surrounding the os
Vaginal mucous glands, discharge	Absent	Present; physiological leukorrhea usually begins at SMR 2–3
Normal vaginal flora	Gram-positive cocci and anaerobic gram-negative bacteria; gonorrhea and chlamydia focally infect vagina	Lactobacilli; yeast part of normal flora; gonorrhea and chlamydia commonly infect cervix
Vaginal length	4–5 cm	11–12 cm
External genitalia	Thin labia, rigid, nonelastic, thin-walled vagina	Thicker labia; thicker, more elastic, wavy, or redundant hymen; more elastic vagina

SMR, Sexual maturity rating.
Data from Hall JE. Disorders of the female reproductive system: normal pubertal development in girls. In: Jameson J, Fauci AS, Kasper DL, Hauser SL, Longo DL, Loscalzo J, eds. *Harrison's Principles of Internal Medicine, 20e*. McGraw Hill; 2018. Smith C, Reirden DH, Nyquist A. Sexually transmitted infections. In: Bunik M, Hay W W, Levin MJ, Abzug MJ, eds. *Current Diagnosis & Treatment: Pediatrics, 26e*. McGraw Hill; 2022.

P_1–Tanner 1. (preadolescent). No growth of pubic hair

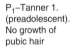
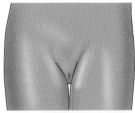

P_2–Tanner 2. Initial, scarcely pigmented straight hair, especially along medial border of the labia

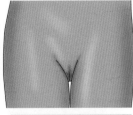

P_3–Tanner 3. Sparse, dark, visibly pigmented, curly public hair on labia.

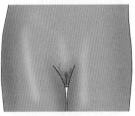

P_4–Tanner 4. Hair coarse and curly, abundant but less than adult.

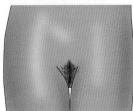

P_5–Tanner 5. Lateral spreading; type and triangle spread of adult hair to medial surface of thighs.

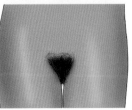

P_6–Tanner 6. Further extension laterally, upward, or dispersed (occurs in only 10% of women).

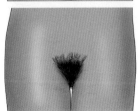

FIGURE 17.6 Sexual maturity rating in females.

pediatric populations.[5] Earlier onset is considered *precocious puberty* and should be investigated. Development and amount of pubic and general body hair can vary based on ancestry; therefore, this alone does not always correlate with sexual maturity. A recent worldwide systematic review found that geographic location played a major part in the onset of puberty.[6] Table 17.3 correlates pubic hair development and *sexual maturity rating* (SMR) or *Tanner Stage*, which includes both breast development (see Chapter 16) and pubic hair distribution. The external genitalia and internal structures—labia majora, labia minora, hymen, vagina, ovaries, uterus—are developing under the influence of increasing estrogens, but they are not included as part of the SMR.

Menarche, the commencement of the menstrual cycle, occurs approximately 2 years following the onset of *thelarche*, at an average age of 12 to 13 years old.[5] With increasing estrogenization during puberty, the presence of *leukorrhea*, or nonpathogenic vaginal discharge, may occur and is a typical finding preceding *menarche*. *Leukorrhea* is composed of cervical fluids and vaginal epithelial cells and changes in color, character, and consistency with cyclical hormonal shifts.[7] Unlike pathological vaginal discharge that is indicative of infection, physiologic *leukorrhea* is not associated with vulvovaginal itching or burning, pelvic pain, or a strong foul odor.[7] In early *menarche* menstrual cycles are generally anovulatory and may be irregular for the first 1 to 2 years; however, there is still a slight risk for pregnancy. Menstrual cycles typically normalize by late adolescence with the onset of regular ovulation.[8]

SPECIAL CONSIDERATIONS DURING GENITAL ASSESSMENT

Many adolescent patients may choose to remove pubic hair through shaving or waxing. This may make the determination of SMR

TABLE 17.3	SEXUAL MATURITY RATING (TANNER STAGES)	
Sexual Maturity Rating (SMR)	Pubic Hair Development	Genital Changes Due to Estrogenization[a]
1	No growth of pubic hair	Thicker, more elastic labia minora and hymen, change from columnar (red) to squamous (pink) epithelium in vagina (SMR 1–2)
2	Downy, scarcely pigmented straight hair, especially along medial border of labia majora	Physiologic leukorrhea (SMR 2–3)
3	Sparse, visibly pigmented curly pubic hair on labia (presentation may vary based on ancestry)	Physiologic leukorrhea (SMR 2–3)Onset of menses (SMR 3–4)
4	Hair coarse, curly, abundant, but less so than adult (presentation may vary based on ancestry); no extension onto medial thighs	Onset of menses (SMR 3–4)
5	Lateral spreading, triangle distribution with some spread onto medial thighs	—

[a]Not part of classic SMR, but important to note in exam findings and for anticipatory guidance.

SMR, Sexual maturity rating.

Data from Hall JE. Disorders of the female reproductive system: normal pubertal development in girls. In: Jameson J, Fauci AS, Kasper DL, Hauser SL, Longo DL, Loscalzo J, eds. *Harrison's Principles of Internal Medicine, 20e*. McGraw Hill; 2018. Smith C, Reirden DH, Nyquist A. Sexually transmitted infections. In: Bunik M, Hay WW, Levin MJ, Abzug MJ, eds. *Current Diagnosis & Treatment: Pediatrics, 26e*. McGraw Hill; 2022.

based on pubic hair distribution challenging in certain individuals. Teens may also present with body modifications such as genital piercings in various locations on the vulva, which is an increasingly common practice among adolescents. Common locations for genital piercings on the vulva are the labia majora, labia minora, clitoral hood, and surface piercings of the mons pubis area.

Female genital mutilation, also known as female cutting, or more rarely as female circumcision, is prevalent in many parts of the world, particularly in some African and Middle Eastern countries, and is considered a rite of passage and a prerequisite for marriage in some cultures. The procedure varies, but may consist of surgically removing part or all of the clitoris, the labia minora, and/or suturing closed the labia majora so that only a small exit remains for urine and menses.[9] The procedure is not legal in the United States or Canada, but females from other geographic areas may have had the procedure performed before migration or during a visit back to their country of origin.[9,10] It is estimated that as many as 513,000 females in the United States may have had this procedure performed.[10] Complications include infection, hemorrhage, tetanus, posttraumatic stress disorder (PTSD), difficulty in urination, sexual dysfunction, childbirth complications,

and infertility.[9,10] There is evidence the acceptability of female genital mutilation is decreasing in some countries and with immigrant populations in the United States; however, second-generation females may be at risk.[11]

In addition to variations in genital development and appearance, some transgender adolescents may experience *gender dysphoria* (see Chapter 16) as secondary sexual characteristics become obvious and are incongruent with their gender identity. The provider should maintain an open dialogue with the adolescent patient and their caregiver about feelings associated with puberty milestones and new physical changes. *Menarche,* or the time during puberty preceding *menarche,* is a time when adolescents and their families may present with questions about *puberty blockers* (see Chapter 16). Providers should be knowledgeable about these conversations and ready to engage in dialogue about the best course of action for adolescents experiencing *gender dysphoria.*

SYSTEM-SPECIFIC HISTORY

The Information Gathering table reviews information gathering on preadolescent and adolescent menstrual history and adolescent sexual history. For more on the approach to adolescent information gathering and obtaining sensitive health information, see Chapter 4.

INFORMATION GATHERING FOR GENITALIA AND INTERNAL PELVIC STRUCTURES AT KEY DEVELOPMENTAL STAGES

Age Group	Questions to Ask
Preadolescent and adolescent	*Menstrual history.* Age at menarche, regularity of cycles, any spotting or bleeding between cycles, dysmenorrhea, family history of menstrual problems? *For primary amenorrhea:* Age of thelarche and adrenarche, presence or absence of secondary sex characteristics? *For secondary amenorrhea:* Any weight loss attempts, including restriction, binging, purging? Significant physical or emotional stress? Other chronic health conditions? Drug use?
Adolescent	*Sexual history:* Any prior sexual activity, including number and gender of partners, types of activity, use of contraception and/or barrier protection? Coerced or unwanted sexual activity? Sexual pleasure and/or readiness to engage in sex? History of prior examinations, prior infections or prior vaginal procedures or surgery? Other prescription medications? Use of over-the-counter medications and cosmetic products or douches? Piercing, shaving, waxing, or use of depilatories for pubic and thigh hair?

PHYSICAL ASSESSMENT

Examination of the Newborn and Infant

Inspection and Palpation

In the newborn, assess presence and size of the clitoris, patency of the vaginal orifice, presence and location of urethra, and distance between the posterior fourchette and the anus. The labia majora should be palpated for the presence of gonads or hernias, even if the vulva appears normal. Any palpable gonads are likely to be testes because ovaries rarely descend below the inguinal ring. The labia should also be gently parted and inspected for adhesions. Reassurance of a healthy vaginal examination or prompt communication of any atypical or concerning physical findings is an important part of building a trust relationship between the caregiver and health care provider.

Examination of the Prepubertal Child

Positioning

Most young children can be examined in the *frog-leg position:* supine, with knees apart and feet touching in the midline (Fig. 17.7). For an apprehensive young child, the parent or caretaker can sit in a chair or on the examination table in a semireclined position (feet in or out of stirrups) with the child's legs straddling their thighs. Older children can be placed

in adjustable stirrups. In cases of suspected trauma or abuse, a foreign body in the vagina, or other suspected structural abnormalities, *knee-chest position* can be used in a child older than 2 years of age (Fig. 17.8). Have the child rest their chest on the exam table and support their weight on bent knees, which are positioned 6 to 8 inches apart. The child's buttocks will be held up in the air, and their back and abdomen will fall downward. In this position, using a penlight or an otoscope head for magnification and light, the examiner can visualize the lower vagina, and in prepubertal females often the upper vagina.

Examination

Lateral separation of the labia will be required to visualize the hymen (Fig. 17.9). The child

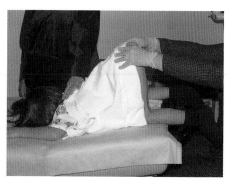

FIGURE 17.8 Knee-chest positioning. (From Gall JA, Boos SC, Payne-James JJ, et al.: *Forensic Medicine*, London, 2003, Churchill Livingstone.)

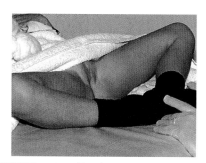

FIGURE   17.7 Frog-leg   positioning.   (From McCann JJ, Kerns DL. *The child abuse atlas*, Evidentia Learning, 2018, www.childabuseatlas.com; In Kliegman, RM, et al. *Nelson Textbook of Pediatrics*, ed 21, Philadelphia, Elsevier.)

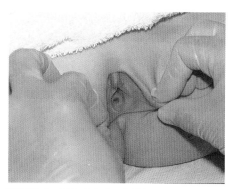

FIGURE 17.9 Anterior labial retraction. (From Gall JA, Boos SC, Payne-James JJ, et al. *Forensic Medicine*, London, 2003, Churchill Livingstone.)

can be asked to take a deep breath for distraction and to open the hymen. Discharge for wet mounts, potassium hydroxide (KOH) exams, Gram stains, or culture should be collected with a small Dacron-tipped swab moistened with saline. Avoid touching the hymen, which causes pain in a prepubertal child. Rarely, in cases of suspected abnormalities, a rectoabdominal examination may be performed following inspection of the vaginal area by placing the gloved and lubricated index finger or little finger of one hand into the rectum and placing the other hand on the abdomen. The cervix and uterus may be felt as a "button," and ovaries are not palpable. As the examiner withdraws the finger, the vagina can be gently milked to elicit discharge, a foreign body, or in rare cases, a polypoid tumor.

Young children are curious about their bodies and often explore the vaginal area. It is not uncommon for young children to insert foreign objects—crayons, beads, coins, batteries, small parts of toys, and other small objects—into their vagina. It is also common for toilet tissue to ball up and enter the vagina. Children with developmental delay who are diapered may have stool pushed into the vaginal vault. Foreign bodies can remain in the vagina for an extended period and cause inflammation and vaginal discharge, often foul smelling, or bleeding. A foreign body should always be considered when a prepubertal child presents with vaginal or urinary symptoms. If the examiner sees a foreign body, it may be removed by using a moistened cotton swab or by gently irrigating the vagina with normal saline. If the foreign body cannot easily be retrieved, or if the child has a significant amount of distress with the exam, referral for removal under anesthesia will be necessary. There is no indication for a speculum exam in the prepubertal child. Any invasive exams or procedures should always be performed under anesthesia by a pediatric gynecologic specialist.

Examination of the Adolescent

There are currently few indications for a pelvic exam in an adolescent. Regardless of history of sexual activity, only a symptomatic patient may be a potential candidate for a pelvic exam until age 21 when a *Papanicolaou (Pap) smear* is indicated.[12] Many examiners will consider an initial evaluation of vaginal complaints in adolescents with careful inspection of the external genitalia and specimen collection of vaginal discharge from the introitus and a vaginal swab for *sexually transmitted infection* (STI) testing if the patient reports sexual activity. The vaginal specimen can be obtained through the patient obtaining a self-swab or can be collected by the examiner. This preliminary process can be followed by a full pelvic exam if indicated. The presence of *trichomonas*, a common bacterial STI, on wet mount indicates the need for a full pelvic exam to evaluate the reproductive tract for pelvic inflammatory disease (PID). In the case of *primary amenorrhea* or absence of the onset of menstrual periods, abnormal vaginal bleeding, abnormal vaginal discharge, or lower abdominal pain, a pelvic exam and/or ultrasound imaging may be appropriate.[13] Adolescents who have experienced sexual abuse, have had negative experiences with health care providers, or who are experiencing *gender dysphoria* may have increased discomfort with pelvic exams. Taking the time to ask patients about preferred language for their anatomy, talking through the exam, and limiting the exam as much as possible can help make the experience easier for these populations. Table 17.4 reviews current indications for pelvic exams and alternatives to the recommended exam for adolescents who refuse or are unable to tolerate the pelvic examination.

The following description of the pelvic examination should be considered a supplement to careful supervision and mentoring of the novice examiner by the more experienced health care provider. Proper clean technique is more easily demonstrated, and specific procedures for collecting specimens for the *pap smear* and testing of STIs vary among clinics and laboratories.

TABLE 17.4 INDICATIONS FOR PELVIC EXAMS AND ALTERNATIVES		
Indications	**Recommended Exam**	**Alternatives**
Sexually active adolescent, asymptomatic, ≤21 years of age	Pelvic exam and Pap smear at age 21, then every 3 years if normal Urine or high vaginal specimen for gonorrhea and chlamydia screen using NAAT technology annually or with every new sexual partner	Pap smear not indicated <21 years Urine or high vaginal specimen for gonorrhea and chlamydia screen using NAAT technology annually or with every new sexual partner
Adolescent at age 21, asymptomatic, no history of sexual activity	Pelvic exam and Pap smear	Pap smear using a "blind technique" for youth whose disability precludes performing a speculum exam without sedation
Sexually active adolescent, asymptomatic, desires start of hormonal contraception	History, weight, and BP check Urine or high vaginal swab for NAAT STI screen, urine β-hCG if indicated	May defer STI screen and if menstruating at time of visit, schedule for STI screening after menses
Adolescent desires start of hormonal contraception, no history of sexual activity	History, weight, and BP check, Urine β-hCG if indicated based on type of contraceptive method (e.g., IUD)	—
Vaginal discharge without abdominal pain, no history of sexual activity	Vaginal swab for wet mount, KOH prep, STI screen if indicated by microscopic exam	Teen may insert vaginal swab, place in test tube with saline; wet mount, KOH prep
Vaginal discharge without abdominal pain, sexually active adolescent	Urine or high vaginal swab for NAAT STI screen, vaginal swab for wet mount, KOH prep; if wet mount findings consistent with STI, perform pelvic exam, Pap smear if due	Teen may insert vaginal swabs for STI screen and wet mounts
Adolescent with lower abdominal/pelvic pain; no history of sexual activity	Urine β-hCG, bimanual exam, speculum exam if indicated by history or presence of discharge or bleeding; ultrasound if results unclear	Urinalysis, urine β-hCG, urgent ultrasound
Sexually active adolescent with lower abdominal/pelvic pain	Pelvic exam, including speculum exam and bimanual, wet mount/KOH prep, and STI screening	Full exam essential; however, adolescent should not be examined against their will Abdominal exam and U/S imaging may be substituted in patient unable to tolerate pelvic exam

β-hCG, Beta human chorionic gonadotropin; *BP*, blood pressure; *KOH*, potassium hydroxide; *NAAT*, nucleic acid amplification test; *STI*, sexually transmitted infection; *U/S*, ultrasound.

Data from: Practice Bulletin No. 168. Cervical Cancer Screening and Prevention. *Obstet Gynecol* 128(4):e111–e130, 2016; Abells D, Kirkham YA, Ornstein MP. Review of gynecologic and reproductive care for women with developmental disabilities. *Curr Opin Obstet Gynecol* 28(5):350–358, 2016.

Preparing for the Exam

Explain the pelvic exam carefully, using a plastic pelvic model, diagram, or internet module and video (see http://www.sexualityandu.ca/sexual-health/going-to-doctor/first-pelvic-exam) that enables the adolescent to gain a concrete understanding of the examination process. It is useful to show the adolescent the speculum and specimen collection instruments in advance to dispel any anxiety or fear of the unknown. Clearly define for the patient whether the exam must be completed with some urgency (e.g., to rule out PID) or can be performed when the patient feels prepared (e.g., as part of an evaluation of primary amenorrhea). Some adolescents may want to have a parent, friend, or partner present for the pelvic examination to provide support. The adolescent may be provided a mirror, if desired, to observe the examination in progress. Encourage the adolescent to empty their bladder before the exam. If any specimens are needed, such as for urine pregnancy test, urinalysis, or urine for STI screening tests, they can be collected at this time. The exam should never be forced or coerced, and the adolescent should be informed that they can change their mind about the exam at any point. With sufficient preparation and explanations, most adolescents can tolerate the examination well. However, adolescents who have been sexually abused, have suffered other trauma, or who are particularly anxious may be helped by specific visualization and relaxation techniques.[14] Some adolescents find it helpful to gently place their open hand on the examiner's hand as they insert the speculum. Each provider and patient must work together to make the examination as comfortable as possible while maintaining safety and cleanliness.

Positioning

Adjust stirrups appropriately for the leg length. The adolescent can leave socks on to make the stirrups more comfortable. Ask the patient to move their buttocks forward to the very edge of the exam table, while the feet are in the stirrups. Although many adolescents are uncomfortable with this position, it is necessary for proper visualization and manipulation of the speculum. Avoid touching or pulling the patient; encourage them to move on their own. Some larger patients may need to move down farther than expected to allow the buttocks to come down over the edge of the exam table, allowing for more ease in visualizing the vaginal walls and cervix.

Most adolescents prefer to have a sheet draped over their abdomen and thighs, but the drape should be positioned so that the examiner can maintain eye contact with the adolescent. The knees should be abducted as far as possible. To have the patient's active participation, encourage them to push their knees apart as if they were doing an exercise in stretching, or to imagine a butterfly opening its wings. It is important for the clinician to be cognizant of their language and to avoid any references that could remind the patient of sexual activity. The adolescent should be encouraged to take slow, even breaths, to avoid tensing the abdominal muscles, and to keep the buttocks relaxed and down on the exam table. Stopping the exam to take breaks if the patient appears nervous or uncomfortable is important, and a regular check-in including consent to proceed should be obtained at each step of the exam.

Inspection

Note the condition of the clitoris, urethra, labia majora, labia minora, hymen, and introitus (Fig. 17.10). Inspect for swelling, lesions such as inflamed pubic hair follicles or condyloma (venereal warts), clitoral hypertrophy, presence or absence of estrogenization, or discharge. The external structures can be visualized more completely if the examiner gently separates the

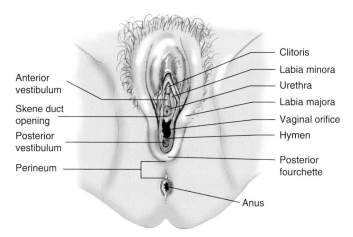

FIGURE 17.10 External female genitalia.

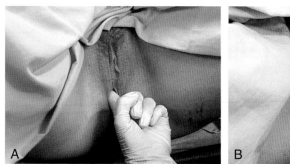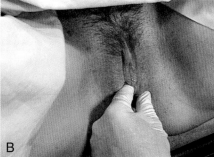

A   B

FIGURE 17.11 Examination of the **(A)** Skene and **(B)** Bartholin glands. (From Ball JW et al. Seidel's Guide to Physical Examination: An Interprofessional Approach, 10th ed., St. Louis, MO, 2023, Elsevier.)

labia majora to note the vaginal structures and anal area.

Palpation

Palpation of the *Skene glands* (Fig. 17.11A) and *Bartholin glands* (Fig. 17.11B) is usually avoided in the adolescent unless the adolescent presents with a complaint of pain or swelling in the labial or vaginal area or the examiner notes abnormalities upon inspection.

Speculum Exam

Choosing the Speculum

A vaginal speculum will assist with the internal examination by allowing you to visualize the vagina and cervix. Choosing the correct size should be based on the patient's age, BMI, sexual activity, width, and length of the vagina, and introital size.[15]

- A Huffman (Huffman-Graves) speculum (½ × 4½ inches) should be used if the hymenal opening is small, as to not cause discomfort to patients who have never or have infrequently experienced vaginal insertion (e.g., tampons or vaginal intercourse). This speculum may also be helpful for patients who have experienced sexual abuse or trauma, or who have *vaginismus*, or pain and uncontrollable tightening of the vagina upon attempted insertion of an instrument.
- A pediatric or child speculum (⅝–⅞ × 3 inches) is not optimal for use in postpubertal adolescents because of the excessive width and inadequate length.

- A Pedersen speculum (⅞ × 4½ inches) is most commonly used in adolescents without a prominent hymen. This speculum type is generally ideal for patients who are more comfortable with vaginal insertion (e.g., tampon use or vaginal intercourse).
- A Graves speculum (1¾ × 3¾ inches) is rarely used in adolescents but may be used for parous patients or if needed when a Pederson speculum does not provide for adequate visualization of the vaginal canal and cervix.
- *Light source:* Some plastic specula have a built-in light source (Fig. 17.12). Otherwise, angle the light over the examiner's shoulder to illuminate the introitus. Warn the patient the light may feel warm. If the lamp needs readjustment after speculum insertion, remember to change gloves before touching the neck of the light.
- *Inserting the speculum:* The speculum should be warmed and lightly lubricated, if possible, before insertion. The examiner should develop an approach to insertion that works for them to maintain clean technique. Some examiners double glove, others change gloves after inspection of the external genitalia and insertion of the speculum. Using the fingers of the non-dominant hand to separate the labia, one finger, lubricated with water or a scant amount of lubricating jelly, can be inserted into the introitus, pressing down on the posterior fourchette to facilitate easy insertion of the speculum. Use the dominant hand to gently insert the speculum, angled toward the sacrum, with slight downward pressure to avoid irritating the urethra. Be careful not to pinch the labia minora or to catch pubic hair in the speculum blades. Fig. 17.13 illustrates the steps of speculum insertion.
- Avoid putting pressure on the hymen if present.
- An alternate method of speculum insertion is to use the second and middle fingers of the nondominant hand to separate the labia, then press in gently on either side of the lower introitus to relax the fourchette tissues without direct pressure.
- Have the patient take in a deep breath or perform a *Valsalva maneuver* to help relax the introitus to insert the speculum.
- To locate the cervix, use a slight side-to-side motion; if the cervix does not come into view, it may cause less discomfort to withdraw the speculum and use one finger to locate the cervix rather than to move the speculum excessively.
- After the speculum is in place and the cervix is in view, secure the speculum in the open position, and remove the first glove on the hand that separated the labia (if double-gloved) or change the glove on the hand that contacted the labia/introitus; then proceed with specimen collection.

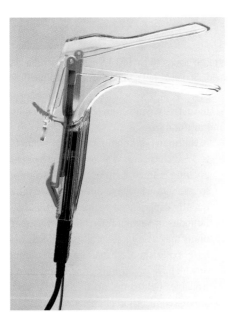

FIGURE 17.12 A vaginal speculum. (From Harkreader H, Hogan MA, Thobaben M. *Fundamentals of Nursing: Caring and Clinical Judgment*, ed 3, St. Louis, 2008, Saunders.)

Inspection of the Vagina and Cervix

Inspect the walls of the vagina, and note the presence, color, and consistency of any discharge. Carefully inspect the cervix for color,

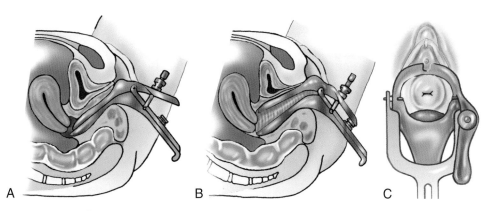

A   B   C

FIGURE 17.13 Female genital examination. **(A)** Insertion of closed speculum. **(B)** Open speculum and locate cervix. **(C)** When cervix is in view, secure speculum.

TABLE 17.5	ATYPICAL FINDINGS ON PELVIC EXAM
Findings	Descriptions
Vulvar and vaginal abnormalities	Imperforate hymen, hematocolpos, vaginal agenesis or signs of a transverse vaginal septum (caused by congenital incomplete fusion of upper and lower vagina), external condyloma or other lesions, signs of trauma, erythema, and discharge
Cervical abnormalities	Reddened, friable (bleeds with insertion of cotton swab into os), visible condyloma, petechiae ("strawberry spots" rarely seen with trichomoniasis), erosions, double cervix (associated with uterus didelphys), absence of cervix
Pelvic masses	Masses resulting from intrauterine or ectopic pregnancy or from pelvic infection (salpingitis or tuboovarian abscess); adnexal torsion secondary to cyst (which presents with twisting sensation, intermittent bouts of severe pain separated by generalized aching, can be surgical emergency); functional, corpus luteum or dermoid, or other complex ovarian cysts; endometriosis Uterine tumors (such as leiomyomas) are rare in the adolescent; ovarian cancers comprise approximately 1% of all childhood cancers, but they are the most common genital tract cancer in adolescents All adnexal masses should be imaged, first with ultrasound, then (if needed) with computed tomography or magnetic resonance imaging

lesions, and any discharge at the *cervical os.* The *cervical os,* the opening of the cervix into the endometrial canal, is round in a *nulliparous* adolescent but may be slit-like in a *parous* adolescent. Physiologic variations of the cervix include *nabothian cysts,* which are small, white, or yellow, raised, smooth, round nodules on the cervix; and an *ectropion cervix,* a visible ring of redder, glossy columnar epithelium protruding out and surrounding the os of the cervix.

Table 17.5 presents atypical findings of the female genitalia.

Specimen Collection

Generally, a Pap smear is not indicated for patients under 21 years of age. If a Pap smear does need to be collected, the recommended order of specimen collection is to start with the Pap smear then follow with the collection of specimens for STI screening. It may be reasonable to collect STI specimens first in some adolescents if there is a copious amount of discharge or purulent discharge from the cervical os, because the exudate needs to be removed before specimen collection for the Pap smear.

- Use a spatula and cytobrush for Pap smear collection. Follow laboratory instructions for liquid cytology (which has replaced the conventional Pap smear as the gold standard) in which the cells are collected and placed in a liquid medium. Be sure to sample the squamocolumnar junction, which may be on the *ectocervix*, or *external os*, in some adolescents. In some individuals with disabilities, collection of the Pap smear by means of a speculum exam may not be a viable option due to spasticity or other conditions that preclude a standard pelvic exam. The option to obtain a Pap smear using a "blind technique" (without using a speculum, palpate the cervical os using a finger then slide the cytobrush over the finger to obtain the endocervical sample) is an acceptable alternative to ensure appropriate and timely cancer screening.[16]
- Next collect vaginal swabs for chlamydia and gonorrhea—the preferred specimen source due to the highest sensitivity of nucleic acid amplification test (NAAT),[17] unless using urine for STI screening.
- Use a moistened cotton-tipped swab or plastic or wooden spatula to collect some vaginal secretions for wet mount and KOH preparations from both the vaginal pool and the vaginal wall, unless there is significant blood present. If scant or light bleeding is present, attempt to gather a sample free from blood. If excessive blood is present, microscopy may be difficult due to obscuring red blood cells in the field, and the patient may have to return for the wet mount and KOH testing if still indicated when bleeding has subsided.
- Testing vaginal pH is a valuable adjunct to the wet mount and KOH prep exams. Vaginal pH is typically 6.5 to 7.5 in prepubertal

girls and 3.5 to 4.5 in pubertal girls. Vaginal discharge adhering to the speculum blades can be collected for pH testing before the speculum is discarded or placed in cleaning solution. Alternatively, a swab of vaginal secretions can be applied to a pH tape or strip. Be advised that the presence of blood, lubrication, or semen on the test strip may be mistaken for an abnormally high vaginal pH due to infection.

- Before withdrawing the speculum, release the locking mechanism. Avoid pinching the cervix and vaginal walls as you allow the blades to close. Maintain downward pressure of the speculum to avoid trauma to the urethra. Turn the speculum to a 45-degree angle to enable the blades to pass through the hymenal ring.

The Bimanual Exam

The purpose of the bimanual exam is to assess the cervix, the corpus of the uterus, and the adnexa. This exam is not recommended for routine screening in nonpregnant people. However, a bimanual exam may be indicated to assess complaints of pain, irregular bleeding, or infection symptoms.[18] The adolescent should be encouraged to relax the abdominal muscles by breathing slowly and steadily, or performing a Valsalva maneuver, which may facilitate insertion of the examiner's fingers. The examiner applies lubricant to the middle and index fingers of a gloved hand and then inserts the fingers into the vagina, keeping the pressure against the posterior fourchette and the pubococcygeal muscle and away from the delicate anterior structures of the clitoris and urethra (Fig. 17.14). In younger adolescents or in adolescents with prominent hymenal tissue, it may be possible to insert only one finger. If the need for a bimanual exam is indicated, the examiner should consider the alternative option of a *rectoabdominal exam* for adolescents who request to avoid vaginal penetration for cultural or religious reasons.

- **Palpate the cervix**: Note consistency of the cervix, normally firm and shaped like the tip of a nose. Note presence of any bumps on the cervix, such as *nabothian cysts*, 3- to 8-mm smooth, nontender, firm lumps, which result from blockage of endocervical gland ducts.

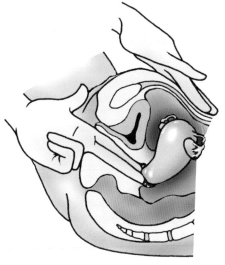

FIGURE 17.14 Bimanual exam.

- **Palpate the uterus**: Press down on the abdomen with the other hand while supporting the cervix. Assess the size, shape, consistency, mobility, and tenderness of the uterus and any palpable masses. The position of the uterus varies from anteverted, anteflexed, midposition, and retroverted to retroflexed (Fig. 17.15). The normal uterus is shaped like an upside-down small pear and is approximately 7.5 cm long and 2.5 cm thick.
- **Assess for cervical motion tenderness**: The examiner gently wiggles the cervix side-to-side and forward and backward between the palpating fingers. In a normal exam the movement of the uterus creates an unusual and uncomfortable sensation in the pelvis for an adolescent. Ask the adolescent to distinguish between pain and discomfort or an unusual feeling. Tenderness or pain on exam is a symptom of pelvic infection.
- **Assess the adnexae and ovaries**: Place the examining fingers in the vagina first at the right lateral fornix then at the left lateral fornix, posteriorly and high. Begin with the

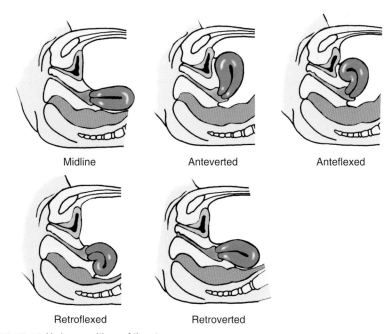

Midline   Anteverted   Anteflexed

Retroflexed   Retroverted

FIGURE 17.15 Various positions of the uterus.

opposite hand on the abdomen just below and medial to the iliac crest and move diagonally toward the symphysis pubis. Apply a firm, steady sweeping motion with the hand on the abdomen as you palpate briefly. Normal ovaries are smooth and almond shaped, slightly tender to deep palpation, and approximately 3 × 1.5 × 1 cm. Tenderness or fullness of the adnexae is abnormal and may indicate infection, ectopic pregnancy, or endometriosis.

- **Rectovaginal exams**: This exam is usually omitted in adolescents, unless there is a suspicion of abnormality or an extremely retroflexed uterus, or the hymenal ring is too tight to adequately assess for the cervix and uterus. It is performed with the index finger in the vagina, the middle finger in the rectum, and the opposite hand on the abdomen. The *rectovaginal septum* should be thin, pliable, and free of masses. The patient should be reassured that feeling the urge to defecate is a normal sensation during this exam, but once the exam is over the urge will pass.

- **Sizing an intrauterine pregnancy**: Recognizing a pregnancy in the adolescent can aid in the swift diagnosis of the cause of complaints ranging from fatigue and nausea to secondary amenorrhea, abdominal fullness, or a mass. The health care provider should maintain a high index of suspicion for pregnancy, even in the youngest adolescents who deny a history of sexual activity. Adolescents may be reluctant to disclose early or unwanted sexual activity. Point of care urine testing for β-hCG is invaluable. The weeks of pregnancy are counted from the first day of the last menstrual period, even though ovulation generally occurs 2 weeks after the beginning of menses (Box 17.1). Fundal height provides a guide for estimating uterine size (Fig. 17.16).

Wrapping up the Examination

The patient should be handed some tissues, so that they may wipe off the lubricant used.

BOX 17.1   SIZING AN INTRAUTERINE PREGNANCY

Nulliparous uterus: 7.5 × 2.5 cm (size of small lime on bimanual exam)

8-week uterus: 9–11 cm × 5 cm (size of orange on bimanual exam)

12-week uterus: 12–14 cm × 7 cm (size of grapefruit, very soft, sometimes difficult to palpate on bimanual exam); just palpable, abdominally at level of symphysis pubis

16-week uterus: Palpate abdomen, felt halfway between symphysis pubis and umbilicus

20-week uterus: Palpate abdomen, felt at umbilicus

More than 20 weeks: Measure from symphysis pubis to height of fundus (number of centimeters—approximate number of weeks)

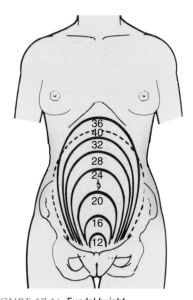

FIGURE 17.16 Fundal height.

The examiner should stay in the room long enough to ensure that the adolescent does not feel dizzy upon sitting up and then leave while they dress. Results of the exam should be given while the patient is dressed, and any abnormalities should be thoroughly explained. To ensure confidentiality, present and discuss results with the adolescent alone.

Suspicion of Sexual Abuse

In cases of suspected child sexual abuse, the patient history and behavioral observations are crucial. Any history of abuse disclosed to the health care provider that occurred within the previous 72 hours (up to 120 hours in some states) requires immediate referral for a forensic examination with possible collection of evidence. Guidelines recommend collection of DNA evidence within 24 hours for prepubertal children and 72 hours for adolescents; however, some regions using DNA amplification will collect DNA evidence over a longer time span, and providers should be familiar with local resources and recommendations.[19] Most sexually abused prepubertal children will have normal findings on physical exams because of the following:

- Delays in disclosure
- Rapid healing of genital and anal tissue in prepubertal children
- Predominance in this age group of sexual abuse involving fondling or oral-genital contact, which does not leave physical signs

It is important to remember that most children reporting sexual abuse will have no abnormal findings in a genital exam.[1] Furthermore, variation in skin color of the genitals due to ancestral background may confound signs of sexual abuse. Providers could potentially miss signs of injury in the vulvovaginal/perianal area in patients with darker skin.[20,21] A variation in anatomy, such as a hymenal tag, may also be mistaken for signs of sexual abuse in an infant (Fig. 17.17).[22] Providers must be vigilant in their assessment of the pediatric patient any time sexual abuse is suspected. The following physical findings in prepubertal children should raise suspicion of sexual abuse and prompt referral for an exam by specially trained practitioners[19]:

- Hymenal irregularities or absence of hymen, including notches, transections, or thin, rounded edges, posterior from the 4- to 8-o'clock position with the child supine, should be confirmed in knee-chest position, because an apparent notch may be a fold in a redundant hymen
- Acute trauma to the hymen or posterior fourchette, or laceration of vaginal mucosa, particularly extending to the rectal mucosa
- Confirmed STI, including human papillomavirus (HPV) infection in a child ≥ 2 years old

Other possible findings include increased erythema, irritation, and vaginal discharge, which may or may not be signs of sexual abuse. Failure or delay of fusion of the median *raphe* between the posterior fourchette and the anus is often mistaken for trauma or sexual abuse. However, it is essential for health care providers to keep in mind they should not solely rely on physical findings when considering a diagnosis of sexual abuse. The examiner should keep the possibility of sexual abuse in mind whenever other nonvenereal infections, chemical irritation, foreign bodies, and/or poor hygiene are included in the differential diagnosis. Additionally, the provider must pay close attention to the behavior and nonverbal communication from the child or adolescent during the visit. Safety should always be assessed during the visit via routine questioning and history taking, and if abuse is suspected, the provider must report it to investigating authorities according to state law.

Conditions of the Vulva and Vagina

Table 17.6 presents common conditions and findings of the prepubertal and pubertal vulva and vagina. The prepubertal vagina is hostile to yeast, and vulvovaginal candidiasis is rare except in cases of diabetes mellitus, recent

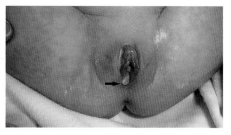

FIGURE 17.17 Hymenal tag. (From Leung AK, Lam JM. Hymenal tags in girls:not to be mistaken for sexual abuse. *Cureus* 2021;13(9):e17931.)

TABLE 17.6	CONDITIONS OF THE VULVA AND VAGINA
Condition	Description
Labial adhesions	Adherence of labia minora or majora, primarily seen in females 3 months to 6 years of age; adhesion may persist until puberty, or may separate spontaneously; treatment is controversial if opening is large enough for normal urinary flow and vaginal drainage
Labial abscesses	Usually caused by *Staphylococcus aureus* and *Streptococcus pyogenes*
Labial lipoma	May be initially mistaken for a hernia
Clitoral lesions	Edema of clitoris, with hypoproteinemia, in conditions such as nephrotic syndrome Hypertrophy of clitoral hood and clitoris, caused by neurofibromatosis, rhabdomyo-sarcoma, increased androgens Hemorrhages around clitoris caused by lichen sclerosis or trauma (see later)
Urethral prolapse	Presents with bleeding and friable, red-blue doughnutlike annular mass that may be visible in perineum ("hemorrhagic cranberry")
Lichen sclerosis	Uncommon; presents with atrophic, hypopigmented, parchmentlike friable skin around vulva and anus, often in an "hourglass" configuration, with inflammation and subepithelial hemorrhages
Vulvar irritation	Often results from irritants such as bubble bath, poor hygiene, candidal overgrowth caused by antibiotics or diaper occlusion; rarely scratching can occur secondary to pruritus from a pinworm infestation
Vulvovaginitis	Vaginal discharge may be caused by bacteria (e.g., *Streptococcus, Shigella*) or overgrowth of normal flora; foreign body in vagina (typically toilet paper); poor hygiene; sexually transmitted infection (STI)
Straddle injuries to vulva	Straddle injuries (as in playground falls) generally cause trauma to anterior vulvar structures and rarely cause trauma to posterior portion of hymen or posterior fourchette; in addition, injury is usually somewhat asymmetrical and not penetrating in nature

antibiotic usage, compromised immune system, or diaper use in infants or children with special health care needs. Sexually transmitted pathogens, such as *Neisseria gonorrhoeae* and *Chlamydia trachomatis*, infect the columnar epithelium of the vagina rather than the *cervix* in sexually active adolescents. Bacterial infections, such as *Streptococcus* and *Shigella*, can cause purulent or even bloody vaginal discharge in infected individuals.

TELEHEALTH TIPS

Examination of the vulva, vagina, and internal pelvic structures should be done at an in-person visit to maintain privacy, comfort, and professionalism. However, a telehealth visit via phone or video can be a valuable way to collect history and triage common dermatological or gynecological concerns in pediatric and adolescent patients. For example, an adolescent may give a history and list of symptoms that is consistent with candidiasis, and a provider may elect to treat the condition presumptively via telehealth while instructing the patient to follow up within a specific time frame in person if symptoms worsen or persist.

SUMMARY OF EXAMINATION

- The genital exam in the asymptomatic child and adolescent includes an assessment of the external genitalia only.
- SMR in females is based on breast development and pubic hair distribution.
- Secondary sexual development must be assessed in the context of overall growth and development.
- The norms for SMR are based on data collected on children of European ancestry. Children of other ancestry may not have pubic hair development that matches SMR.
- There are currently few indications for a pelvic exam in an adolescent; it is not necessary for STI screening in asymptomatic, sexually active adolescents.
- Most children who report sexual abuse will not have atypical findings on the genital exam.

- Providers should be aware of variations of vulvar appearance and the causes of the variations; whether a variation of normal anatomy, or signs of abuse including sexual abuse or cultural practices like female genital mutilation.

DOCUMENTATION

Sexually Active Adolescent
External Genitalia: No lesions, rashes or discharge. SMR stage 4 to 5 pubic hair distribution.
Internal Exam: Vaginal mucosa pink, moist, and rugated. Cervix pink, no lesions, scant blood at cervical os, scant mucoid discharge in vault.
Bimanual: Cervix smooth, firm, mobile. No cervical motion tenderness. Uterus midline, anteverted, firm, smooth, nontender; not enlarged. Ovaries not palpable. No adnexal tenderness or masses.

REFERENCES

1. Jenny C, Crawford-Jakubiak JE. The evaluation of children in the primary care setting when sexual abuse is suspected. *Pediatrics.* 2013;132(2):e558–e567.
2. Carlson BM. *Human Embryology and Developmental Biology: With STUDENT CONSULT Online Access.* 5th ed. Philadelphia: Saunders; 2014.
3. French A, Emans J. Vulvovaginal problems in the prepubertal child. In: Emans, Laufer, Goldstein's *Pediatric and Adolescent Gynecology.* 7th ed. Philadelphia: Lippincott Williams & Wilkins; 2019.
4. Kremen J, Chan YM, Holm I. Ambiguous genitalia in the newborn and disorders of sex development. In: Emans, Laufer, Goldstein's *Pediatric and Adolescent Gynecology.* 7th ed. Philadelphia: Lippincott Williams & Wilkins; 2019.
5. Hall JE. Disorders of the female reproductive system: normal pubertal development in girls. In: Jameson J, Fauci AS, Kasper DL, Hauser SL, Longo DL, Loscalzo J, eds. *Harrison's Principles of Internal Medicine, 20e.* McGraw Hill; 2018.
6. Eckert-Lind C, Busch AS, Petersen JH, et al. Worldwide secular trends in age at pubertal onset assessed by breast development among girls: a systematic review and meta-analysis. *JAMA Pediatr.* 2020;174(4):e195881.
7. Smith C, Reirden DH, Nyquist A. Sexually transmitted infections. In: Bunik M, Hay WW, Levin MJ, Abzug MJ, eds. *Current Diagnosis & Treatment: Pediatrics, 26e.* McGraw Hill; 2022.

8. Carlson LJ, Shaw ND. Development of ovulatory menstrual cycles in adolescent girls. *J Pediatr Adolesc Gynecol.* 2019;32(3):249–253.
9. Nowak B. The school nurse's role in addressing female genital mutilation. *NASN School Nurse (Print).* 2016;31(5):286–291.
10. Goldberg H, Stupp P, Okoroh E, Besera G, Goodman D, Danel I. Female genital mutilation/cutting in the United States: Updated estimates of women and girls at risk, 2012. *Public Health Rep.* 2016;2016(131):1–8.
11. Puppo V. Female genital mutilation and cutting: an anatomical review and alternative rites. *Clin Anat.* 2016;30:81–88.
12. Practice Bulletin No. 168 Cervical Cancer Screening and Prevention. *Obstet Gynecol.* 2016;128(4):e111–e130.
13. French A, Emans J. Office evaluation of the child and adolescent. In: Emans, Laufer, Goldstein's Pediatric and Adolescent Gynecology. 7th ed. Philadelphia: Lippincott Williams & Wilkins; 2019.
14. O'Laughlin DJ, Strelow B, Fellows N, Kelsey E, Peters S, Stevens J, Tweedy J. Addressing anxiety and fear during the female pelvic examination. *J Prim Care Community Health.* 2021;122150132721992195.
15. Taylor GA, McDonagh D, Hansen MJ. Improving the pelvic exam experience: a human-centered design study. *Des J.* 2017;20(sup1):S2348–S2362.
16. Abells D, Kirkham YA, Ornstein MP. Review of gynecologic and reproductive care for women with develop-

mental disabilities. *Curr Opin Obstet Gynecol*. 2016;28(5): 350–358.

17. Papp J, Schachter J, Gaydos C, Van Der Pol B. Recommendations for the laboratory-based detection of Chlamydia trachomatis and Neisseria gonorrhoeae—2014. *MMWR Recomm Rep*. 2014;63(RR-02):1–19.

18. Qin J, Saraiya M, Martinez G, Sawaya GF. Prevalence of potentially unnecessary bimanual pelvic examinations and Papanicolaou tests among adolescent girls and young women aged 15–20 years in the United States. *JAMA Intern Med*. 2020;180(2):274–280.

19. Adams JA, Kellogg ND, Farst KJ, et al. Updated guidelines for the medical assessment and care of children who may have been sexually abused. *J Pediatr Adolesc Gynecol*. 2016;29(2):81–87.

20. Rossman L, Solis S, Rechtin C, Bush C, Wynn B, Jones J. The effects of skin pigmentation on the detection of genital injury from sexual assault. *Am J Emerg Med*. 2019;37(5):974–975.

21. Sommers MS, Regueira Y, Tiller DA, et al. Understanding rates of genital-anal injury: role of skin color and skin biomechanics. *J Forensic Leg Med*. 2019;66:120–128.

22. Leung AK, Lam JM. Hymenal tags in girls: not to be mistaken for sexual abuse. *Cureus*. 2021;13(9):e17931.

MUSCULOSKELETAL ASSESSMENT

Keely E. Giss; Carrie T. Chan

Assessing the musculoskeletal system is challenging for pediatric health care providers due to the variations in growth and development and the normal range of rotational changes in the extremities in children from birth to young adulthood. Increasing knowledge about the normal developmental changes in the musculoskeletal system is key to accurate assessment and limiting over referral. Performing appropriate physical assessment techniques assists in diagnosis of common orthopedic conditions and prompt referral when indicated for children with intentional or unintentional injuries.

EMBRYOLOGIC DEVELOPMENT

The rudimentary skeletal system forms as early as the fourth week of gestation, when the development of the vertebrae begin, and the upper extremities begin as buds on the fetus. By the eighth week of gestation, a cartilaginous skeleton is formed, which serves as the scaffold for bone development.[1] During the ninth week of gestation, bone cells called *osteoblasts* begin forming bone through a process called *ossification*. This begins in the primary ossification centers in the vertebrae and the center of long bones. The hand pads develop from the extremity buds by days 33 to 36, and the finger rays begin to form on days 41 to 43.[2] It is during this period of gestation that *polydactyly*, the presence of extra digits, or *syndactyly*, the webbing or fusing of the digits, occurs along with other deformities of the extremities. The position of the fetus in utero has the greatest

impact on the skeletal system, and the most common variants present at birth.

Muscle structures, including the tendons, ligaments, cartilage, and joints, originate from the embryonic *mesoderm*. Muscle fibers are developed by the fourth or fifth month of gestation. They increase in size along with changes in muscle and fat proportions throughout childhood and adolescence.

DEVELOPMENTAL VARIATIONS

At birth, the *epiphyses* at the ends of the long bones are composed of hyaline cartilage. Shortly after birth, secondary ossification centers begin to replace the cartilage in the epiphyses. The replacement of cartilage by bone is known as *endochondral ossification*. This creates an epiphyseal plate, or *physis*, of remaining cartilage between the primary and secondary ossification centers that serve as the growth plate. The physis continually creates new hyaline cartilage while the older cartilage is calcified in the *metaphysis*, the wide portion of long bones where longitudinal growth occurs. Longitudinal growth creates the shaft of the long bones called the *diaphysis*[1] (Fig. 18.1). Growth along the physis continues until the cells in the growth plate mature and stop dividing in puberty, and closure of the growth plate occurs in young adulthood when the metaphysis and the epiphysis fuse.

Several factors influence the healthy development of the skeletal system and normal growth at the physis. Trauma during childhood can cause separation of the epiphysis

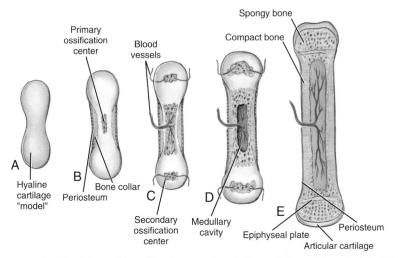

FIGURE 18.1 Growth plates and transition from cartilage to bone at the epiphyseal plate. **(A)** Hyaline cartilage "model." **(B)** Periosteum and bone collar form. **(C)** Blood vessels and osteoblasts infiltrate primary ossification centers. **(D)** Osteoclasts form medullary cavity. **(E)** Ossification is complete. Hyaline cartilage remains as articular cartilage and in the epiphyseal plate. (From Applegate E: *The Anatomy and Physiology Learning System*, ed 4, St. Louis, 2011, Saunders.)

and the blood vessels to rupture, resulting in cessation of bone growth and a shortened extremity.[2] Nutritional factors, such as adequate protein in the diet, the amount of calcium intake daily, and adequate intake of vitamin D, which regulates the adsorption of calcium and phosphorus in the intestines, impact bone growth. Adequate levels of vitamin D, particularly important in the breastfed infant, may also have a role in improving muscle and immune function in childhood. Parents are advised to apply sunscreen and limit direct sun exposure for infants and children due to long-term risks of skin cancer, therefore reducing vitamin D synthesis from the skin. Balancing safe sun exposure and maintaining adequate levels of vitamin D in infants and children is important to maintaining bone strength. *Rickets* is a deficiency of vitamin D in which the growth plate is impaired by calcification of newly formed bone on the metaphyseal plate. Alterations in thyroid or growth hormones can also impact normal patterns of growth in childhood.[2]

ANATOMY AND PHYSIOLOGY

Head and Neck

Assessment of the head and neck area is reviewed in Chapter 13 and Chapter 19.

Upper Extremities and Torso

The *clavicle* lies in a horizontal plane above the first rib and rotates between the *sternum* and the *acromion* at the anterosuperior surface of the *scapula* (Fig. 18.2). The scapula, a large, flat triangular bone, lies posterior on the upper back and forms the posterior portion of the upper extremity. The superolateral process of the scapula, the *glenoid*, articulates with the rounded head of the *humerus*, the long bone of the upper arm. The distal end of the humerus is divided into the *medial epicondyle, the lateral condyle, the trochlea, and the capitellum*. The *ulna* articulates proximally with the humerus at the trochlea and is the medial (little finger side) of the two long bones in the forearm. The *olecranon* is the posterior, rounded surface of the ulna. The

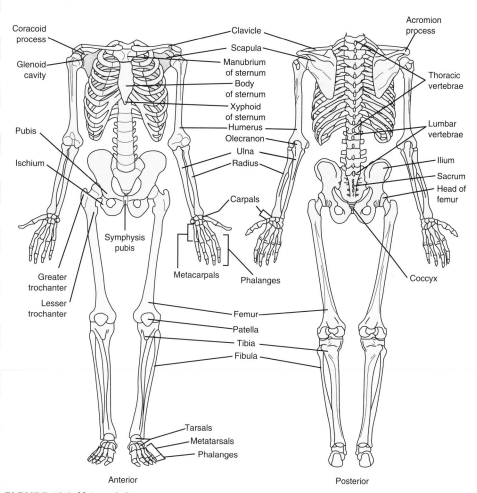

FIGURE 18.2 **Mature skeleton.**

distal end of the ulna is small and articulates with the *radius* at the wrist at the *distal radi-oulnar joint*. The lateral (thumb side) forearm bone, the radius, articulates proximally with the capitellum of the humerus and distally with the ulna as well as the carpal bones of the hand to form the wrist. The radius enables rotation of the forearm.

The hand consists of eight carpal and five metacarpal bones. Many of the carpal bones are cartilaginous at birth. A radiograph of a child's hand at 2.5 years of age illustrates ossi-fication of only the *capitate* and *hamate* bones in the midhand. Development and ossification of the hand continues until 11 years of age, when all the carpal bones are ossified except for the small *pisiform* bone, which develops by 12 years of age. Fingers are composed of three *phalanges* each except for the thumb, which is made up of only two phalanges. Abnormal-ities of the fingers such as *syndactyly*, web-bing or fusion between adjacent digits of the hands or feet, may be an isolated anomaly or associated with additional anomalies and syn-dromes (Fig. 18.3A). *Polydactyly*, the presence of supernumerary digits, is a more common variant and is not usually associated with other congenital anomalies (Fig. 18.3B).

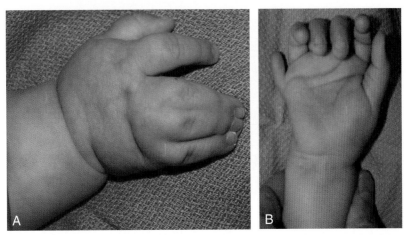

FIGURE 18.3 **(A)** Syndactyly. **(B)** Polydactyly. ([A] From Davis P, Cladis F, Motoyana E: *Smith's Anesthesia for Infants and Children*, ed 10, Philadelphia, 2022, Elsevier. [B] Chung, KC: Hand and upper extremity reconstruction with DVD: A volume in the procedures in reconstructive surgery series. Philadelphia, 2009, Saunders.)

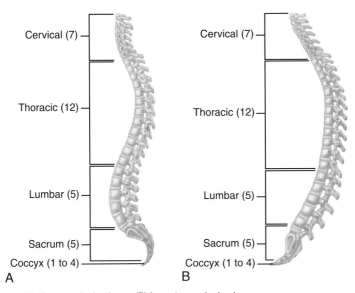

FIGURE 18.4 **(A)** Mature spinal column. **(B)** Immature spinal column.

Spine

The infant has a C-shaped spinal curve at birth in comparison with the S curvature that is present in late adolescence (Fig. 18.4). The secondary cervical curve in the neck is present by 3 to 4 months of age, when the infant begins to hold up their head. The lumbar curvature in the low back begins to form as the infant bears weight and begins to walk. The young child often has an exaggerated thoracic-lumbar curvature and a protuberant abdomen until 3 years of age, when gait and balance become more normal. The *sacrum* below the lumbar spine is composed of five separate bones at birth and by 18 to 20 years of age is fused into one large bone. The *coccyx* at the bottom end of the spine consists of three or four small bones that begin to ossify between the first and fourth years of life and fuses into one bone by 25 years of age.

Pelvis

The pelvis has three distinct parts in childhood, which are later fused in the adult. The *ilium* is the superior, broad, flat surface of the pelvis. The *ischium* is the strongest portion of the pelvis and contains a portion of the *acetabulum* that forms the articulating surface of the pelvis for the femur, and the opening or *foramen* (Fig. 18.2). The *pubis* contains the medial portion of the acetabulum and joins medially to form the complete pelvic girdle.

Lower Extremities and Feet

The *femur* is the longest and strongest bone in the body that makes up the thigh. The head of the femur becomes ossified during the first year of life, but the shaft of the femur does not become completely ossified until 14 years of age. The long bones of the extremities continue to grow from the physis (or multiple physes) throughout childhood and adolescence; peak bone mass is achieved by young adulthood.

The *patella*, or kneecap, is the small triangular bone that lies over the junction of the femur and the tibia. The health of the patella during growth and development depends not only on strong bone growth but also on the strength of the ligaments and tendons supporting the patella.

In the lower leg, the larger, medial bone is the *tibia*, or the shin bone. The proximal tibia closer to the knee articulates with the femur and the distal end closer to the ankle forms the medial border of the ankle joint, the *medial malleolus*, as well as the joint surface of the ankle. The *fibula* is the smaller, lateral bone in the lower leg. The distal end of the fibula forms the lateral border of the ankle, the *lateral malleolus*.

The seven tarsal bones and five metatarsal bones of the foot undergo dramatic ossification during the first year of life. The ossification of the bones in the foot follows the normal development of the gross motor milestones. The *talus* is ossified by the seventh month of life and, along with the distal tibia, forms the ankle joint. The *metatarsal* bones continue to form during the latter half of the first year of life. The three phalanges of each toe, two at the great toe, continue the ossification process through adolescence.

The lower limbs go through a continuous process of growth and rotational change until approximately 8 to 10 years of age.[3] The torsional development of the skeletal system is a process that begins in infancy and progresses from sitting to crawling (though not all infants crawl), then standing, cruising, and finally walking with an exaggerated gait and a wide base of support. The laxity in the ligaments and fetal positioning in the intrauterine environment contribute to the normal torsional variations in the lower extremities during childhood. Torsional variations and musculoskeletal abnormalities are hereditarily linked and often show a strong family tendency.

Monitoring Growth

During growth, bone has the remarkable capacity to remodel itself. Bone is deposited in areas subjected to stress and reabsorbed in areas where there is little stress. This physiologic process explains the ability of children to remodel residual deformity after fractures and demonstrates the biologic plasticity of growing bones. The rate of bone growth is greatest in the lower extremities before and around the onset of puberty, and the *distal* (furthest from the center of the body) extremities reach adult size in early puberty. This is often reflected in shoe size in preadolescents. The trunk and *proximal* (closest to the center of the body) extremities exhibit the dominant growth during puberty and into young adulthood. Longitudinal bone growth is complete once all the physes have closed, typically in late adolescence or early adulthood, although peak bone mass is not achieved until 35 years of age.

Monitoring the velocity of growth is a key focus of routine well-child visits and when following children with chronic health conditions,

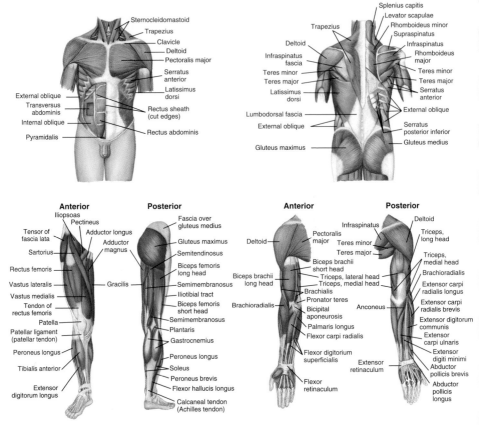

FIGURE 18.5 Muscular system, front and back. (From Mourad LA: *Orthopedic Disorders*, St. Louis, 1991, Mosby.)

particularly cardiac conditions. For the child with slow growth or delayed onset of puberty, obtaining past growth charts and evaluating the progression of the growth curve along with familial patterns of growth and pubertal development is critical to assessing an abnormal growth pattern. See Chapter 2 for more information on assessment of growth.

Muscle Development

The rate of muscle growth and development increases rapidly beginning at age 2 years. Early muscle growth is balanced by a normal decrease in adipose tissue in early childhood.[2] The growth and maturation of the muscles continues along with the ossification of the

skeletal system (Fig. 18.5). *Muscle tone* is the state of normal tension of the muscles, and term infants normally have strong muscle tone at birth. Abnormalities in muscle tone in an infant may be noted shortly after birth when an infant is floppy. Less than normal muscle tone is described as *hypotonia;* rigidity or increased muscle tone is known as *hypertonia;* and *spasticity* is resistance to the range of motion of the muscles, including flexion and extension. Musculoskeletal terminology is presented in Box 18.1. Normal muscle function requires the normal function of the *lower motor neurons* (LMNs) in the spinal cord and the normal reflexivity of the muscle fibers. Normal muscle tone requires the normal function of the spinal

BOX 18.1	MUSCULOSKELETAL TERMINOLOGY
Distal	Away from a reference point
Proximal	Near a reference point
Medial	Toward the midline or median plane
Lateral	Farther from the midline or median plane
Anterior (ventral)	Near the front
Posterior (dorsal)	Near the back
Supine/supination	Lying on back facing upward, palmar surface facing upward
Prone/pronation	Lying face downward/palmar surface facing downward
Flexion	A decrease in the angle of the resting joint in the upper or lower extremities
Extension	An increase in the joint angle
Hyperextension	An increase in the angle of the joint beyond the usual arc
Plantarflexion	Extension of the foot/ankle downward
Dorsiflexion	Flexion of the foot/ankle upward
Abduction	Movement away from the midline
Adduction	Movement toward the midline
Rotation	Movement around a central axis
Circumduction	Rotation or circular movement of the limbs
Inversion	Turning inward/movement toward the body
Eversion	Turning outward/movement away from body
Varus	Toward midline of body
Valgus	Away from midline of body

cord stretch reflex and the balance of the *upper motor neurons* (UMNs) and LMN function. Lesions on the UMNs result in increased tone, and LMN lesions result in decreased tone.

PHYSIOLOGIC VARIATIONS

Table 18.1 presents physiologic and developmental changes in the musculoskeletal system from the newborn through adolescence.

SYSTEM-SPECIFIC HISTORY

Obtaining a complete history or a symptom-related history of the musculoskeletal system is key to accurate assessment in children and adolescents. The Information Gathering table reviews the pertinent areas for each age group and developmental stage of childhood.

PHYSICAL ASSESSMENT

Preparation for the Examination

For a thorough and complete assessment of the musculoskeletal system, infants must be undressed except for the diaper, and children must be dressed in clothing that allows visualization and examination of the spine, upper, and lower extremities such as shorts or a gown to provide modesty. The skeletal positions, planes of the body, and movements are presented in Fig. 18.6.

Inspection and Palpation

Initial inspection of the musculoskeletal system in the child from birth to adolescence begins with inspection of skin for color and

TABLE 18.1	PHYSIOLOGIC VARIATIONS OF THE MUSCULOSKELETAL SYSTEM AT KEY DEVELOPMENTAL STAGES
Age Group	**Variation**
Preterm infant and newborn	Lower extremities in external rotation and flexion at hips; upper femur is anteverted and knees are flexed; tibias are internally rotated; ankles are dorsiflexed
Infancy	Internally rotated tibias gradually begin to rotate externally toward midline by 12 months of age; flat feet (common due to flexibility and presence of fat pad) and bowed legs until walking is firmly established
Early childhood	Stance with wide base of support, hyperflexion of hips and knees with disjointed (toddling) pattern when walking; arms held abducted and elbows extended; intoeing is common; normal arm swing and heel-toe walking generally begin by 18 months of age; longitudinal arch not present in infant but begins to develop by 2.5 years of age. At 3 years of age, children exhibit mature pattern of motion and muscle action; resolution of intoeing and marked torsion of lower extremities often disappear by school entry
Middle childhood	*Genu valgum* may be present until 7 years of age; adult alignment typically achieved by 8–10 years of age
Adolescence	Hormonal changes impact ligaments and tendons; laxity of knees is particularly common in adolescent females, making them vulnerable to injury

INFORMATION GATHERING FOR ASSESSMENT OF THE MUSCULOSKELETAL SYSTEM AT KEY DEVELOPMENTAL STAGES

Age Group	Questions to Ask
Preterm infant	History of lack of oxygen (hypoxia) in early neonatal period? Any history of bleeding in the brain, seizures, or injuries to the brain (intraventricular insult)? Need for resuscitation or ventilation in immediate newborn period? Presentation at birth? Breech or shoulder injury at birth? Time spent in the neonatal intensive care unit (NICU)? Any history of exposure to prenatal substance use? When did prenatal care begin?
Newborn	History of exposure to prenatal chronic health conditions or infection? Any trauma sustained at birth? Need for resuscitation or ventilation in immediate newborn period? Presentation at birth? Breech or shoulder injury at birth? Time spent in the NICU; why? Family history of skeletal deformities or genetic disorders? Getting vitamin D supplement if breastfeeding?
Infancy and First Year	Family history of bone or joint disorders? Getting vitamin D supplement if breastfeeding? Any delay in achieving gross motor milestones? Does infant roll over? Sit without support? Crawl? Stand alone? Walk without support? Does the child tend to walk on their toes?
Early childhood	Any delay in achieving gross motor milestones? Do you think your child is clumsier or falls more often than other young children? Is the child's gait normal? Is there a family history of feet turning in or out when walking? Family history of bone or joint disorders?
Middle childhood	Involved in organized/competitive sports? Any pain that awakens child at night? Any pain that impedes activity? Any complaint of pain when walking/running? History of joint stiffness or swelling? Any complaint of back pain? Does the child carry a heavy backpack? Is there a good ergonomic desk set up at home? History of prolonged steroid use with chronic conditions?

INFORMATION GATHERING FOR ASSESSMENT OF THE MUSCULOSKELETAL SYSTEM AT KEY DEVELOPMENTAL STAGES —CONT'D

Age Group	Questions to Ask
Adolescence	Involved in organized/competitive sports? Single sport or multi-sport involvement? Involved in the same sport year-round? Any limited range of motion of joints? History of fractures, sprains, or trauma? Any complaint of back pain? Is posture normal when standing? Does adolescent carry a heavy backpack? Is there a good ergonomic desk set up at home? Family history of skeletal deformities? Start of menstrual periods? Regular menstrual periods?
Environmental risks	Contact with chemical cleaning agents, hazardous smoke, or chemicals? Exposure to toxic pesticides? History of elevated lead level?

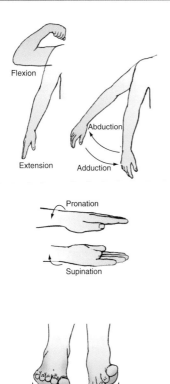

FIGURE 18.6 Skeletal positions.

temperature and noting of scars, unusual pigmentation or lesions, swelling, and any bruising. Erythema, swelling, tenderness, or temperature changes should also be noted over the joints. Bruising is the most common sign of physical abuse and intentional injury in children. Bruising over bony prominences such as the shins, knees, and forehead are common in children and usually the result of active play. However, bruising seen on the buttocks, neck, face, and earlobes should be considered suspect and require further information gathering and assessment for signs of abuse (Fig. 18.7).[4]

Observation of posture when standing and sitting, assessing the proportion of upper extremities to lower extremities, and noting any obvious gait abnormalities are all part of a complete musculoskeletal assessment. Palpation for bone or joint tenderness, and any unusual prominence, thickening, and/or indentations in the bony skeleton should be noted. Muscle tone, muscle strength, and symmetry should be evaluated. Assessment of the mobility of the spine and range of motion of the joints and extremities are included in a thorough and complete assessment of the musculoskeletal system.

Joints

Joints in the body have a slightly moveable to freely moveable motion throughout the period of growth and development. Types of joints include hinge (elbow), pivot (atlantoaxial), saddle (thumb CMC), condyloid (knee), ball and socket (hip), and plane or acromioclavicular joint (AC) (Fig. 18.8). The *hinge joint*, between the humerus and the ulna, permits motion in one plane, whereas the *pivot joint*, between the atlas and the axis in the neck, allows rotation only. *Saddle joints*, such as at the carpometacarpal joint of the thumb, form a concave-convex fit to achieve motion. The

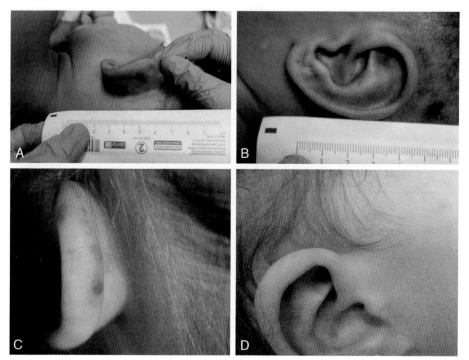

FIGURE 18.7 Facial bruising concerning for abuse. (From Zitelli BJ, et al.: *Zitelli and Davis' Atlas of Pediatric Physical Diagnosis*, ed 8, Philadelphia, 2023, Elsevier.)

condyloid joint between the femoral and tibial condyles in the knee allows flexion, extension, adduction, abduction, and circumduction. The hip and shoulder joints are examples of *ball-and-socket joints*. Finally, the *plane joints* allow a gliding motion between two flat or nearly flat surfaces, such as between the acromion process and clavicle at the shoulder, as well as between the carpal and metacarpal bones in the hand and the tarsal and metatarsal bones in the feet.

Head and Neck

Assessment of the head and neck is presented in Chapter 13 and Chapter 19. Children presenting with head and neck pain should be evaluated for *nuchal rigidity* to determine if they have pain or resistance when neck is flexed forward when lying supine. See Chapter 13 for further musculoskeletal examination techniques to evaluate head and neck pain in children.

Upper Extremities and Clavicle

In the newborn infant, the clavicles should be fully palpated to detect a possible fracture often associated with a traumatic delivery. Localized tenderness along the clavicle shortly after birth leads to a palpable bony prominence as the fracture heals. A full range of motion assessment of the upper extremities, including the elbows and wrists, must be evaluated to determine any trauma that may have affected the clavicles or shoulders during the birth process. *Erb's palsy*, injury to the fifth and sixth cranial nerves of the brachial plexus, is a form of birth-related brachial plexus injury where no spontaneous abduction of the shoulder muscles or flexion of the elbow is noted on examination (Fig. 18.9). The arm is held at the side, adducted and internally rotated, often with the elbow extended and forearm pronated, with the wrist and fingers in flexion.[3] Normal grip in the hand is present.

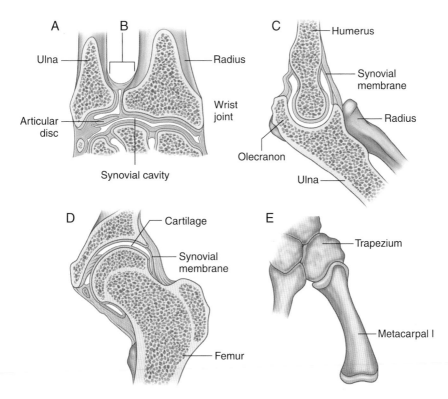

FIGURE 18.8 Skeletal joints. **(A)** Condylar (wrist). **(B)** Gliding (radio-ulnar). **(C)** Hinge (elbow). **(D)** Ball and socket (hip). **(E)** Saddle (carpometacarpal of thumb). (From Drake R, Vogl AW, Mitchell A: *Gray's Anatomy for Students*, ed 4, Philadelphia, 2020, Elsevier.)

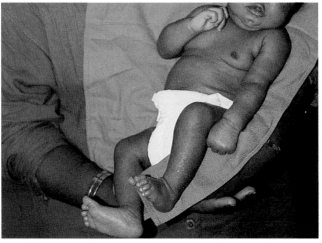

FIGURE 18.9 Erb's palsy. (From Hockenberry MJ, Wilson D: *Wong's Nursing Care of Infants and Children*, ed 10, St. Louis, 2015, Mosby.)

Range of motion should be passively evaluated in infants and young children and assessed actively when children are cooperative with examination. Any limitation of range of motion in joints and extremities or asymmetrical response should be further investigated. Muscle tone and strength should also be evaluated. Laxity of the ligaments in the young child is expected but can predispose them to injury. In early childhood, the proximal radial-ulnar joint is particularly vulnerable. *Subluxation*, or partial dislocation, of the radial head from the capitellum of the distal humerus is referred to as *nursemaid's elbow*. A nursemaid's elbow is painful, as the *annular ligament* becomes partially trapped in between the radius and capitellum and is common in children from 1 to 4 years of age. Often there is no clear history of trauma, but there may be a history of traction injury in which the arms were stretched with the elbow in a straight position such as when a child is being pulled upward or being held by the hand and suddenly falls. A nursemaid's elbow is not sustained during a fall. In cases of a radial head subluxation, the child usually refuses to use the affected arm, holding it with the elbow slightly flexed and forearm pronated.[3] There are simple maneuvers to reduce the radial head subluxation in the outpatient setting, and the child should be pain free within minutes without further need for follow-up.

EVIDENCE-BASED PRACTICE TIP

Supination-flexion technique to reduce radial head subluxation: Hold the child's arm at 90 degrees of flexion with the forearm fully supinated. While applying pressure with the thumb over the radial head, maximally flex the elbow. There may be a click with reduction of the radial head.

Hyperpronation technique: Hold the child's arm at 90 degrees of flexion. Quickly hyperpronate the forearm followed by flexion of the elbow.

Trauma to the upper extremities is common in children and adolescents. Strains, sprains, or fractures can occur with physical activity, falls, motor vehicle or pedestrian injuries, or participation in competitive sports. In children, the bone is weaker than the surrounding soft tissue structures due to the presence of the open growth plate as well as the plasticity of the maturing bone; therefore, fractures are more common than sprains in children. The converse is true as the body approaches skeletal maturity in adolescents and adults. Careful assessment is warranted in the growing child when any history of trauma is obtained. Fractures that are highly suggestive of intentional injury or abuse in children are rib fractures, especially posterior rib fractures, scapular fractures, sternal fractures, fractures of the spinous processes, and metaphyseal lesions.[4] Clavicular fractures and long bone fractures in children older than 1 year of age are common traumatic injuries of childhood, though a high index of suspicion should be maintained especially for nonambulatory children with femur fractures.

Lower Extremities and Feet

Lower extremity range of motion can be assessed at the hip, knee, ankle, and foot while lying supine and/or seated. Muscle tone, muscle strength, and symmetry should be evaluated with the child standing and while observing gait. Leg length is difficult to reliably measure until the child is able to stand with knees extended. With the child standing, the examiner places their fingers on top of the iliac crests (hip bones) while seated or standing behind the child and assesses the symmetry in height of the iliac crests. The clinician may attempt to measure leg lengths on a younger child with them lying supine with hips in neutral extension, knees fully extended, and by using a measuring tape from the anterior superior iliac spine (a bony protrusion at the anterior aspect of the hip) to the medial malleolus of the distal tibia. A discrepancy in length or asymmetrical appearance may indicate an abnormality in hips, long bones, or knees. In infants, leg length discrepancy may indicate developmental hip dislocation. At any age, a length discrepancy or asymmetry in thigh circumference could suggest the possibility of a syndromic diagnosis. Abnormal leg length should be referred to pediatric orthopedics for further evaluation.

Evaluate the shape of the foot. The heel-toe bisector, a vertical line that crosses along the plantar aspect of the foot from the midpoint of the heel through the toes, should cross between the second and third toe webspace. Many neonates and infants have *metatarsus adductus*, which is a flexible kidney bean appearance to the foot (Fig. 18.10). There is adduction of the forefoot with normal hindfoot alignment at the back of the foot with a curved lateral border. In metatarsus adductus, the heel-toe bisector crosses lateral to the second and third toe webspace. This is common, thought to be secondary to intrauterine positioning. A foot that is rigid on manipulation and range of motion requires further evaluation (Fig. 18.11). A mild deformity with a flexible foot may benefit from passive stretching, which consists of supporting the heel dorsiflexed at a right angle to the shin and stretching the forefoot laterally to a straight position. This often resolves as the child grows without intervention, usually by age 4. Metatarsus adductus is the most common cause of intoeing in the younger child.

Assessment of the feet in the infant includes the position and alignment of the forefoot and heels and the range of motion of the ankle and plantar arch. Limited dorsiflexion, or a fixed position of the hindfoot in an equinus (plantar-flexed) position, is abnormal in the newborn. When coupled with a rigid adduction of the

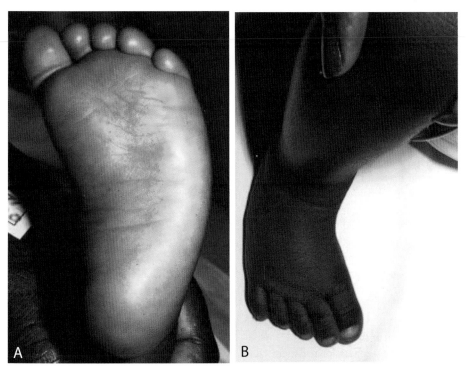

FIGURE 18.10 Metatarsus varus (adduction of the forefoot). **(A)** Ventral view. **(B)** Dorsal view. (From Graham JR & Sanchez-Lara PA: *Smith's Recognizable Patterns of Human Deformation*, ed 4, Philadelphia, 2016, Elsevier.)

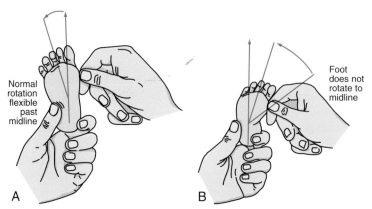

FIGURE 18.11 Examination of the forefoot. **(A)** Typical rotation of foot. **(B)** Fixed position of forefoot.

forefoot, this could be diagnostic of *clubfoot.* Decreased range of motion or pain should be noted on exam and referred for further evaluation. Many clubfoot deformities are initially observed on prenatal ultrasound and require treatment after birth by a pediatric orthopedic specialist.

Infants and toddlers do not develop a longitudinal arch in the foot until the second or third year of life secondary to age-appropriate flexibility. Studies have shown that children have lower arch heights, on average, than adults. These arch heights often increase spontaneously during the first decade of life.[3] Lack of development of a longitudinal arch in the young child may indicate a generalized laxity of the ligaments or flat foot, *pes planus.* Pes planus is often hereditary, and use of orthotics is indicated only if the child is symptomatic. It is important to note that orthotics do not change the natural position of the foot, and they do not result in the formation of an arch; orthotics simply support the arch while the child's foot is in the shoe.[3] Examine the feet with the child standing erect and on tiptoe to determine the longitudinal arch of the foot (Fig. 18.12). Older children may have physiologic flat feet due to laxity of the ligaments with rapid growth, which is a normal variant and may improve with age. Referral may be warranted if the arch

is not evident while the child is standing on their tiptoes, as this could indicate a connection between bones (a fibrous or bony *coalition*) that could cause pain or lead to recurrent ankle injuries.

Inspect the lower leg for evidence of *tibial torsion,* a curving or twisting of the tibia either inward or outward. With the child lying supine in shorts, the examiner should ensure the patella is facing straight upwards to the ceiling, rotating the leg to position it appropriately. The angle at which the toes point (when straight up toward the ceiling is considered 0, or neutral) determines the degree of tibial torsion. Alternatively, the child may be positioned lying prone, and the examiner may evaluate the thigh-foot axis by observing the angle made between a vertical line down the posterior thigh and a vertical line down the center of the plantar aspect of the foot (Fig. 18.13). Internal tibial torsion is the most common cause of intoeing in early childhood. There is an average of 5 degrees internal tibial rotation in infants, whereas the tibia rotates to 10 degrees external by 8 years of age.[3] Thus, internal tibial torsion generally resolves with growth and is common until 4 or 5 years of age. Therefore, reassuring the parent is an important component of anticipatory guidance. The tibia does not rotate significantly after 12 years of age.[3]

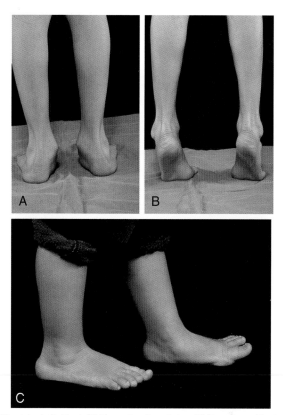

FIGURE 18.12 **(A)** Physiologic flat feet. **(B)** Normal arch on tiptoe. **(C)** Pes planus (flat foot). (From Chaudhry B, Harvey D: *Mosby's Color Atlas and Text of Pediatrics and Child Health*, St. Louis, 2001, Mosby.)

As the child grows, the long bones of the lower extremity continue to rotate. The rotation of the femur is secondary to intrauterine positioning, even years later. Internal rotation of the femur, *femoral anteversion*, is the most common cause of intoeing as children reach kindergarten age. Children with femoral anteversion may want to "W sit" as this position is more comfortable for their alignment (Fig. 18.14). The rotation of the femur should be assessed with the child in shorts, prone on the table. The examiner flexes the knees to 90 degrees and then internally rotates the thigh from the hip, allowing the lower legs to relax outward (off the table). This is compared to the external rotation at the hip, assessed by externally rotating the thigh and allowing the lower legs to relax inward (on the table). A child with femoral anteversion has greater internal than external rotation of the thigh from the hip. Similar to tibial torsion, femoral anteversion often corrects spontaneously by around age 10. Anteversion at the femoral neck decreases from (on average) 30 degrees at birth to 20 degrees by 10 years of age.[3]

Next, inspect the alignment of the legs with the child standing. Standing behind the young child, observe the child walk while wearing only a diaper or underwear. Intrauterine positioning may be a contributing factor to the degree of bowleggedness or *genu varum* in the infant and young child. At birth, the infant typically has significant torsion in the lower extremities. *Genu varum* is a normal condition until 2 years

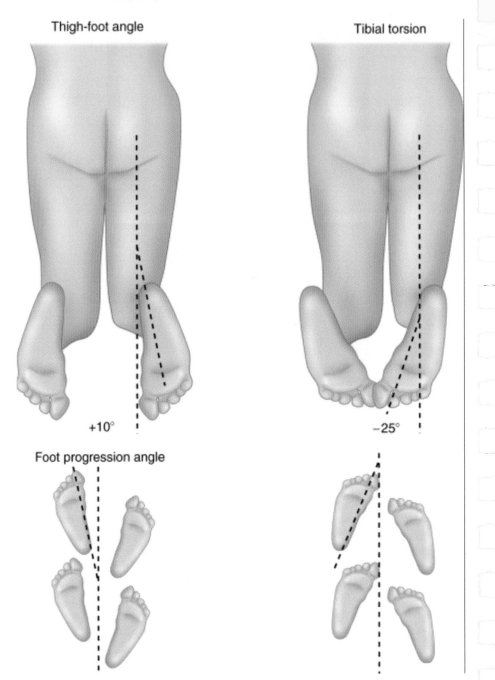

FIGURE 18.13 Assessment of tibial torsion while lying prone. (From Graham JR, Sanchez-Lara PA: *Smith's Recognizable Patterns of Human Deformation*, ed 4, Philadelphia, 2016, Elsevier.)

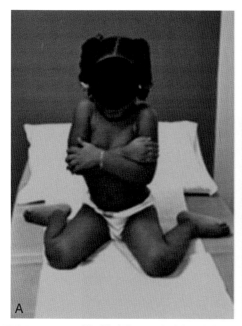
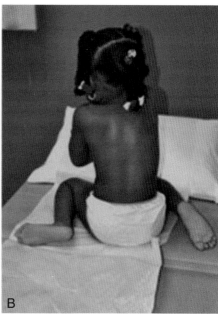

FIGURE 18.14 The W-sitting or television-sitting position with the legs externally rotated. (From Harris, E: The intoeing child. *Clin Podiatr Med Surg* 30(4):531–565, 2013).

of age (Fig. 18.15) and typically resolves with growth.[3] In certain cases, such as poor nutrition, genu varum can be pathologic in early childhood. Genu varum or bowing after 2 years of age that is severe can be the result of nutritional deficiencies or obesity in young children and may require further evaluation.

Genu valgum, or knock-knee, should be evaluated with the child standing and is present if the medial malleoli of the ankles are more than 8 cm apart when the knees are touching. Genu valgum is most common between 3 and 5 years of age and can be normal until 7 years of age. It often resolves in middle childhood with the rotational development of the lower extremities (Fig. 18.16).[3] Persistence of genu valgum may be familial or the result of childhood obesity, skeletal dysplasia, or previous unilateral injury. If persistent, genu valgum could require further evaluation and referral.

Gower sign is a screening test for muscle weakness in children and is an early sign of a neuromuscular abnormality often associated with *Duchenne muscular dystrophy*. Ask the child to stand from a sitting position on the ground. The child with muscle weakness will move from a seated position to standing by using their hands to climb up the legs and hips to push the trunk up until they are erect. A child with good muscle strength will rise to a standing position without using the arms for leverage.[5]

Hip

The examination of the hip in the newborn and growing infant is performed with the infant in the supine position with the knees flexed bilaterally and supported by the thumb and index or middle finger of the examiner, with the pad of the index or middle finger on the bony prominence of the greater trochanter and the thumb near the lesser trochanter. It is best to have the diaper open when examining the hips. Fully abduct the thighs to the examining table to evaluate for symmetry. Decreased abduction on one (or both) sides is concerning for potential

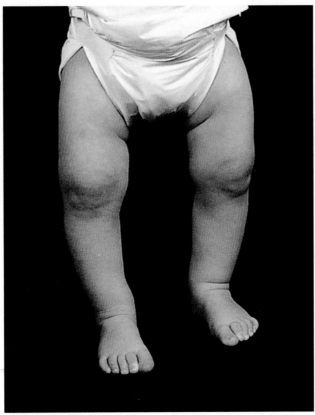

FIGURE 18.15 Physiologic genu varum (bowleggedness). (From Zitelli BJ, et al.: *Zitelli and Davis' Atlas of Pediatric Physical Diagnosis*, ed 8, Philadelphia, 2023, Elsevier.)

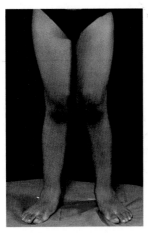

FIGURE 18.16 Genu valgum (knock-knee). (From Chaudhry B, Harvey D: *Mosby's Color Atlas and Text of Pediatric and Child Health*, St. Louis, 2001, Mosby.)

hip dysplasia. Next, again abduct the thighs gently—one at a time—while applying gentle upward/forward pressure to the greater trochanter with the middle finger (Fig. 18.17A).[3] This exam, the *Ortolani* maneuver, may elicit a palpable clunk that signifies a dislocated hip reducing over the posterior lip into the acetabulum of the hip. Therefore, an Ortolani positive hip is a dislocated hip at rest and is considered unstable. After performing the Ortolani maneuver, the examiner should then adduct the thighs—one at a time—while applying gentle backward and outward pressure with the thumb on the inner side of the thigh while the infant is supine with hips flexed. This maneuver is known as the *Barlow* test (Fig. 18.17B). A positive *Barlow* sign would again result in a

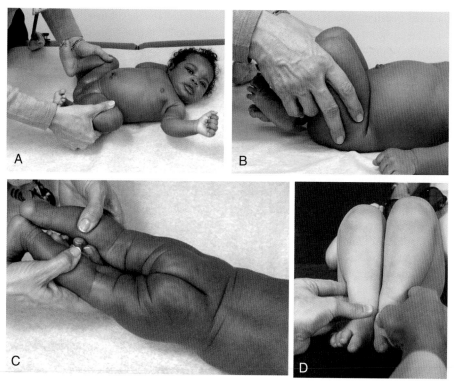

FIGURE 18.17 **(A)** Ortolani sign. **(B)** Barlow sign. **(C)** Inspecting thigh folds. **(D)** Galeazzi sign. ([D] From Azar FM & Beaty JH: *Campbell's Operative Orthopaedics*, ed 14, Philadelphia, 2021, Elsevier.)

palpable clunk, this time signifying the femoral head slipping out, or dislocating posteriorly, over the posterior lip of the acetabulum.[3] A Barlow positive hip is also considered unstable, indicating that the hip is located at rest but is able to be dislocated. Ortolani and Barlow tests become negative by about 3 months of age due to increased adductor and/or flexor muscle strength and contractures, so they are most useful in the neonatal period.[3] A click can occur during the maneuvers that may radiate from the knee and is often associated with crepitus of the joint, which is a normal finding. With the infant prone, inspect for the symmetry of the thigh folds (Fig. 18.17C). Asymmetry should be noted, but it is not highly correlated with hip abnormality. *Galeazzi* or *Allis sign* is also used to detect unequal leg length or hip dislocation. With the infant supine on the examining table, knees flexed to 90 degrees and the feet stabilized on the examining table, inspect for

symmetry of height of knees. The knees should be equally aligned. Any asymmetry of the knees is abnormal and may indicate a subluxated or dislocated hip that requires further evaluation (Fig. 18.17D). Examination of the hips is indicated until an infant is walking independently without support and gait is normal.

Developmental dysplasia of the hip (DDH) is a congenital or acquired condition involving an improper alignment of the head of the femur and the acetabulum. DDH is associated with a range of conditions. The incidence of DDH in infants remains controversial due to the changing development of the femoral head in the acetabulum. DDH is the most common hip disorder in children, affecting between 0.1% and greater than 10% of live births.[6] In infants with a positive clinical examination in the early neonatal period, DDH resolves in 60% to 80% by 2 to 8 weeks of age.[7] Major risk factors for DDH include breech positioning at any point throughout gestation, infants assigned female at birth, first-born infants, preterm infants, and infants with a positive family history of DDH. Additional risk factors include prenatal oligo-hydramnios, torticollis, lower limb deformity, and metatarsus adductus.[3]

Screening for DDH leads to earlier detection in affected infants but can lead to over-treatment. Therefore, the recommendation for routine clinical examination and screening remains controversial.[8] The American Academy of Pediatrics (AAP) recommends periodic newborn physical exam surveillance throughout infancy; universal ultrasound screening is not routinely recommended, though there is a moderate recommendation for obtaining an ultrasound for infants less than 6 months of age with one or more risk factors for DDH. There is a universal recommendation to avoid tight swaddling of infant legs, such as putting the hips in tight adduction, which increases the risk for DDH.[8] Regardless of additional risk factors, ultrasound evaluation should be performed at 6 weeks of life for any infants who were breech throughout their gestation.[8] Obtaining a routine screening ultrasound earlier than 6 weeks of life could lead to false positives due to immaturity of the hip. Ultrasound is a safe modality, so a screening exam may be performed for any infant about whom the examiner has concerns, whether they may be based on history or exam. Nine percent of all primary hip replacements and up to 29% of hip replacement in adults up to 60 years of age are related to DDH, so detecting and referring the infant with persistent misalignment of the femoral head in the acetabulum remains important to prevent premature degenerative joint disease in adulthood.[9]

Examination of the hip in middle childhood and adolescence begins with observation of the standing posture. The height of the iliac crests should be level or equal, and the child should be able to stand on one foot without any tilting of the pelvis.[8] A positive *Trendelenburg sign* is noted when the iliac crest drops on the nonstanding leg, indicating weak hip abductor muscles on the weight-bearing side. The range of motion of the hips should be evaluated with the child or adolescent in shorts, lying supine. The examiner may evaluate for asymmetry or limitation in hip flexion, abduction, and internal or external rotation. Any child with abnormal findings, pain on examination, and/or presenting with a limp should be further investigated and referred if indicated.

Among older children and adolescents, a critical diagnosis of concern is *slipped capital femoral epiphysis (SCFE)*. SCFE is a displacement of the capital or proximal femoral epiphysis from the femoral neck through the epiphyseal plate. SCFE is the most common adolescent hip disorder, estimated to affect 1/10,000 adolescents in the United States. Presenting symptoms are limp, external rotation of the affected hip and/or lower extremity, and hip, groin, or thigh pain that can radiate to the knee.[10] This commonly presents in early puberty during rapid growth. SCFE requires urgent orthopedic consultation and referral.

Knee

The knee is a common site for both overuse and injury in middle childhood and adolescence. With the child standing, note any swelling in the knee, limp, inability to bear weight, and/or pain with weight bearing. The remainder of the knee examination should be performed with the child seated and lying supine on the exam table. Inspect the knee for any obvious deformity, erythema, edema, effusion (extra joint fluid), ecchymosis, or skin breakdown. The patella should be evaluated for any abnormal tilt or alignment from the midline. The examiner should take care to observe for any evidence of effusion in the joint or *ballottement*. Effusion is an indicator of intra-articular injury and should be further evaluated. Next, palpate the landmarks of the knee. Notably, medial or lateral joint line tenderness or pain may indicate a *meniscal tear*.[11] Knee range of motion, flexion and extension, should be assessed and compared bilaterally. Hyperextension at the knee may be a sign of ligamentous laxity. Any child with a knee effusion, locked knee, inability to flex and extend the knee completely, ligamentous instability, fracture or osteochondral (bony and/or cartilage) lesion, or inability to bear weight on the affected side should be referred to orthopedics.[12]

A common complaint of adolescent athletes is anterior peripatellar pain with exercise or prolonged sitting and pain or buckling when ascending or descending the stairs. Pain may be elicited on exam; however, findings may also be relatively normal. Patellofemoral pain syndrome affects 30% of adolescents and often presents as complaints of anterior knee pain aggravated by ascending or descending stairs, running, jumping, squatting, or occasionally after prolonged sitting.[12]

Sudden traumatic injury of the knee in the young athlete is unfortunately common and requires imaging as well as specialty examination techniques. Box 18.2 presents the physical examination of the knee and assists with decision-making regarding the need for imaging and referral. The knee maneuvers should be performed bilaterally beginning with the non-injured knee with the child or adolescent lying supine on the examining table. Some variation in the flexibility and laxity of the joints is within normal. Acute injuries can be treated with RICES: rest, ice, compression, elevation, and stabilization.[12]

Spine

The spine should be inspected and palpated in infancy to note any congenital abnormalities, such as hair tufts, dimples, a sacral sinus, or hemangiomas, as these could indicate spinal abnormalities. Young children develop a normal curvature of the spine with *lordosis* of the neck and lumbar region and *kyphosis* of the thorax. An exaggerated lumbar lordosis is normal in the young child. Inspection of the spine in the child and adolescent begins with the examiner behind the standing child. Assess for the contour of the back, the symmetry of the shoulders, the symmetry and/or

---

BOX 18.2 EXAMINATION OF THE KNEE

All knee examination techniques should be compared for symmetry with the contralateral knee, noninjured knee tested first. Some individuals have more laxity than others; therefore, what may feel to be excessive movement may actually be typical for the child, rather than a positive test.

Lachman Test
- To assess anterior cruciate ligament (ACL), knee should be flexed 20–30 degrees with child or adolescent lying supine; stabilize the lower thigh/femur with one hand while pulling the upper tibia anteriorly with the dominant hand[30]; feel resistance at firm endpoint and note how far tibial tubercle moves anteriorly compared with the unaffected knee (See Fig. 18.22).
- **Positive finding:** Increased movement compared to the other knee with abnormal "soft" endpoint. Increased movement of tibial tubercle anteriorly or forward from neutral position suggests possible ACL injury and need for referral.

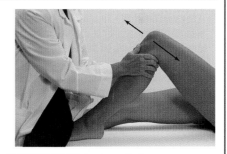

FIGURE 18.22 Lachman test

Anterior/Posterior Drawer Test
- To assess the ACL and posterior cruciate ligament (PCL) for injury, hips should be flexed to 45 degrees and knees flexed to 90 degrees with child or adolescent lying supine; foot should be stabilized on exam table in neutral position with examiner sitting on the child's foot. The examiner grasps the upper (proximal) tibia with both hands, both thumbs on the joint line, and

---

Continued

BOX 18.2   EXAMINATION OF THE KNEE—CONT'D

pulls the tibia forward (anterior drawer) and then pushes backward (posterior drawer). Thumbs on joint line aid to better assess the displacement of the tibia.[13] (See Fig. 18.23.)

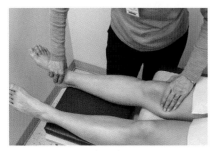

FIGURE 18.23 Anterior drawer test

- **Positive finding:** Excessive movement of tibia anteriorly from neutral position or lack of firm endpoint suggests ACL insufficiency. Excessive posterior tibial sag suggests PCL insufficiency. Significant laxity on exam suggests injury of ACL or PCL.

Varus/Valgus Stress Test
- To assess the stability of medial collateral ligament (MCL) and lateral collateral ligament (LCL), with the child lying supine, leg should be extended. The examiner uses one hand to elevate the extended leg off the table at the ankle. Apply valgus stress at the lateral knee with the other hand to evaluate the LCL and then varus stress at the medial knee to assess the MCL. Then repeat the same process again, with the knee flexed to 30 degrees (Fig. 18.24).

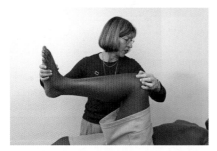

FIGURE 18.24 Varus/valgus stress test with knee extended

- Note: For valgus stress, push on the lateral knee, stabilizing at medial malleolus. For the varus test, push on medial knee while stabilizing lateral malleolus.
- **Positive finding:** Lateral knee pain or excessive varus movement of tibia indicates injury to LCL. Medial knee pain or increased valgus movement with lack of a firm endpoint indicates injury to MCL. Laxity or opening in the joint space suggests tear of MCL or LCL.

McMurray Test
- Assess the medial and lateral meniscus with child lying supine, flex knee to 90 degrees, and hold the knee at the medial and lateral joint lines with thumb and forefinger with one hand (see Fig. 18.25). Using other hand to hold the foot, place the knee into valgus external rotation and gradually extend the leg from the knee to assess for medial meniscus injury. Repeat while placing the knee into varus and internal rotation to assess for lateral meniscus injury.[13]
- **Positive finding:** Any click or pain.

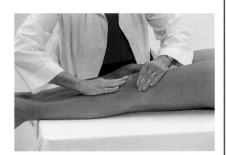

FIGURE 18.25 McMurray test

Ballottement of Patella Test
- With child lying supine and knee fully extended, examiner squeezes suprapatellar pouch to push fluid underneath patella; then push the patella downward against the femur with index finger of contralateral hand[13]).
- **Positive finding:** A feeling of the patella "floating" in the effusion.

Data from Abdelgawad A, Genrich CM: Sport injury: Lower extremity. In: Abdelgawad A, Naga O, Abdou M, eds. *Pediatric Orthopedics and Sports Medicine*. Cham: Springer; 2021.

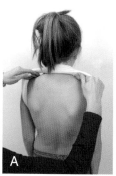
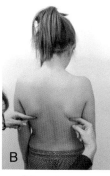
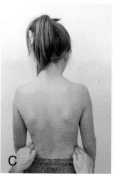
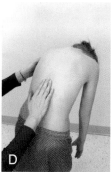

FIGURE 18.18 Assessment of the spine. **(A)** Testing shoulder symmetry. **(B)** Scapular symmetry. **(C)** Iliac crest symmetry. **(D)** Beginning Adams forward bend test.

prominence/shape of the scapula and ribs, and the symmetry of the waistline and the iliac crests (Fig. 18.18A–C). The head should be aligned directly over the sacrum; any deviation from the midline may indicate scoliosis or another spinal deformity. Next, viewing the child or adolescent standing from the side allows the examiner to evaluate normal sagittal alignment (kyphosis, lordosis). Range of motion of the spine is evaluated by asking the child or adolescent to bend forward (flexion), backward (hyperextension), to the side (lateral bending), and bilateral rotation. The *Adams forward bend test* begins with the child or adolescent standing with knees straight and feet together. Ask the child to bend forward at the waist and to touch the toes with hands dangling or in a diving position (Fig. 18.18D). An elevated or prominent scapula, uneven iliac crests, waistline asymmetry, or the presence of a rib rise on forward bend indicates a positive finding (Fig. 18.19). A *scoliometer* can be used to assess the magnitude of trunk rotation (Fig. 18.20). Place the scoliometer on the trunk at the peak of the curvature to evaluate alignment. A rotation of 5 to 7 degrees on scoliometer correlates with a radiographic scoliosis curve of 15 to 20 degrees; therefore, scoliometer readings of 7 degrees or greater warrant further evaluation via x-ray and referral.[3] Approximately 1% to 3% of adolescents between 10 and 16 years of age have scoliosis curves of greater than 10 degrees.[14]

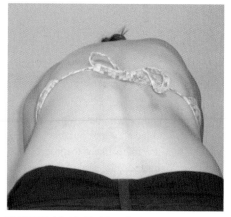

FIGURE 18.19 Positive rib rise. (From Skirven T, et al: *Rehabilitation of the Hand and Upper Extremity*, ed 7, Philadelphia, 2021, Elsevier.)

Routine screening for scoliosis remains controversial, and the U.S. Preventive Services Task Force (USPSTF) concludes that the current evidence is insufficient and that the balance of benefits and harms of screening for adolescent idiopathic scoliosis cannot be determined.[14] If scoliosis screening is undertaken, the American Academy of Orthopaedic Surgeons (AAOS), Scoliosis Research Society (SRS), Pediatric Orthopaedic Society of North America (POSNA), and AAP agree that females should be screened twice, at 10 and 12 years of age (grades 5 and 7), and boys once, at age 13 or 14 (grades 8 or 9). Adolescents who are in

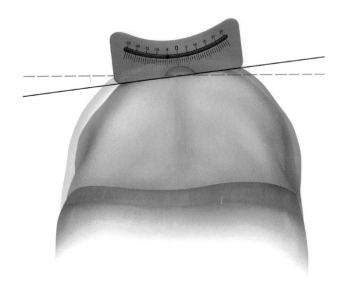

FIGURE 18.20 Scoliometer measuring inclination angle of thoracic spine. (From Horne JP, Flannery R, Usman S: Adolescent idiopathic scoliosis: diagnosis and management. *Am Fam Physician* 89:193–198, 2014.)

a period of rapid growth, have a positive family history, and have a more notable curve on presentation are more likely to progress and require imaging and referral. Evaluation of *sexual maturity rating (SMR) or Tanner stage* is key to determining skeletal and spinal maturity when diagnosing scoliosis in adolescents. When there is question of skeletal maturity, an x-ray of the hand may be obtained to assess the individual's bone age.

DIAGNOSTIC PROCEDURES

Concern remains over the relationship of frequent cumulative exposure to radiologic diagnostic procedures, particularly computed tomography (CT) scans, and later health effects including cancer in children and adults. Pediatric health care providers have continued to adhere to the policy, "As Low As Reasonably Achievable" (ALARA), and an "Image Gently" approach, in most pediatric health care settings.[15]

Ultrasound is used to evaluate soft tissue masses and to diagnose and/or monitor DDH until 4 to 6 months of age, due to incomplete ossification of the femoral heads in early infancy.[16] *X-ray* is utilized to evaluate and treat fractures as well as bony anomalies or deformities. We have seen the emergence of low-dose radiation x-ray machines over the past 15 years, which allow certain x-rays to be obtained at 45 times less than conventional x-ray.[17] *Magnetic resonance imaging* (MRI) is often used for higher anatomic detail for soft tissue or bony masses, with and/or without contrast, but may require sedation, especially for the younger child.[16] *CT scans* may be warranted to understand more complex fracture patterns and may be utilized by the specialist to determine whether surgical intervention is indicated. *Bone age* radiographs of the secondary ossification centers at the end of the long bones are used to assess growth rate in children who lag behind in height velocity compared with the norm or who have delayed onset of puberty. A skeletal series of radiographs is indicated to detect occult fractures when serious physical abuse is suspected, or to evaluate further when a suspicious fracture is identified, especially in children under 2 years of age.[4] A

CT *scanogram* or x-ray orthoroentgenogram is often used to diagnose and evaluate unequal leg length in childhood, though the low-dose x-ray machines discussed above are able to perform the same imaging with less radiation exposure.[17]

PREPARTICIPATION SPORTS PHYSICAL

Preparticipation Sports History

The primary purpose of the preparticipation sports physical exam is to promote the health and safety of athletes during training and competition.[18] It can also be used to screen for injuries and illness. The *preparticipation physical evaluation (PPE)* may be the healthy adolescent's only contact with a pediatric health care provider during an important period of physical and psychosocial growth and development.

Therefore, the PPE should incorporate routine health maintenance and confidential psychosocial screening, especially if incorporated into a well-child or well-adolescent exam. It is important to evaluate any risks related to sports participation and use the encounter as an opportunity for anticipatory guidance and encouraging positive health behaviors.[18] There is, however, no standard requirement for PPE prior to athletic participation and no standard interval between examinations.[18]

The PPE is also an opportunity for the pediatric health care provider to evaluate risky health practices related to participation in sports, particularly unhealthy weight loss or weight gain (Box 18.3). Sports such as wrestling, boxing, and martial arts are graded by weight class, which creates significant pressure on the young athlete to maximize body strength and bulk. There are also powerful

---

BOX 18.3 FOCUSED HISTORY FOR PREPARTICIPATION PHYSICAL EVALUATION FOR THE MIDDLE CHILDHOOD AND ADOLESCENCE

CURRENT MEDICAL HISTORY	PAST MEDICAL HISTORY	FAMILY HISTORY	DIETARY HISTORY
• Sport youth intends to play, including position and weight class if relevant • Any medications used by the youth, including diet supplements, creatine, anabolic steroids and their analogs, *macrolide* antibiotics, *tricyclic* antidepressants, *neuroleptics* • Any chronic illnesses, including asthma, how well controlled, and any exacerbations during exercise	• Any previous experience in the same or other sports • Any history of previous injuries, especially injuries requiring exclusion for >1 week • Any history of shortness of breath, syncope, or chest pain during exertion • History of seizures, including type, frequency, controlling medication, and past complications • *As appropriate:* Age of menarche, regularity of menses, and any prior disturbances of menses during sports	• Family history of cerebrovascular accident (CVA) or myocardial infarction (MI) before age 50 years • Any family history of sudden, unexplained death in adolescent or young adult relative • Family history of hypertrophic cardiomyopathy (HCM), prolonged QT syndrome, Marfan syndrome, or other cardiac/circulatory abnormalities	• Are you happy with current weight? Want to gain or lose for sport? • Fruits/vegetables daily? Milk or calcium intake? • Fluids for hydration (water, sports drinks, sodas, caffeine intake)? • Supplements, medications for weight loss, weight gain, muscle gain?

pressures on dancers, distance runners, and gymnasts to maintain a low weight. By contrast, youth playing positions such as linebacker in football may want to increase weight gain, even if their body mass index (BMI) is greater than the 95th percentile for age. Information gathering during the PPE should include satisfaction with or concerns about weight and body image. Athletes should also be questioned about such practices as severe food restriction, binging or purging, weight loss, or muscle-enhancing supplements, including medications containing *ephedra, creatine*, and anabolic steroids or their analogs. Tables 18.2 and 18.3 present a review of systems and medical conditions related to participation in competitive sports.

To perform the PPE, the young athlete should be examined in clothing that allows visualization and examination of the spine, upper, and lower extremities such as shorts or a gown to provide modesty. Appropriate clothing should allow a thorough assessment of the joints and muscles. A 13-step orthopedic exam is included in the PPE to assess the athlete's musculoskeletal health (Fig. 18.21). The components of the 13-point orthopedic examination are as follows:[18]

1. With the athlete standing, facing toward examiner, assess for symmetry of trunk, shoulders, and extremities.
2. Assess neck forward flexion, extension, lateral flexion side to side, and rotation to evaluate range of motion of cervical spine.
3. Assess trapezius strength by having the young athlete shrug shoulders against resistance from the practitioner.
4. Assess deltoid strength by having the young athlete abduct the shoulders against resistance from the practitioner.
5. Assess internal and external rotation of shoulder to evaluate range of motion of the glenohumeral joints.

TABLE 18.2	REVIEW OF SYSTEMS FOR PREPARTICIPATION PHYSICAL EVALUATION FOR MIDDLE CHILDHOOD AND ADOLESCENCE
System	**Disorders**
Head, eyes, ears, nose, and throat (HEENT)	Use of corrective lenses? Visual difficulties? Otitis externa, frequent otitis media (OM), allergic rhinitis, hearing difficulties?
Respiratory	Shortness of breath (SOB), wheezing with exercise, chronic cough?
Cardiovascular	SOB, chest pain, dizziness, syncope with exertion, palpitations with exertion?
Gastrointestinal	Pain or reflux with exercise? Current/chronic problems with diarrhea, constipation?
Genitourinary	*(As appropriate)* History or symptoms of hernias, lumps or masses in groin or testicles? Menstrual history (menarche, length, regularity of cycles, missed cycles during sports)? Last menstrual period (LMP)?
Musculoskeletal	Instability of any joints (especially shoulder, knee, ankle)? Any pain with exercise? Swelling of joints? Any weakness?
Neurologic	Headaches, dizziness, seizures, history of concussions, recent injuries, weakness, difficulties with sleep, cognitive function, emotional regulation, balance, or gait?
Dermatologic	*Lesions:* Recent history of herpes, fungal infections, bacterial infections? Sunscreen protection? Eczema, reaction of skin to perspiration or athletic equipment?

TABLE 18.3	MEDICAL CONDITIONS AND LEVEL OF SPORTS PARTICIPATION

Condition	Level of Sports Participation and Rationale
Bleeding disorder	Qualified yes[a]
Cardiovascular disease	No
Carditis (inflammation of the heart)	May result in sudden death with exertion
Hypertension (high blood pressure)	Qualified yes[a] Qualified yes[a] Those with mild forms may participate fully; those with moderate or severe forms or those who have undergone surgery need further evaluation
Congenital heart disease (structural heart defects present at birth)	
Dysrhythmia (irregular heart rhythm)	Qualified yes[a] Those with symptoms (chest pain, syncope, dizziness, shortness of breath) or evidence of mitral valve regurgitation (leaking) needs further evaluation; all others may participate fully
Heart murmur	Qualified yes[a] If innocent, full participation is permitted; otherwise, the athlete needs further evaluation
Cerebral palsy	Qualified yes[a]
Diabetes mellitus	Yes Blood glucose concentration should be monitored every 30 min during continuous exercise and 15 min after completion of exercise
Diarrhea	Qualified no[a] Unless mild, no participation is permitted, may increase risk of dehydration
Eating disorders	
Anorexia nervosa	Qualified yes[a]
Bulimia nervosa	Qualified yes[a]
Fever	No Increases cardiopulmonary effort, reduces maximum exercise capacity, makes heat illness more likely, and increases orthostatic hypertension during exercise
Hepatitis/HIV	Yes All sports may be played that athlete's state of health allows; skin lesions should be covered properly, and universal precautions used when handling blood or body fluids with visible blood
Musculoskeletal disorders	Qualified yes[a]
Neurologic disorders	Qualified yes[a]
History of serious head or spine trauma, severe or repeated concussions, or craniotomy	Research supports conservative approach to management of concussion, with cognitive rest and gradual step-return to play only when asymptomatic. Athletes with multiple concussions may need an extended time away from sports

Continued

TABLE 18.3	MEDICAL CONDITIONS AND LEVEL OF SPORTS PARTICIPATION—CONT'D

Condition	Level of Sports Participation and Rationale
Seizure disorder	
Well controlled	Yes
Poorly controlled	Risk of seizure during participation is minimal
	Qualified yes[a]
	Archery, riflery, swimming, weight or power lifting, strength training, or sports involving heights should be avoided because occurrence of a seizure may pose risk to self or others
Obesity	Qualified yes[a]
Organ transplant recipient	Qualified yes[a]
Respiratory conditions	
Pulmonary compromise, including cystic fibrosis	Qualified yes[a]
Asthma	Yes
Acute upper respiratory infection	Only most severe asthma requires modified participation
	Qualified yes[a]
	Individual assessment required for all but mild disease
Sickle cell disease or trait	Qualified yes[a]
	Carefully condition, acclimatize, and hydrate to reduce any possible risk
Skin disorders	Qualified yes[a]
Boils, herpes simplex, impetigo, scabies, molluscum contagiosum	While contagious, participation in gymnastics with mats; martial arts; wrestling; or other collision, contact, or limited-contact sports is not allowed

[a]Patient needs evaluation for sports clearance.

HIV, Human immunodeficiency virus.

Adapted from Rice SG: Medical conditions affecting sports participation, *Pediatrics* 121(4):841–848, 2008 and McCrory P, Meeuwisse W, Dvorak J, et al.: Consensus statement on concussion in sport – the 5th international conference on concussion in sport held in Berlin, October 2016, *Br J Sports Med* 51:838–847, 2017.

6. Assess range of motion of the elbows by having young athlete perform flexion and extension of the elbows.

7. Assess range of motion of the elbows and wrists by observing pronation and supination of the forearm or wrist.

8. Assess range of motion of the hands and fingers by having the young athlete clench the fist and spread the fingers.

9. Assess symmetry of the posterior body, trunk, and extremities with the young athlete standing, facing away from examiner.

10. Have the young athlete stand with knees straight and then flex forward and bend backward (hyperextending the spine) to assess any discomfort of the lumbar spine that could indicate spondylolysis or spondylolisthesis.

11. Perform Adam's forward bend test by having the young athlete bend forward and touch the toes, if possible, with hands dangling. Assess for rib rise or asymmetry for potential spinal curvature as well as thoracic and lumbosacral spine range of motion and hamstring flexibility.

12. To assess for symmetry of leg musculature, have the young athlete stand facing the practitioner with quadriceps flexed.

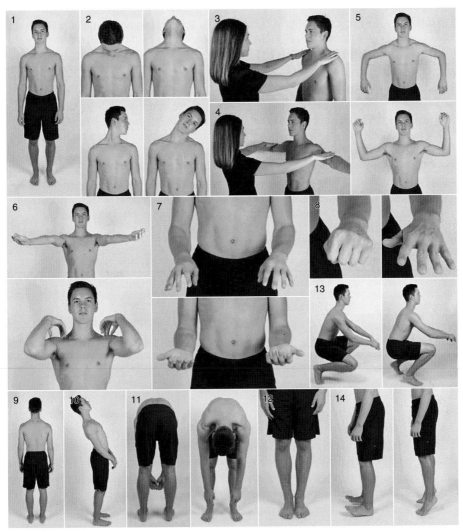

FIGURE 18.21 (From Miller SM, Peterson AR: The sports preparticipation evaluation. Pediatr Rev 40(3):108–128, 2019.)

13. Assess calf strength, symmetry, and balance by having the young athlete stand on heels and then toes.

Cardiac Preparticipation Physical Evaluation

Though the PPE looks at the whole child or adolescent, an important focus is placed on the cardiac portion of the history and exam. Sudden cardiac arrest or death (SCA/SCD) is rare among athletes (estimated 1.25 per 100,000 high school athletes per year), but cardiovascular disorders are the leading cause of sudden death in young athletes during exertion.[18] Therefore, the PPE aims to identify athletes that may be at greater risk for SCD by gathering a detailed personal history and family history to identify asymptomatic young athletes with underlying cardiac disease (Box 18.4).[19]

In regard to personal health history, the American Heart Association (AHA) recommends eliciting any history of exertional chest pain or discomfort, unexplained syncope or near

---

BOX 18.4 AMERICAN HEART ASSOCIATION RECOMMENDATIONS FOR PREPARTICIPATION CARDIOVASCULAR SCREENING OF COMPETITIVE ATHLETES

Personal History
1. Exertional chest pain/discomfort
2. Unexplained syncope/near-syncope[a]
3. Excessive exertional or unexplained dyspnea/fatigue, associated with exercise
4. Prior recognition of a heart murmur
5. Elevated systemic blood pressure

Family History
6. Premature death (sudden and unexpected, or otherwise) before age 50 years due to heart disease, in ≥1 relative
7. Disability from heart disease in a close relative <50 years of age

8. Specific knowledge of certain cardiac conditions in family members: hypertrophic or dilated cardiomyopathy, long QT syndrome or other ion channelopathies, Marfan syndrome, or clinically important arrhythmias

Physical Examination
9. Heart murmur[b]
10. Femoral pulses to exclude aortic coarctation
11. Physical stigmata of Marfan syndrome
12. Brachial artery blood pressure (sitting position)[c]

[a] Judged not to be neurocardiogenic (vasovagal); of particular concern when related to exertion.
[b] Auscultation should be performed in both supine and standing positions (or with Valsalva maneuver), specifically to identify murmurs of dynamic left ventricular outflow tract obstruction.
[c] Preferably taken in both arms.
Parental verification is recommended for high school and middle school athletes.
Adapted from Maron BJ, Friedman RA, Kligfield P, et al.: Assessment of the 12-lead ECG as a screening test for detection of cardiovascular disease in healthy general populations of young people (12-25 years of age): a scientific statement from the American Heart Association and the American College of Cardiology, *Circulation* 130(15):1303–1334, 2014.

---

syncope, excessive exertional or unexplained dyspnea/fatigue associated with exercise, prior recognition of a heart murmur, or elevated systemic BP.[18] Family history questions should include: premature death before age 50 years caused by heart disease in one or more relative, disability from heart disease in a close relative younger than 50 years, and specific knowledge of family members with cardiac conditions known to cause SCD in athletes.[18]

Physical exam consists of auscultation for heart murmurs, palpation of femoral pulses, examination for the physical stigmata of Marfan syndrome, and a brachial artery BP taken while the individual is seated.[18]

In young athletes, *hypertrophic cardiomyopathy*, a cardiovascular condition caused by an asymmetrical left ventricular hypertrophy and a nondilated left ventricle with impaired diastolic function, is the leading cause of SCD.[20] In general, no evidence of cardiac disease is present before SCD. Other cardiac conditions implicated in SCD include anomalous coronary arteries, Marfan syndrome, prolonged QT interval, and cardiac dysrhythmias. The use of screening tests such as electrocardiography (ECG) or echocardiography is a topic of debate, and therefore not recommended routinely by the AHA during the PPE.[18] With any concerning findings, the athlete may benefit from referral to pediatric cardiology for further evaluation and clearance for sports participation.

SPORTS INJURIES

Sports injuries can be classified as traumatic (*macrotrauma*), usually from collision or contact sports, such as basketball, football, or soccer, or as overuse (*microtrauma*). Athletes are at risk for repetitive motion and overuse injuries to the shoulder, knee, elbow, or shin (tibia). When gathering history about sports injuries in young athlete, the pediatric health care provider should assess the level of participation in recreational play versus competitive sports to guide whether decision-making related to returning to play is indicated. Young athletes should also be screened for history of previous concussion (see Chapter 19), fractures, and ligament damage.

A young athlete's Tanner stage/SMR is also relevant to injury and the mechanism for injury. Rapid growth during adolescence results in decreased strength at the growth plates and greater strength in ligaments compared to bones, leading to greater potential for fractures relative to older adolescents and adults.[21] Rapidly growing athletes with relatively good muscle strength yet incomplete ossification of the growth plate are predisposed to physeal (growth plate) fractures. Because injuries may recur from season to season, young athletes with a history of repetitive injuries such as frequent ankle sprain might benefit from further evaluation by pediatric orthopedics. They may benefit from physical therapy or could be given strengthening exercises at the time of the PPE to help prevent future injury. Early sports specialization may lead to overuse injuries, and cross-training in young athletes is recommended.[22] For most adolescents, the physical and social benefits of carefully monitored sports participation outweigh the risks, including adolescents with chronic health conditions and special health care needs.

PEDIATRIC PEARLS

Ligaments are stronger than bones until adolescence; therefore, injuries to long bones and joints in the preadolescent are more likely to cause fractures (some of which may not be easily visible on x-ray, whether nondisplaced or through the cartilaginous physis) rather than sprains.[3]

Evaluation of sports-related concussions and recommendations for return to play are presented in Chapter 19.

Relative Energy Deficiency in Sports

When assessing adolescent athletes, an in-depth history should include assessment for *Relative Energy Deficiency in Sports* (RED-S). Whether by decreased caloric intake and/or excessive energy expenditure, RED-S is a syndrome that can disrupt a number of different body systems, including reproductive, bone, endocrine, metabolic, hematologic, growth and development, physiological, cardiovascular, gastrointestinal, and immunological.[23] As a result of an energy deficit, the body goes into a state of stress, activating the HPA and autonomic nervous system; this occurs to save energy for vital functions.

In individuals assigned female at birth, decreased energy availability secondary to over exercise and/or insufficient intake can cause menstrual disturbances, causing a negative influence on GnRH with resultant FSH/LH changes and lower estradiol and progesterone. In individuals assigned male, there may be a decrease in testosterone.[24] RED-S also causes changes in bone metabolism, largely by effects of energy deficiency on estrogen, IGF-1, leptin, and T3. Higher risk for fracture and impaired healing can result. Decreased bone mineral density and decreased bone strength may occur especially in individuals assigned female. Other changes observed with RED-S may include a decreased resting metabolic rate, iron deficiency, increased growth hormone resistance, lipid elevations, lower resting heart rate and/or blood pressure, decreased immune system function, and mental health challenges. Poor performance in sports may also be a result of RED-S.[24]

History may include questions about nutrition, dietary changes, food security, exercise frequency/duration/intensity, sleep hygiene, stress, menstrual cycle regularity (where appropriate), and traumatic or stress fractures. Treatment for RED-S is multimodal and may involve an interdisciplinary team of mental health professionals, dietitians, coaches, physical therapists, and clinicians.

MUSCULOSKELETAL CONDITIONS

Table 18.4 presents the most common abnormal orthopedic conditions seen in infants, children, and adolescents by the pediatric health care provider.

TELEHEALTH TIPS

Many orthopedic visits may occur via telehealth using video with a parent or guardian present. Some of these visits include gait evaluation for younger children, initial orthopedic evaluations, or injury follow-ups. If indicated during the visit, x-rays can be ordered during the visit and

TABLE 18.4	MUSCULOSKELETAL CONDITIONS
Condition	Description
Clubfoot (congenital talipes equinovarus)	• Rigid congenital equinovarus position of the foot consisting of muscle contractures and bony deformity • Treatment is casting, possible Achilles tendon release, and bracing
Talipes calcaneovalgus	• Eversion and dorsiflexion of hindfoot, an intrauterine positioning "packaging problem" • Treatment is stretching and possibly casting
Metatarsus adductus	• Increased adduction abnormality of forefoot at the tarsometatarsal junction, an intrauterine "packaging problem" • Ankle and hindfoot are normal • Lateral border of foot is curved rather than straight, usually shaped like a "kidney bean" • Line drawn medially from heel often intersects third toe or more lateral; no treatment versus stretching or casting
Torticollis	• Persistent head tilt due to abnormal sternocleidomastoid muscle contraction • Treatment is stretching and referral as indicated
Pes planus/planovalgus (flat feet)	• Flattening of longitudinal arch in school-age child when standing erect with full weight bearing on feet bilaterally with or without a valgus hindfoot and forefoot abduction • Often related to ligamentous laxity • Flat feet are developmentally normal until 3 years of age and often are accentuated by a fat pad on ventral surface of foot • Arch heights often increase during second decade of life; no treatment necessary if asymptomatic • Orthotics provide support if symptomatic but do not change development or position of foot
Tibial torsion, internal or external	• Inward or outward twisting of tibia, often a variation of normal rotational development, an intrauterine "packaging problem" • Internal tibial torsion is the most common cause of intoeing children <3 years of age • Resolves with normal growth (tibia twists from 5 degrees inward to 10 degrees outward by 8 years of age), observation recommended with surgical intervention rarely indicated only for older children with persistent deformity, braces/straps/special shoes do not change natural history • Continued reassurance to parent is important
Femoral anteversion	• Increased internal rotation of the femur due to anteversion of the femoral neck relative to the femur, an intrauterine "packaging problem" • Common cause of intoeing between 3 and 6 years of age • Resolution usually occurs by 11 years of age (femoral neck anteversion decreases from 30 degrees at birth to 20 degrees at 10 years of age), observation recommended with surgical intervention rarely indicated only for older children with persistent deformity, braces/straps/special shoes do not change natural history • Continued reassurance to parent is important
Genu varum	• Normal physiologic bowed leg appearance in children less than 2 years of age; • Observation recommended with surgical intervention indicated only for older children with persistent deformity, braces/straps/special shoes do not change natural history
Blount's disease (tibia vara)	• Progressive abnormal ossification of the proximal tibia leading to pathologic genu varum in children 2–5 years old • Treatment is bracing versus surgery

TABLE 18.4   MUSCULOSKELETAL CONDITIONS—CONT'D

Condition	Description
Genu valgum	• Normal physiologic knock-knee appearance in children between 3 and 7 years of age • Observation recommended with surgical intervention indicated only for older children with persistent deformity, braces/straps/special shoes do not change natural history
Developmental dysplasia of the hip (DDH)	• Abnormal hip development resulting in a spectrum of acetabulum dysplasia and hip subluxation, possible dislocation secondary to capsular laxity and mechanical instability • Risk factors include breech positioning in utero, female infant, first born, positive family history for DDH, prematurity, maternal oligohydramnios • Screening recommended via ultrasound < 4 months and x-ray > 4 months of age with risk factors and/or positive Barlow/Ortolani/Galeazzi exams and/or limited abduction • Treatment may include observation versus abduction bracing versus surgery
Slipped capital femoral epiphysis (SCFE)	• Displacement of the capital or proximal femoral epiphysis from the femoral neck through the physeal plate • Presenting symptoms are limp, external rotation of the affected hip and/or lower extremity, and hip, groin, or thigh pain that can radiate to the knee • Common presentation in early puberty during rapid growth period • Requires urgent orthopedic consultation and referral
Legg-Calvé-Perthes	• Blood supply to femoral capital epiphysis is disturbed and produces avascular necrosis of femoral head; affects children 3–12 years of age, with peak incidence from 4–8 years of age • Children may have history of intermittent painless limp and present with or without diffuse pain in hip, knee, or upper thigh • On examination, child has limited abduction and internal rotation of affected hip • Treatment is observation with activity restrictions under 8 years of age, surgical intervention over 8 years of age
Toxic, or transient, synovitis (commonly at the hip)	• Inflammation of the synovium at the hip often after a recent URI or viral illness • Often presents in children 3–10 years old as hip, groin, or thigh pain with or without refusal to weight bear • Diagnosis of exclusion, may require labs (including WBC/CRP/ESR) to rule out septic arthritis • Referral as indicated
Osteomyelitis	• Infection within bone with or without abscess • Most commonly secondary to spread of bacteria from skin lesion, local trauma, or infection with subsequent bacteremia • Presents as limp or refusal to bear weight, with or without fever, edema/erythema/warmth in the area, mean age 6–7 years old • Evaluated with x-ray, labs, and referral as indicated
Septic arthritis (of the hip or knee most common)	• Intra-articular infection that affects younger children in the first few years of life that causes articular surface damage and bony destruction • May be caused by trauma/surgery, hematogenous spread of infection, extension from adjacent bone infection • Presents with acute pain, fever/systemic symptoms, limp or refusal to bear weight, significant pain with passive hip motion • Diagnosed with labs, vital signs, imaging, immediate referral as indicated • Requires emergent irrigation and debridement

Continued

TABLE 18.4	MUSCULOSKELETAL CONDITIONS—CONT'D

Condition	Description
Osgood-Schlatter syndrome	• Overuse type inflammation, pain, bony bump formation at the tibial tubercle due to traction stress from the patellar tendon that inserts distally at the tibial tubercle secondary growth center • Presents with activity-related pain that is relieved with rest and NSAIDs, also commonly a bony bump (enlarged tibial tubercle) that is tender to palpation • Common finding in adolescent athletes with peak occurrence from 8–15 years of age, waxes and wanes until growth center closes between 14–18 years of age
Sinding-Lars-en-Johansson syndrome	• Overuse type pain, inflammation at the secondary growth center at the inferior pole of the patella due to traction stress where the patella tendon attaches proximally • Presents with activity-related pain around the inferior patellar pole that is relieved with rest and NSAIDs • Common finding in adolescents, waxes and wanes until growth center closes
Sever's apophysitis	• Overuse type pain, inflammation at the secondary growth center of the calcaneus due to traction stress from the Achilles tendon that inserts in the area • Presents as activity-related pain at the posterior calcaneus • Common finding in younger adolescents, waxes and wanes until growth center closes; may benefit from stretching/physical therapy • May consider heel cups or orthotics
Osteogenesis imperfecta	• An inherited connective tissue disorder and deficiency of type I collagen but has multiple phenotypes resulting in brittleness of bones characterized by spontaneous fractures, and short, bowed extremities • Associated with scoliosis, bluish sclera, and hearing loss
Marfan syndrome	• Inherited connective tissue disorder characterized by excess linear growth of the long bones and hypermobility of joints, arachnodactyly (long/slender fingers/toes), pectus deformities, hindfoot valgus, longer extremities in proportion to trunk • May be associated with serious cardiac manifestations (increased risk of aortic enlargement and mitral valve prolapse)

obtained afterward. Alternatively, the child could be referred to an orthopedic specialist or even the emergency department for urgent concerns.

First, a thorough history should be obtained from the child or adolescent and their parent. The child or adolescent should be dressed in shorts so that the examiner is able to see the area of concern. The child's parent or guardian or adolescent can manipulate the camera so the examiner is able to get a full view of the area of concern. The child or their parent may palpate landmarks for tenderness with the examiner's direction. The child may demonstrate range of motion of the joint as directed by the examiner. For gait concerns or lower extremity pain, the visit should take place in a hallway in the home that will enable the child or adolescent to walk, jog, and hop.

There are times when an evaluation on telehealth may indicate the need for a follow-up visit in person or at the emergency department. If there are findings that require a physical examination to determine the treatment plan (such as special maneuvers to evaluate for particular injury or pathologic process), these should be done in a follow-up in-person evaluation. If findings suggest an injury that requires immobilization with a splint or cast, these should be referred to an orthopedic specialist or the emergency department. Additionally, if there is concern for an urgent pathologic process such as infection or open fracture, this should be referred urgently to an orthopedic specialist or emergency department.

SUMMARY OF EXAMINATION

- Nutritional factors, such as adequate protein in the diet, the amount of calcium intake daily, and adequate intake of vitamin D, which regulates the absorption of calcium and phosphorus in the intestines, impact bone growth.
- Growth along the epiphyseal plate (physis) continues until the cells in the growth plate mature and stop dividing in puberty, and closure of the growth plate occurs in young adulthood.
- Evaluating progression of the height growth curve is critical to assessing normal and abnormal growth patterns, along with familial patterns of growth and pubertal development.
- Note any obvious gait abnormalities; observe posture when standing and sitting; assess proportion of upper extremities to lower extremities. Standing behind the child, or adolescent, observe their walk to evaluate alignment variations of genu varum and genu valgum.
- Assess for torsional variations throughout childhood: metatarsus adductus, tibial torsion, and femoral anteversion, which are typical developmental findings and rarely require referral, though require significant family reassurance.
- Evaluate range of motion of joints and assess muscle tone of trunk and extremities.
- Evaluation of the lower extremities includes assessment of flexion/extension, adduction/abduction, and internal/external rotation.
- Assessment of the hip in the young infant is performed in supine position with the knees flexed bilaterally and thumb and middle finger of examiner on the bony prominence of greater trochanter. Ortolani sign tests for a dislocated hip at rest and Barlow maneuver evaluates for a hip that is aligned at rest but is dislocatable. Galeazzi test may help to identify a dislocated hip.
- Knee assessment maneuvers should be performed bilaterally beginning with the noninjured knee. Some variation in the flexibility and laxity of knee joints is normal.
- Assess for contour of back, symmetry of shoulders, shape and/or prominence of scapula and ribs, and symmetry of iliac crests.
- Observe for alignment of spine with child or adolescent in forward bend position. Note any curvature, asymmetry, or rib rise from the rear, front, and sides of the back. A scoliometer may be used, as indicated, to quantify spinal rotation.
- To perform the PPE, a 13-step orthopedic exam is included to assess the athlete's musculoskeletal health.
- The AHA recommends the PPE include (1) auscultation for heart murmurs; (2) palpation of femoral pulses; (3) evaluation for Marfan syndrome; and (4) blood pressure evaluation.
- Many orthopedic visits may occur via telehealth with a parent or guardian present including gait evaluation for younger children, initial orthopedic evaluations, or injury follow-ups. Refer to an orthopedic specialist or emergency department for urgent concerns when indicated.

DOCUMENTATION

A Healthy Young Child

Extremities and Back: Spine straight with mildly exaggerated lumbar lordosis. Full active spine ROM (range of motion) with flexion/hyperextension/bilateral bending/bilateral rotation. Mild internal tibial torsion with thigh-foot axis 15 degrees internal, and intoeing bilaterally R > L with foot progression angle 5–10 degrees internal.

DOCUMENTATION

14-year-old PPE

Extremities and Back: Spine straight while standing. No significant asymmetry/rotation on Adams forward bend. Full active ROM (range of motion) and strength throughout upper and lower extremity joints bilaterally. 13 pt. exam WNL.

REFERENCES

1. Yang T, Grover M, Joeng KS, Lee B. Human fetal and neonatal bone development. In: Bilezikian JP, Bouillon R, Clemens T, eds. *Primer on the Metabolic Bone Diseases and Disorders of Mineral Metabolism.* 9th ed. Wiley-Blackwell; 2018.

2. Norris TL. *Porth's Essentials of Pathophysiology.* Fifth edition. Philadelphia: Wolters Kluwer; 2020.

3. Weinstein S, Flynn J, Crawford H, eds. *Lovell and Winter's Pediatric Orthopaedics.* 8th ed. Philadelphia: Wolters Kluwer Health/Lippincott Williams & Wilkins; 2021.

4. Horner G. Medical evaluation for child physical abuse: What PNP needs to know. *J Pediatr Health Care.* 2012;26: 163–170.

5. Ball JW, Dains JE, Flynn JA, Solomon BS, Stewart RW. *Seidel's Guide to Physical Examination.* 10th ed. St. Louis: Elsevier; 2023.

6. Young J, Anderson M, O'Connor C, Kazley J, Mantica A, Dutt V. Team approach: Developmental dysplasia of the hip. *JBJS Reviews.* 2020;8e20.00030–e20.00030.

7. U.S. Preventative Service Task Force Screening for developmental dysplasia of the hip: a metanalysis. *Pediatrics.* 2006; 117:898–902.

8. Yang S, Zusman N, Lieberman E, Goldstein R. Developmental dysplasia of the hip. *Pediatrics.* 2019;143:e20181147.

9. Pun S. Hip dysplasia in the young adult caused by residual childhood and adolescent-onset dysplasia. *Curr Rev Musculoskelet Med.* 2016;9:427–434.

10. Skaggs DL, Flynn JM, Kocher MD, Noonan KJ, Vitale MG. *Staying Out of Trouble in Pediatric Orthopedics.* 2nd ed. Philadelphia: Wolters Kluwer; 2021.

11. Yen YM. Assessment and treatment of knee pain in the child and adolescent athlete. *Pediatr Clin North Am.* 2014;61: 1155–1173.

12. Crowther MJ, Duffaut CJ. General management of pediatric knee injuries. In: Coleman N, ed. *Common Pediatric Knee Injuries.* Cham: Springer; 2021.

13. Abdelgawad A, Genrich CM. Sport injury: Lower extremity. In: Abdelgawad A, Naga O, Abdou M, eds. *Pediatric Orthopedics and Sports Medicine.* Cham: Springer; 2021.

14. U.S. Preventive Services Task Force (USPSTF) Final recommendation statement: Adolescent idiopathic scoliosis: Screening. *JAMA.* 2018;319:165–172.

15. Tomà P, Bartoloni A, Salerno S, et al. Protecting sensitive patient groups from imaging using ionizing radiation: effects during pregnancy, in fetal life and childhood. *Radiol Med.* 2019;124:736–744.

16. Piccolo CL, Galluzzo M, Ianniello S, et al. Pediatric musculoskeletal injuries: role of ultrasound and magnetic resonance imaging. *Musculoskelet Surg.* 2017;101(Suppl 1): 85–102.

17. Melhem E, Assi A, El Rachkidi R, et al. EOS® biplanar X-ray imaging: Concept, developments, benefits, and limitations. *J Child Orthop.* 2016;10:1–14.

18. American Academy of Family Physicians, American Academy of Pediatrics, American College of Sports Medicine, American Medical Society for Sports Medicine, American Orthopaedic Society for Sports Medicine, American Osteopathic Academy of Sports Medicine. *Preparticipation Physical Evaluation.* 5th Ed. American Academy of Pediatrics Publishing Staff; 2019.

19. Maron BJ, Friedman RA, Kligfield P, et al. Assessment of the 12-lead ECG as a screening test for detection of cardiovascular disease in healthy general populations of young people (12-25 years of age): A scientific statement from the American Heart Association and the American College of Cardiology. *Circulation.* 2014;130:1303–1334.

20. Schmied C, Borjesson M. Sudden cardiac death in athletes. *J Intern Med.* 2014;275:93–103.

21. Browne GJ, Barnett P. Common sports-related musculoskeletal injuries presenting to the emergency department. *J Pediatr Child Health.* 2016;52:231–236.

22. Jayanthi N, Schley S, Cumming SP, Myer GD, Saffel H, Hartwig T, Gabbett TJ. Developmental training model for the sport specialized youth athlete: A dynamic strategy for individualizing load-response during maturation. *Sports Health.* 2022;14:142–153.

23. Coelho AR, Cardoso G, Brito ME, Gomes IN, Cascais MJ. The female athlete triad/relative energy deficiency in sports (RED-S). *Rev Bras Ginecol Obstet.* 2021;43:395–402.

24. Mountjoy M, Sundgot-Borgen JK, Burke LM, et al. IOC consensus statement on relative energy deficiency in sport (RED-S): 2018 update. *Br J Sports Med.* 2018;52:687–697.

CHAPTER 19

HEAD AND NEUROLOGICAL SYSTEM

Bridget Ward Gramkowski

The nervous system provides the vital motor, sensory, and cognitive functions that sustain human life and comprise human behavior. It is important for the pediatric provider to remember that beyond all the cellular and structural entities that influence neurologic health and normative expectations for attainment of milestones, lies the essential experience of the child in their world. Social determinants of health (SDH),[1] including influences of the child's housing, neighborhood, schools, and community, powerfully shape neurologic development from fetal origins to beyond adolescence. Assessment of neurological health must be done holistically and includes evaluation of the child's environment in addition to their physical function. Clinicians can harness this assessment to maximize a child's development and detect opportunities for caregiver support.[2]

EMBRYOLOGIC DEVELOPMENT

The head and brain begin a period of rapid growth during the third to fifth week of embryonic life. By the eighth week, the embryo is humanlike in form, although the disproportionate head size constitutes 50% of the body length. Head growth then slows between the 9th and 12th weeks of fetal development, while spine growth accelerates. During the 13th week, ossification of the cranium begins in the skull, one of the primary ossification centers of the skeletal system. As the bones of the cranium grow medially from the ossification centers, sutures form at the junctions of the calvaria or skullcap, and *fontanels* form at the intersection of the sutures. During the second and third trimesters of fetal growth, head size becomes proportional to the body.[3,4]

Between the 9th and 12th week of fetal development, hair follicles first appear with facial lanugo on the eyebrows, upper lip, and chin. The hair patterns on the scalp develop during the 13th through 16th week, and the scalp hair present in the term infant is established by the 20th week of gestation. Hair patterns are unchanged from birth to death, and differences in hair whorl (direction of hairs on the scalp around an axis) placement and number are associated with neurologic differences and genetic syndromes.[5–7]

Nervous system formation develops from the ectoderm layer as a thickened layer or "neural plate" of poorly differentiated cells in a 14-day-old embryo. In a rapid series of closures, the "neural tube" is formed by the 26th day of embryonic development. The end of the neural tube is a group of cells that come from both the ectoderm and mesoderm "caudal cell mass" where the cauda equina, sacrum, filum terminale, and conus medullaris form. Errors in this region result in tethered cord, sacral pits, and other sacral tracks. During the fifth week of fetal development, the anterior portion of the neural tube enlarges to form the segments of the cerebral hemispheres, and axons migrate to link these hemispheres forming the corpus callosum. Within the brain itself, regions develop that will further grow into specialized brain structures. These include: *rhombencephalon* (hindbrain), *mesencephalon* (midbrain), and *prosencephalon* (forebrain). Brain growth is rapid throughout the first and second trimester of gestation. By the 18th gestational week, the fetal brain can be imaged using in vivo magnetic resonance imaging (MRI).[3,4]

The *neuron* is the basic unit of the nervous system, and each neuron contains numerous dendrites and one axon. Dendrites are the protoplasmic branches of the cell body. Neural impulses enter the cell body through the dendrites and leave through the single axon. They then connect by a series of synapses with another dendrite of the next axon. At the synaptic junction, neurons also release specific neurotransmitters (such as GABA, glutamate, acetylcholine, norepinephrine, dopamine, serotonin, and histamine) that regulate brain and body functions. *Myelin*, a lipoid material surrounding cell fibers, covers the axons and allows for rapid and smooth transmission of nerve impulses. However, only a portion of the axons contain myelin at birth. By 24 weeks of gestation, the fetus has developed most of the nerve cells, or neurons, needed for the formation of the neural pathways.[3,4]

DEVELOPMENTAL VARIATIONS

Head

Normal skull growth depends on placental function, genetics, growth potential within the uterus, and optimum nutrition during pregnancy and early childhood (Fig. 19.1). Insufficient vitamin D supplementation during pregnancy and insufficient intake in early infancy are associated with an increased risk of skull deformity in first year of life.[8] The contour of the cranium of the newborn reflects fetal positioning and the effects of the delivery presentation. The cranial bones are pliable and are loosely connected by the sutures and the *fontanels*, which allow the head to be molded during delivery (Fig. 19.2). Depressed skull fractures are rare, but they can occur with forceps delivery or vacuum-assisted vaginal

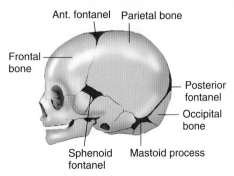

FIGURE 19.1 Anatomy of the skull in the newborn.

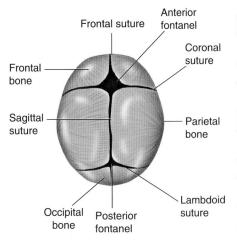

FIGURE 19.2 Fontanels and sutures.

births. If intrauterine growth retardation does occur as a result of either intrinsic or extrinsic factors in fetal growth, skull growth and brain development are impacted and result in long-term consequences of delayed growth and development in the infant.[8]

Head and neurologic growth are closely linked. Head circumference (HC) increases sixfold in the first year of life and is the best proxy measure of normal brain growth. Early detection of *microcephaly* and *macrocephaly* in infants will lead to improved treatment outcomes. The American Academy of Pediatrics (AAP) and World Health Organization (WHO) recommend HC measurements at every well-child visit through the age of 2 years. HC is significantly correlated with academic performance; for example, lower school performance has been correlated with *microcephaly*, and improved reading scores with larger head sizes.[7,9–11]

Several developmental variations in facial features can point to genetic differences requiring additional clinical attention. *Cleft lip*, with or without cleft palate, is the most common facial finding, occurring in about 1 in every 700 births. The causes of cleft lip or palate are multifactorial, including syndromic differences in 3% to 4% of those affected. *Micrognathia* (small mandible and receding chin) is associated with a range of chromosomal differences. The formation of the orbit is composed of seven different facial bones, and *hypertelorism* (greater distance between the orbits) or *hypotelorism* (shortened distance between medial walls and between inner and outer canthal distances) are associated with many chromosomal differences.[3,4,6,7]

Neurologic System

The location of closure errors along the neural tube will lead to specific disorders, for example: anencephaly (problem with anterior closure), encephalocele (partial problem with anterior closure), and *spina bifida* or *myelomeningocele* (problem with posterior closure).[3]

Brain growth is rapid after birth and is influenced by both genetics and environmental factors. The brain's plasticity changes throughout the lifespan, correlating with developmental stages. Fifty percent of postnatal brain growth is achieved by 1 year of age. By 2 to 3 years of age, the brain is 80% of adult size.[7] Exposure to a variety of therapeutic or other substances can impact fetal neurologic development. In the case of prenatal substance use, alcohol and nicotine use has been measured to impact fetal neurologic development even more severely than drugs such as cocaine.[12] Environmental exposures to teratogens, lead, and air pollution also contribute to impaired neurologic growth; these exposures are often directly linked to the health of neighborhoods and lack of resources.[13] Changes in our climate are also exposing more children to wood smoke from forest fires, found to correlate with neurologic problems in growth and development.[14] Brain development continues to be impacted throughout the pediatric lifespan both by chemical and substance exposures, including throughout the sensitive adolescent period of neurologic maturation.

Myelination, the deposit of the protective fatty substance around the axons, continues in the brain throughout the first 2 years of life, and in the preterm infant continues into the third year of life. Myelination proceeds from head to toe (*cephalocaudally*) beginning with the spinal cord and cranial nerves and then from midline to fingertips (*proximodistally*) followed by the brainstem, corticospinal tracts, and sensory pathways. Preterm or very low birth weight (VLBW) infants may develop from toe to head, which is associated with persistent hypertonia in the lower extremities. The control of motor functions in infancy and early childhood is closely associated with the normal myelination of the nerve fibers.[7] The rapid increase in myelination in the brain in the first 2 years of life is followed by a decrease in brain growth and maturation during early childhood. The growth of gray matter in the brain continues throughout childhood into adolescence and early adulthood in a nonlinear pattern. SDH such as stress, sleep, and adequate nutrition, as well as genetic factors, affect the volume of gray matter and brain growth.[3,7]

There is now a strong understanding of the impact of chronic stress on the developing brain, such as increased activity in the amygdala (fear, vigilance) and reduced development in areas such as the hippocampus (memory).[15] These neurophysiologic changes result in increased difficulty regulating emotions, making decisions, and managing stress, which can directly impact the ability to learn and interact with others. We are still learning more about how we can protect and promote neurologic resiliency in the face of these damaging exposures.[16]

ANATOMY AND PHYSIOLOGY

Head

At birth, there are seven movable and separate skull plates, or bones, joined together by sutures that accommodate brain growth (Figs. 19.1 and 19.2). The *fontanels* are the membranous spaces between the frontal and parietal bones and the parietal and occipital bones. The *anterior fontanel* lies along the *coronal, sagittal, and frontal* or metopic sutures. The *posterior fontanel* lies at the juncture of the *sagittal* and *lambdoidal* sutures. There are smaller *fontanels* located bilaterally in the lower skull. The sphenoid fontanel is located at the lower juncture of the frontal and parietal bones superior to the ear and along the coronal suture. The mastoid fontanel is posterior to the ear at the juncture of the occipital and posterior parietal bones. The cranium is supported by the first cervical vertebra, the *atlas*, a solid vertebra, and rests on the second vertebra, the *axis*. These bones form the rotational bones of the skull. Ossification of the skull continues throughout infancy and childhood and into adulthood.[17]

The facial bones are also pliable at birth, except for the *maxilla* and the *mandible*, which are very small and underdeveloped in the newborn. The facial skeleton consists of the larger bones of the frontal area, *zygomatic processes*, maxilla, and mandible (Fig. 19.3). The two nasal plates and the *lacrimal, ethmoid*, and *sphenoid* bones comprise the smaller bones in the head. The maxillary and ethmoid sinuses are present at birth but are small, and the sphenoid and frontal sinuses develop during infancy and childhood. The muscular structure of the head is an intricate part of the underlying fascia of the cranium and neck structures. The connections between the muscular fascia and the facial orifices control facial expressions such as smiling, raising the eyebrows, and wrinkling the forehead.

Slow progression of closure of the *anterior fontanel* occurs during the first year of life. In many infants, closure of the *anterior fontanel* (Fig. 19.2) occurs by 18 months of age, and 98% to 100% are closed by 24 months of age. Head growth in the first year is not determined by the size of the fontanel but by the normal increase of the occipital-frontal circumference (OFC) of the head. *Microcephaly*, a small head for gestational age, is defined as 1 to 2 standard deviations (SD) below the norm for age and size, and *macrocephaly*, a large head for gestational age, is 1 to 2 SD *above* the norm for age and size.[7,18,19]

Cephalhematoma is a soft, fluctuating effusion of blood trapped beneath the pericranium caused by rupture of the blood vessels over the parietal area (Figs. 19.4 and 19.5). It is usually unilateral and does not cross the sagittal suture. The bleeding into the periosteum of the cranium may occur slowly and, therefore,

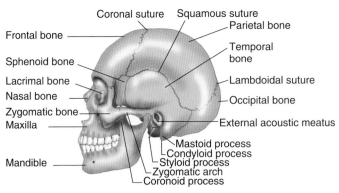

FIGURE 19.3 Facial skeleton.

may not be apparent until the infant is 24 to 48 hours old. A cephalohematoma may be a risk factor for hyperbilirubinemia due to the additional need for breakdown of blood cells. Resolution of a cephalhematoma may be slow, and it may persist until 6 weeks to 2 months of age.[3,18] See Chapter 6 for further discussion of cephalohematoma.

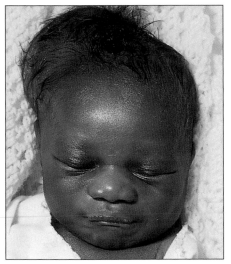

FIGURE 19.4 Cephalohematoma. (From Lissauer TM, Carroll W. *Illustrated Textbook of Paediatrics.* 6 ed. London: Elsevier Ltd.; 2022.)

CENTRAL NERVOUS SYSTEM

Cerebrum

The outermost part of the brain is the *cerebral cortex*, which is often referred to as "gray matter" because the neurons are unmyelinated. The outer layer of the brain is composed of fissures and grooves, or sulci, and the ridge between grooves is the gyrus. The newborn infant has fewer convolutional surfaces, or *sulci*, in the cerebral cortex and more pliable skull bones. The sulci of the brain deepen throughout childhood and continue to mature into young adulthood.[3,4]

The *cerebrum* is the largest part of the brain and is covered by the *cerebral cortex*. The cerebrum is divided into two hemispheres, the left and right. The right hemisphere controls the functions of the left side of the body, and the left hemisphere controls the functions of the right side of the body. Infants should use both hands equally and generally prefer to use the hand on the same side as the desired object.[6] The preference for handedness should not be observed before the age of 12 months.

The cerebral hemispheres are connected by a bridge of 190 million myelinated axons, the *corpus callosum*, which lies between the

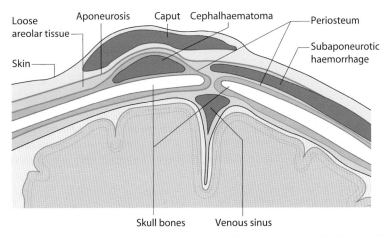

FIGURE 19.5 Location of extracranial hemorrhages. (From Lissauer TM, Carroll W. *Illustrated Textbook of Paediatrics.* 6 ed. London: Elsevier Ltd.; 2022.)

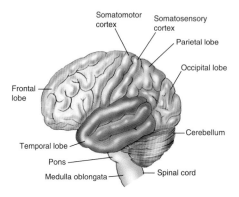

FIGURE 19.6 Regions of the cerebral cortex.

fissures of the left and right hemispheres. The corpus callosum controls and integrates motor, sensory, language, and higher intellectual functions. The right and left hemispheres are divided into four lobes—*frontal, parietal, temporal*, and *occipital*—with arbitrary borders. Each lobe controls particular bodily functions and behaviors (Fig. 19.6).[3,4]

- **Frontal lobe:** Considered the "personality center" of the brain, and is responsible for higher cognitive functions. Movement of the flexor muscles of hands and feet initiates here. The Broca area in the frontal lobe controls the ability to articulate speech. The prefrontal area controls thought processes for anticipation and prediction of behavior, and the frontal region is involved in complex learning, movement patterns, and writing. Damage to the frontal region causes *expressive aphasia*, motor weakness, or personality changes.[20]
- **Parietal lobe:** Controls processing and interpretation of sensory input—visual, auditory, smell, taste, and touch sensations, including pain and temperature; perceives where a stimulus or pressure is and on which part of the body, and provides *proprioception*, the sense of the position of the limbs of the body. It has an important role in language processing and symbol interpretation, including reading and numbers. Damage to the parietal region results

in sensory loss, spatial disorientation, or receptive language deficits like *agnosia*, an inability to recognize or perceive the meaningfulness of an object, persons, sounds, shapes, or smells.[21]

- **Temporal lobe:** Primary center for the perception and interpretation of sounds and auditory association and perception, and episodic memory; also involved in integration of taste, smell, and balance. Several critical regions are located within the temporal lobe. The *Wernicke area* is related to speech production and perception. The hippocampus is where "declarative memories" are formed—about specific occasions, times, and places – and is essential to learning. The amygdala is also located here, which is responsible for powerful emotions such as fear, in addition to sexual and eating behaviors.[22]
- **Occipital lobe:** Primary visual cortex in the brain and the center for both receiving and interpreting visual data. This includes recognition of colors, objects, faces, depth perception and, also has a role in creating memories.[23]

The *basal ganglia* are a cluster of neurons deep in the subcortical layer that process connections between the cerebral motor cortex and the upper brainstem. It has been called the "gate keeper" of initiation or inhibition of motor movements. The maturation of the basal ganglia occurs in early childhood with the development of fine motor skills and, in childhood, process movement functions such as arm swinging during walking and running and throwing a ball overhand. Dysfunction of the basal ganglia has clinical significance, often manifesting as involuntary movements ranging from tremor to tics to chorea (abrupt irregular unpredictable nonstereotyped movements). Dopamine plays an important role in basal ganglia function. Dysfunction of the basal ganglia can result in abnormal postural movement patterns as in dyskinetic *cerebral palsy* (CP), Parkinson's disease, and *Huntington's disease*.[24]

Cerebellum

The *cerebellum* is located in the posterior cranium and has been called "a neuronal learning machine"[25]; it has a critical role in a diverse array of functions. The *cerebellum* maintains the body's equilibrium and coordinates both voluntary and involuntary movements of the limbs, trunk, head, larynx, and eyes. The motor cortex in the *cerebrum* relays signals to the cerebellum, which results in precise muscle movements, requiring a high level of fine motor dexterity. It is the portion of the brain that processes sensory input from the musculoskeletal system, as well as from the visual, auditory, and touch receptors, and it transmits signals to the motor system to direct reflexes, muscle tone, posture, and balance. The *cerebellum* has many "closed-loop circuits" to various regions of the *cerebral cortex* that provide learning pathways for cognitive functions, voluntary muscle movements, emotional control, and speech. Dysfunction in these cerebro-cerebellar circuits plays an essential part in neurodevelopmental disorders, including autism spectrum disorder, attention deficit hyperactivity disorder, and developmental dyslexia. Damage to the *cerebellum* in childhood causes more significant damage than damage that is sustained in adulthood, which underscores the importance of this region in development. *Cerebellum* damage can also cause *ataxia*, loss of coordination of motor movement, inability to perform rapid alternating movements, and a wide-based gait. Abnormal development or dysfunction of the cerebellum in preterm infants can result in hypotonia, nystagmus, and language deficits.[25]

Brainstem and Cranial Nerves

The *brainstem* is also called the "primary vertebrate brain" and is found in the central core of the brain. The brainstem contains the sensory and motor tracts that connect the brain and spinal cord and is the location for most of the twelve cranial nerves. The brainstem has three divisions: the pons, medulla oblongata, and midbrain (Fig. 19.7). The *pons* acts as

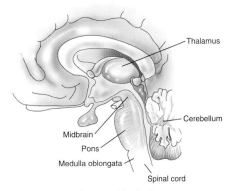

FIGURE 19.7 Brain and brainstem.

the neural transmission center from all parts of the central cortex and supports ascending and descending nerve fibers. It controls basic bodily functions—breathing, eating, and motor functions. Cranial nerve V (trigeminal nerve), cranial nerve VI (abducens nerve), and cranial nerve VII (facial nerve) arise from the pons. Dysfunction or damage of the peripheral pons is associated with a loss of outward or lateral motion of the eye muscles causing strabismus and may also cause a loss of sensory or motor function of the facial and mouth area. The medulla oblongata, which lies between the pons and the *cerebellum*, is a continuation of the spinal cord. The *medulla oblongata* processes impulses from the hypoglossal, vagal, spinal accessory, glossopharyngeal, and the vestibular and acoustic cranial nerves. It also aids in the life functions of respiration and circulation and controls involuntary reflexes such as coughing, sneezing, and yawning. Dysfunction or damage of the medulla causes weakness in the shoulder muscles, affects tongue muscles and salivary function, decreases gastrointestinal motility, alters swallowing and speech functions, causes nerve deafness, and diminishes cardiovascular and respiratory functions. The *midbrain* controls the integration of basic bodily functions and contains the neural fibers of cranial nerve III (oculomotor) and cranial nerve IV (trochlear) that come from the spinal cord and merge into the thalamus and hypothalamus. The midbrain also contains the reticular activating system that regulates wakefulness and arousability.[26]

The *diencephalon* is the extension of the brainstem and lies embedded in the cerebral cortex (Fig. 19.8). It contains the thalamus, hypothalamus, pituitary gland, and the pineal gland—an endocrine gland that produces melatonin, a hormone that regulates the sleep-wake cycle. Parts of the third ventricle and the nuclei of the cranial nerve II (optic nerve) and retina arise from the *diencephalon*.[26,27]

- **Thalamus:** Gray matter region that acts as the brain's relay station and receives input from the sensory and motor systems of the body and dispatches input from the pons and cerebellum to the cerebral cortex. It also plays a role in consciousness and alertness. Clinical conditions impacting the thalamus are rare; however, a genetic condition termed "fatal familial insomnia" impacts the thalamus causing severe insomnia that leads to death.[28]
- **Hypothalamus:** Controls and regulates the body's internal environment—body temperature, metabolic processes including appetite and weight, and involuntary response activity such as fever.[29,30]
- **Pituitary gland:** Responsible for hormonal control of growth, reproductive function, and assists in regulating thyroid gland function, lactation, and metabolism. The posterior pituitary gland produces vasopressin, which regulates the balance of water and sodium in the body.[29,30]

The *limbic system* is the group of subcortical structures in the diencephalon including the hypothalamus and hippocampus. The *hypothalamus* is the regulator of our circadian rhythms and manages the sleep-wake cycle.[30] The *hippocampus* is essential to forming new memories. This is the area of our brains that is most active when we dream.[31]

Ventricular Nervous System

The brain and spinal cord are lubricated by *cerebrospinal fluid* (CSF), which provides protection from stretching and compression forces that are typically generated by head movement. CSF regulates intracranial pressure and transports centrally acting hormones. It also excretes waste products. Taken together, the CSF is an essential element in maintaining physiology and is a key agent responding to a variety of pathologies. CSF is produced by specialized tissue called choroid plexus, which line the ventricles of the brain and spinal cord. It flows from the lateral ventricles to the third and fourth ventricles through a series of foramens. The fourth ventricle, which lies in the medulla, contains three openings that allow the cerebrospinal fluid to pass into the subarachnoid space. Approximately 500 mL of cerebrospinal fluid is produced daily in adolescents and young adults and is continually being reabsorbed in the brain. Any disruption in the circulation or absorption of CSF causes a build-up in the ventricles, resulting in hydrocephalus.[32]

The brain is covered by protective layers that cushion and lubricate the outer surface (Fig. 19.9). The *dura mater* lies just beneath

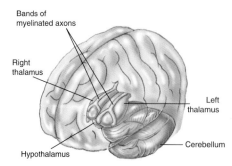

FIGURE 19.8 **The diencephalon.**

Bands of myelinated axons

Right thalamus

Left thalamus

Cerebellum

Hypothalamus

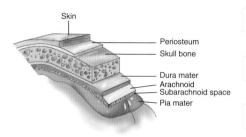

FIGURE 19.9 **The meningeal layers.**

Skin

Periosteum
Skull bone

Dura mater
Arachnoid
Subarachnoid space
Pia mater

the skull bone and periosteum and consists of layers of fibrous connective tissue. Adjacent to the dura mater is the arachnoid, the avascular, weblike membrane that cushions the cortex. The dura mater is separated from the arachnoid by the subdural space. The pia mater is the highly vascular area of the cortex that attaches directly to the gray matter or irregular surface of the brain. The subarachnoid area and a cushion of cerebrospinal fluid separate the arachnoid from the *pia mater*.[33]

Spinal Nerves

There are 31 pairs of spinal nerves that innervate the upper and lower torso, extremities, skin, and muscles—8 cervical, 12 thoracic, 5 lumbar, 5 sacral, and 1 coccygeal (Fig. 19.10). These spinal nerves form complex nerve networks called *plexuses*. There are four major plexuses in the peripheral nervous system— the cervical, brachial, lumbar, and sacral plexuses—and the body surface that is innervated by the plexus of a spinal nerve is called a *dermatome*. Although dermatomes map specific segments of the body surface, spinal nerve sensation can be transmitted to adjacent dermatomes. The sensory pathways of the spinal nerves carry sensations of touch, temperature, and pain; the motor fibers activate reflexes and impulses that control skeletal muscles and the involuntary muscles of the viscera. The spinal nerves function as part of the lower motor neurons and become dysfunctional in the presence of spinal cord lesions.[33]

Spinal Cord

The spinal cord is an extension of the medulla oblongata and is composed of gray and white matter extending to the lumbar region. The gray matter runs laterally along the spinal cord and protects the myelinated and unmyelinated fibers of the white matter. *Proprioceptors*, the specialized nerve endings in muscles, tendons, and joints, are located in the white matter and are sensitive to changes in the tension of muscles and tendons. Temperature, pain, touch, and equilibrium are transmitted through the proprioceptors to the brainstem.[33,34]

Peripheral Nervous System

The spinal nerves originate in the spinal cord and exit from the intervertebral spaces. They contain sensory and motor fibers and with the cranial nerves and visceral fibers of the autonomic nervous system compose the pathways of the peripheral nervous system. The *autonomic nervous system* carries impulses to and from the central nervous system (CNS). It is divided into the sympathetic and parasympathetic nervous systems and is made up of unmyelinated nerves. The *sympathetic nervous system* activates in times of stress and provides increased energy for needed bursts of activity. The *parasympathetic nervous system* balances the activities of the *sympathetic nervous system* by restoring stability and maintaining reserve energy for daily bodily functions such as digestion and elimination.

Upper and Lower Motor Neurons

Upper motor neurons are located within the CNS and convey impulses from the motor areas of the cerebral cortex to the lower motor neurons in the spinal cord. They can influence the function of the *lower motor neurons*, as evidenced in conditions such as CP. The *lower motor neurons* are located primarily in the *peripheral nervous system* and provide pathways for nerve fibers to translate movement of the muscles into action.

Muscle wasting can be the result of dysfunction in the anterior horn cells of the upper motor neurons. Dysfunction in the lower motor neurons can cause wasting of localized muscle groups and a soft rather than firm tone to the muscle mass. Acquired atrophy of the muscles accompanied by a wide-based gait and muscle weakness when arising from a sitting position is characteristic of *muscular dystrophy*, a developmental muscle wasting condition with onset in early childhood.

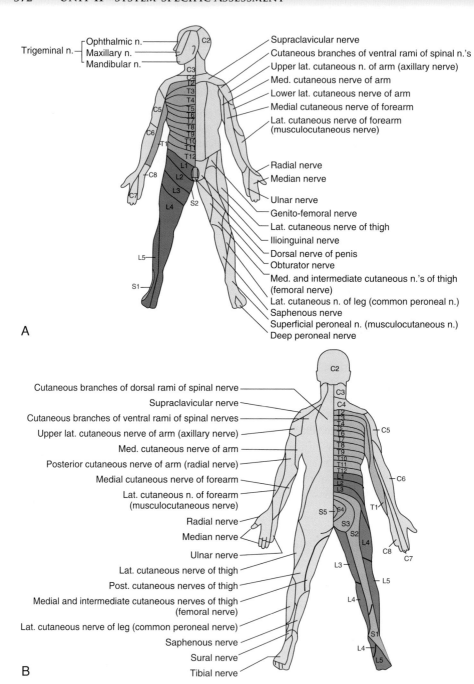

FIGURE 19.10 The spinal nerves and dermatomes. **(A)** Ventral view. **(B)** Dorsal view.

Spinal Reflexes

A *reflex* is an expected response between a stimulus and an elicited motor response. The *reflex arc* operates outside the level of conscious control and is the basic defense mechanism of the nervous system (Fig. 19.11). *Superficial reflexes* occur at the at the insertion of specific muscles (biceps, brachioradialis,

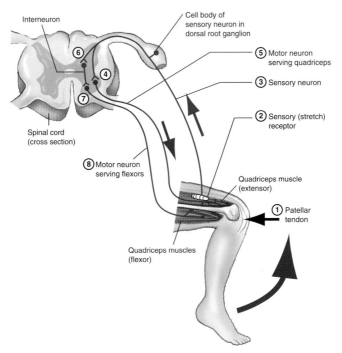

FIGURE 19.11 Reflex arc.

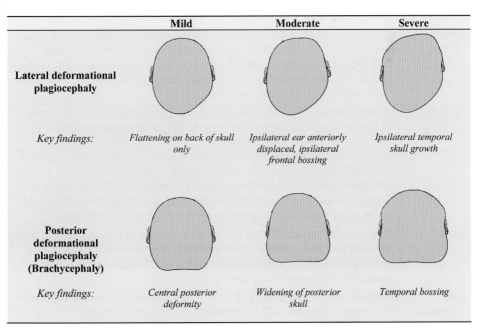

	Mild	Moderate	Severe
Lateral deformational plagiocephaly			
Key findings:	*Flattening on back of skull only*	*Ipsilateral ear anteriorly displaced, ipsilateral frontal bossing*	*Ipsilateral temporal skull growth*
Posterior deformational plagiocephaly (Brachycephaly)			
Key findings:	*Central posterior deformity*	*Widening of posterior skull*	*Temporal bossing*

FIGURE 19.12 Deformational plagiocephaly. View of infant's head from crown. (From Looman WS, Kack Flannery AB. Evidenced-based care of the child with deformational plagiocephaly, Part I: assessment and diagnosis. *J Pediatr Health Care.* 2012;26(4):242–250.)

triceps, patellar, and ankle), corneal (blink), abdominal, cremaster, and plantar reflex. *Visceral reflexes* include the anal (wink) and bulbocavernosus. Reflexes help the body maintain appropriate muscle tension and react to painful or harmful stimuli. A stimulus, for example, the tap of a reflex hammer, creates an impulse that is transmitted instantaneously outward by the motor neurons of the spinal cord via the spinal nerve and peripheral nervous system to produce a brisk muscle contraction (Fig. 19.11).

PHYSIOLOGICAL VARIATIONS

Plagiocephaly refers to an asymmetrical flattening or deformity of the skull. It occurs when external forces are applied to the developing skull of an infant and it becomes misshapen, often resulting in asymmetry of the ears and face. *Deformational* or positional plagiocephaly occurs in 20% to 50% of children[18] and is most commonly seen on the lateral and central side of the occiput (Fig. 19.12). It is more common in infants with a lower level of motor activity and with *congenital torticollis* or head tilt. *Deformational plagiocephaly* may be prevented by varying the head position frequently when putting the very young infant down to sleep on the back and by giving supervised tummy time when awake. It is important to differentiate *deformational plagiocephaly* from premature fusion of the lambdoid suture, a rare condition with an incidence of only 0.003%.[18] *Lambdoid synostosis* is a surgical diagnosis and should be expeditiously referred to a craniofacial specialist.

Table 19.1 reviews the physical, developmental, and cognitive variations that occur

INFORMATION GATHERING FOR HEAD AND NEUROLOGIC ASSESSMENT AT KEY DEVELOPMENTAL STAGES

Age Group	Questions to Ask
Family History	History of neurologic, neuromuscular, or developmental conditions?
Preterm infant	Access to prenatal care? Neurologic insults such as: bleeding, infection, hypoxia, drugs, or trauma. Exposure to substance use or perinatally acquired infections (syphilis, HSV, cytomegalovirus [CMV], varicella, parvovirus B19, coxsackie virus, COVID-19, or others)? History of intraventricular hemorrhage? Developmental screening completed, as recommended by gestational age at birth?
Newborn	Access to prenatal care? Fetal movement during pregnancy? Age of mother and father at time of infant's birth? Vaginal or cesarean birth? Prolonged third stage of labor? Vacuum or forceps-assisted delivery? History of birth injury? Shoulder presentation? Need for resuscitation/ventilation in immediate newborn period? Exposure to prenatal infection? Perinatally acquired infection? Neurologic insults such as: bleeding, infection, hypoxia, drugs, or trauma. Large or small for gestational age? Apgar scores (if known)? Congenital abnormalities? Jaundice? Neonatal infections? Newborn screening results? Developmental screening completed, as recommended by age?
Infancy	Difficulty feeding? Protuberant tongue or tongue thrust? Quality of muscle strength, tone, and head control? Any delay in achieving developmental milestones? Delay, slowing, cessation, or regression of developmental milestones? Developmental screening completed, as recommended by age?
Early childhood	Hand dominance (abnormal before 24 months)? Delay, slowing, cessation or regression of developmental milestones? Any stumbling, limping, poor coordination? History of falls, head injury, or concussions? History of seizures/spasms or staring spells? Use of helmet with bike or scooter? Developmental screening completed and assessed, as recommended by age?

Continued

INFORMATION GATHERING FOR HEAD AND NEUROLOGIC ASSESSMENT AT KEY DEVELOPMENTAL STAGES—CONT'D

Age Group	Questions to Ask
Middle childhood	School performance and behavior/friendships? IEP, 504, other school services or interventions? Delay, slowing, cessation or regression of developmental milestones? History of head injury or concussions? History of headaches, including presence of red flags with headache? Use of helmet or other protective sports equipment?
Adolescence	School performance and behavior/friendships? IEP, 504, other school services or interventions? History of headaches, including presence of red flags with headache? History of head injury or concussions? Use of helmet or other protective sports equipment?
Environmental risks	Prenatal or individual exposure to potential chemical or environmental irritants? Location of housing in relation to hazardous exposures? History of elevated lead level? Contact with chemical cleaning agents, hazardous chemicals or smoke? Pesticide exposures?

TABLE 19.1 PHYSIOLOGIC VARIATIONS DURING DEVELOPMENT

Age Group	Physical Variations	Developmental Variations	Cognitive Variations
Preterm infant	Head lag persists for 6 months; myelination of brain continues until 3 years of age	Increased extensor tone in lower extremities; with marked stiffening and toe-pointing	Sensorimotor reflexive response to stimulus
Newborn	Decreased gyral development at birth; cerebral cortex is half the adult thickness	Exhibits primitive reflexes until 3 to 4 months; requires strong stimulus to elicit response	Innate knowledge of environment, evokes survival response such as sucking
Infancy	Head circumference increases sixfold in first year; in term infant, important myelination of brain continues until 2 years of age	Plagiocephaly, asymmetrical head, shape, is common; most often related to sleeping position; normally, resolves by 3 months	Develops mental image of hidden object; imitates sounds by 6 months
Early childhood (1–3 years of age)	Proprioception, awareness of spatial/body positions begins; increased movement and sphincter control	Develops basic self-control and ability to separate from attachment person	Parallel play; independence increases; attention span develops
Early childhood (3–5 years of age)	Slowed growth, minimal change in head circumference; increased connectivity between neurons to initiate complex thought	Hand preference established; rapid fine motor development; gross motor athletic ability	Egocentric; aggressive behavior; one-dimensional understanding; magical thinking
Middle childhood	Brain reaches 90% of adult size by 5–7 years of age; deepening of sulci in brain, increasing complex thought	Transmission of nerve impulses improves, thereby enhancing fine motor and gross motor development	Consequential understanding; concrete operations and objective thought
Adolescence	Neurologic development continues into adolescence	Defines self-concept; role differentiation causes conflict	Develops abstract thinking ability

during the development and maturation of the nervous system in infancy and childhood.

SYSTEM-SPECIFIC HISTORY

The Information Gathering table reviews the pertinent areas for the head and neurologic system for each age group and developmental stage of childhood. Obtaining a complete history of developmental milestones using validated screening tools is key to early identification and effective intervention.

PHYSICAL ASSESSMENT

The examination of the head and neurologic system involves inspection and palpation. In infants and young children, examination of the head and neurologic system may follow the quieter parts of the examination (cardiac and respiratory), while in the older child, the physical examination may proceed from head to toe. Examination of the head and neurologic system require knowledge of expected growth and development throughout the pediatric lifespan to interpret clinical findings. In addition to clinical expertise, providers will need a penlight, an ophthalmoscope (use and exam described in Chapter 10), and a reflex hammer.

Inspection and Palpation of the Head

Inspection of the head includes observation by the health care provider for head movement and head control. Head alignment should be evaluated in the young infant with the head at midline on the examining table and in the older infant and young child while being supported in a sitting position by the parent or caregiver. Persistent head tilt from the normal position may indicate *hypotonia, congenital torticollis*, muscular abnormalities, gastrointestinal reflux, or visual and hearing deficits. Range of motion of the neck and movement of the head should be examined to determine tone and flexibility. In examining the infant younger than 3 months, the provider should move the head passively on the examining table to the left and right to determine mobility and range of motion. At 3 to 4 months of age, the infant can begin to follow a light or small toy to determine the full range of motion of the head and neck and the function of the musculature. Any limited range of motion, head bobbing or jerking, tremors, persistent downward gaze, or involuntary muscle contractions or spasms should be further evaluated and referred when indicated. *Head lag* should be evaluated in all infants in the first 6 months of life as an indicator of muscle tone. *Head lag* when pulling the infant to the sitting position is normal until 3 to 4 months of age in the term infant. Persistent *head lag* between 4 and 6 months of age in the term infant is concerning, and the infant should be monitored closely for the attainment of developmental milestones and referred when indicated.

Observe and palpate the shape and size of the head in the infant and young child. Head shape varies widely in young infants and generally follows a normal growth pattern influenced by familial and genetic patterns. Positional skull patterns typically occur unilaterally on the parietal region, with the clinician taking a "bird's eye view" to observe head shape (Fig. 19.12). If the shape is a "parallelogram," these are reversible *positional plagiocephaly* findings and typically return to symmetric shape by 3 months. If the head has a "trapezoid" shape, or if there are clinical findings on palpation, such as the clinician can lay a finger width in the proximal suture along the *anterior fontanel*, then there is a high concern for *craniosynostosis* or *lambdoid synostosis*, which requires immediate evaluation and referral. In the first few months of life, an infant may have a visible or palpable ridge at the suture lines of the cranium. This is a *metopic ridge* and is normal variant when the head shape appears normal and the OFC is normal. Infants with a wide margin along the sagittal suture may have a communicating *anterior* and *posterior fontanel*, often referred to as a *metopic suture*. Suture lines are normally not palpable after 4 to 6 months of age in the term infant.

Observe and palpate the level of the *fontanels* in the cranium (Fig. 19.13). Normally,

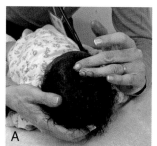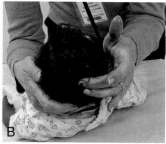

FIGURE 19.13 Palpation of the anterior **(A)** and posterior fontanels **(B)**.

there is a slight pulsation in the *anterior fontanel*, and it is fuller or tenses slightly when the infant is crying but flattens when the infant calms. In the ill infant, a tense, bulging *anterior fontanel* can be a sign of increasing intracranial pressure due to *meningitis* or head trauma and is a medical emergency. Tumors in the brain and meninges can also cause increased intracranial pressure indicated by a bulging *fontanel*. Infants can have a mildly depressed *fontanel*, unaccompanied by other symptoms, which may indicate mild dehydration due to the metabolic demands of growth or fluid lost through heat and perspiration. A sunken *fontanel*, if accompanied by gastrointestinal symptoms, infection, or loss of normal turgor of skin and mucous membranes, may indicate severe dehydration and requires immediate further evaluation and treatment. Note the length and width of the fontanel for infants with unusually large fontanels and monitor the head circumference. If fontanels are closed earlier than 5 months or later than 24 months there is clinical concern for a variety of conditions such as *craniosynostosis*, or genetic syndromes that may present with atypical closure timing; referral under 6 months is essential for minimally invasive treatment options.[18]

Examination of the Neurologic System

The comprehensive assessment of the pediatric neurologic system includes evaluation of mental status, motor and sensory function, cranial nerves, and reflexes. Observation of the child with the caregiver will provide the foundation for your assessment. Clinicians should note:

> **BOX 19.1 PEDIATRIC NEUROLOGIC ASSESSMENT CHECKLIST**
>
> - Infant reflexes (children younger than 1 year)
> - Fontanels (children younger than 18 months)
> - Mental status: Level of alertness or consciousness
> - Cranial nerves
> - Motor function
> - Deep and superficial reflexes
> - Sensory function

head shape, facies, body habitus, position, posture, spontaneous movements, spontaneous vocalizations, and/or quality of cry. In children who are mobile, observing their interaction with the caregiver will yield developmental data and information on strength, coordination, and balance.

Box 19.1 presents the basics of the neurologic examination in infants and young children.

Mental Status

Mental status is assessed using observation of the patient and incorporating elements of pertinent history. Level of function is examined using simple tests with the patient's cooperation. Together, clinical findings in these areas can differentiate between neurologic disease, psychiatric illness causing neurologic symptoms, or psychiatric illness secondary to neurologic disease. Mental status includes documentation of developmentally appropriate:

alertness, appearance, behavior, mood, vegetative symptoms, delusions, hallucinations, and illusions.[35]

Developmental delays in infants may occur in any domain—gross motor, fine motor, language, social/emotional, and/or cognitive—but they are usually first noted in gross motor skills and abilities. Language and all of the developmental domains should be assessed using validated screening tools recommended by the AAP. The process of speech requires hearing, understanding, thought and word finding, voice production, and articulation. *Dysphonia*, often used interchangeably with hoarseness, is the term for disorders of the voice. *Dysarthria* is condition identified by slurred, monotonous, or labored speech pattern.[35] Early referral and intervention services for developmental concerns are directly correlated with improved outcomes. See Chapter 3 for further discussion of developmental assessment.

Testing of higher cerebral functions assesses six domains: attention, memory (immediate, short term, and long term), calculation, abstract thoughts, spatial perception, and visual and body perception. In pediatrics, we adapt these tests for developmental age and cognitive ability as appropriate. Higher function tests are indicated if there are elements of history of concern; this will often necessitate history from caregivers or friends. Documentation of this testing will allow tracking of function over time, will distinguish focal versus diffuse deficits, and reveals the person's ability to function within the community.[35] In the developing child, cerebral function is more challenging to assess than in adults, and again requires a strong understanding of development.

In the child with head trauma, the basic components of the mental status examination can be performed with a targeted screening tool such as the Sports Concussion Assessment Tool 5 (SCAT5).[36] *Concussion* is defined as a traumatic injury to the brain that leads to a temporary impairment of brain function.[37] *Concussions* are common, often unrecognized,

and usually (90%) do not involve loss of consciousness.[37] There has been an increased focus on the immediate and long-term sequelae of concussion as a mild subset of *traumatic brain injury* (TBI) in child and adolescent athletes due to their increased participation in high-impact competitive sports.[38,39] Approximately 45% of sports- and recreation-related TBIs are a result of collision or contact sports in children, including football, soccer, and basketball.[40] *Concussions* may differ from a major TBI in that concussions are not associated with structural abnormalities on traditional imaging.[37] Children and adolescents take longer to recover from concussion than older athletes, potentially with symptoms extending for up to 4 weeks.[38,40] The short sequelae of *concussion* may include *postconcussion syndrome*, which can last for weeks to months. *Second impact syndrome* can occur if a second head injury occurs during the postconcussion period. The long-term sequelae of *concussion* include permanent neurologic deficits, such as decreased cognitive functioning and limiting cognitive potential.[38]

Information gathered during a sports participation physical exam (see Chapter 18) should include screening questions related to prior *concussions* and related symptoms, including any headaches or cognitive, emotional, or sleep impairment. See Box 19.2 for signs and symptoms of concussion. The SCAT5 for evaluation of young athletes 13 years of age and older following history of head injury or concussion, and a Child SCAT5 for children 5 to 12 years of age, can be obtained at: https://bjsm.bmj.com/content/51/11/851.

The Pediatric Glasgow Coma Scale (GCS) is an adapted assessment tool that assesses the level of consciousness for children with impaired arousal.[41] For both preverbal (<2 years of age) and verbal (>2 years of age) children, the Pediatric GCS correlates with the presence of TBI. For infants and young children, the Pediatric GCS assess visual acuity with the ability to open the eye spontaneously (response to speech, to pain, or no response); verbal cues (coos and babbles appropriately,

---

BOX 19.2   SIGNS AND SYMPTOMS OF CONCUSSION

Cognitive Symptoms
- Confusion
- Disorientation
- Inattention
- Mental fogginess
- Slurred speech
- Vacant stare

Headache/Migraine Symptoms
- Headache
- Nausea
- Photosensitivity
- Neck pain
- Photophobia
- Phonophobia

Anxiety-Mood Symptoms
- Agitation

- Flat affect
- Depression
- Labile mood
- Anxiety

Ocular Symptoms
- Blurry vision
- Double vision
- Eye fatigue

Fatigue Symptoms
- Tiredness
- Decreased arousal
- Somnolence
- Difficulty sleeping

Vestibular Symptoms
- Imbalance
- Abnormal visual motion sensitivity

From Pujalte GGA, Dekker TM, Abadin AA, Jethwa TE. *Concussion Management for Primary Care.* Cham: Springer; 2020.

---

irritable cries inconsolable, cries or screams persistently to pain, grunts or moans to pain, or no response); and motor function (normal spontaneous movements, withdraws to touch, withdraws to pain, abnormal flexion, abnormal extension, or no response), which reflect the functional integrity of the major CNS pathways. The Pediatric GCS is available at: https://onlinelibrary.wiley.com/doi/10.1111/acem.13014.

Motor and Cerebellar Function

Motor function is assessed by evaluating gait, coordination, involuntary movements, and individual muscle strength, bulk, and tone. Assessment of cerebellar function includes the evaluation of balance, coordination, cognitive processing, and input from visual, auditory, and touch receptors.

Gait and Coordination

The following simple tests can be performed in children during the physical examination and are fun and effective in assessing cerebellar function:
- **Gait:** Once a child can walk, observing gait is an essential part of the neurologic and developmental assessment. Toddlers have a wide-spaced gait for support and may appear to be high stepped and flat footed with arms outstretched. Heel strike does not appear until about 18 months with reciprocal arm swing. Running and changes in direction occur after the age of 2 years. By 8 years old, children will have adult gait and posture; however, there are diverse familial variations in normal gaits. Clinical observation includes symmetry, size of paces (both length and lateral distance between the feet), posture (marked rotation of the shoulder and pelvis is termed waddling), and arm swing. Around the age of kindergarten, additional types of gait can be assessed including: tandem walking (as if on a tightrope), which tests the steadiness of the gait; walking on heels, which detects foot drop; and walking on toes, which identifies a weak gastrocnemius (calf) muscle.[42]
- **Romberg test** is used to assess joint position sense. This test can be performed with a cooperative 3- or 4-year-old child. Ask the child to stand erect with eyes closed and hands touching the sides. Observe the child's balance for several seconds while

monitoring the child closely. Lesions in posterior column of the spinal cord can cause the child to stagger or fall.

- Clinical tests to assess for coordination include the following:
- **Finger-to-thumb test:** Assesses cerebellar function, coordination, and cognitive processing disorders in middle childhood. Ask the child to touch each finger to the thumb in rapid succession. Test can be performed with one hand at a time and then repeated with both hands.
- **Hopping in place:** Ask the child to alternately hop on one foot and then the other. Test for balance, cerebellar function, intact motor function, and spatial sense.
- **Rapid alternating movements test:** Assesses for cerebellar function, coordination, and cognitive processing disorders in middle childhood. Ask the child to place their hands palm down on the thighs. Then demonstrate the rapid, rhythmic movement of the hands back and forth, asking the child to repeat the movement rapidly for 10 seconds. Next ask the child to perform the rapidly alternating movement with one hand only. Lastly, ask the child to tap each foot rapidly on the floor. Inability to perform the task may indicate cognitive or behavioral dysfunction and requires further evaluation.
- **Finger-to-nose test:** Ask the child to close their eyes and then touch their nose with the first finger of one hand and then with first finger of the other hand. Then, with eyes open, have the child touch their nose with first finger and then touch the examiner's finger held at the edge of the child's reach (causing full extension of the arm). Repeat with both hands. Then increase speed of movements with examiner's finger changing position. Consistent failure of child to point at the finger indicates dysfunction in spatial perception and coordination and is termed dysmetria. The child should be able to perform this by 8 to 9 years of age.

- **Heel to shin test:** Assesses coordination and balance in middle childhood. Ask the child to stand and place the right heel on the left shin below the knee and then slide the heel down the shin to the foot. Repeat with the left leg. The test may be performed with the child lying down or sitting. Inability to perform the task or maintain balance may indicate decreased motor strength, a cerebellar dysfunction, or an alteration in proprioception.

Involuntary Movements

Abnormal involuntary movement can occur throughout the pediatric lifespan, with varying clinical significance. Any spontaneous or involuntary movements throughout the exam should be noted and described. *Tremors*, a rhythmic and oscillatory movement of a part of the body with more or less constant frequency and variable intensity, can be observed intermittently in the term newborn in the first few days after birth and they are generally considered within normal limits. Persistent tremors beyond the newborn period are considered abnormal and require referral and further diagnostic evaluation by a pediatric specialist.[3]

Clonus, rhythmic tonic-clonic movements of the foot elicited by stimulus, can be a normal finding in the newborn; however, beyond infancy this is clinically significant, requiring further diagnostic evaluation and referral. In infants, clonus can be elicited by the examiner's firm touch on the sole of the foot with the finger, while older children can be tested with dorsiflexion of the ankle with a hold to detect any rhythmic contractions.[35]

Chorea is the slow, involuntary, random, twisting movement seen in some children with cerebral palsy and Huntington disease.[3] *Tics* are involuntary movements that can be simple, involving one body part or sound, or complex, involving several body parts.[43] Simple motor *tics* include blinking, facial grimacing, shoulder shrugging, and hand or head jerking. Simple vocal *tics* range from humming or clearing the throat to yelling a word or phrase. Although the precise incidence is unknown, studies have found approximately 19% to 24% of children have *tics* at some point in childhood.[44]

Infantile spasms are a form of epilepsy that can cause irreversible brain damage if not treated.[45] *Infantile spasms* involve the muscles of the neck, trunk, and extremities and present as repetitive flexor/extensor movements with head nod, mixed movements, or as *myoclonic-tonic spasms* or *seizures*. The peak incidence of onset is between 3 and 7 months of age, and 90% of affected children present with symptoms by 1 year of age. The spasms may be subtle, brief, and sudden and may be associated with an underlying disorder. Suspicion of this condition requires urgent referral to a pediatric neurologist.[45]

Muscle Strength, Bulk, and Tone

Muscle strength can be assessed both through functional testing (patient performs movements) and formal testing with an examiner. Upper extremity strength testing includes: chin to chest when supine, raising arms above the head, and when making a fist the knuckles blanch. Lower extremity testing includes standing from a chair without using hands, rising from a squat, stepping onto a chair with one leg, and as described previously, walking on toes and heels. *Pronator drift* is a functional muscle test for the upper extremities, patient holds both hands outstretched, palms up, and eyes closed. Abnormal findings include: one or both arms pronate, the arm rises, or fingers continuously move up and down. Formal muscle testing using a 0–5 scale and push/pull with examiner can also be conducted.[34] Bulk can only be assessed by palpation of the muscles in the extremities; proximal and distal portions should be symmetric on both sides of the body. *Atrophy* is an abnormal finding, describing a loss of muscle bulk.[35]

Muscle tone is the normal degree of tension maintained by muscles while at rest, changes

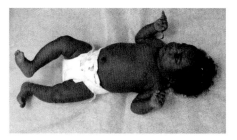

FIGURE 19.14 Normal flexion in term infant.

during the first 2 years of life as myelination of the neuronal pathways proceed, the primitive reflexes disappear, and the cerebral cortex begins to control motor functions. The assessment of muscle tone begins in the young infant by observing the resting posture. In the term infant at birth, arms and legs are in a semiflexed position with the hips slightly abducted (Fig. 19.14). At 2 months old, tone in the neck and trunk is evaluated by gently pulling the infant upward from the exam table, grasping the hands and forearms. Significant *head lag* or inability of the infant to exhibit strength in the neck and shoulders when pulled to sitting may indicate hypotonia, a decrease in the normal resting tension in the muscle. In the term infant 4 to 6 months of age, strength in the extremities and trunk is evaluated by gently pulling the infant to a sitting position; muscle tone can also be evaluated in the standing position while supporting the trunk to assess the strength of the lower extremities. At 9 months of age, gently pull the infant with both arms from a sitting position to standing to evaluate muscle tone and strength.[35]

Neurological disorders often present in early infancy with *hypotonia* and muscle weakness. *Hypotonia* may be caused by lesions in the central or peripheral nervous system, as well as neuromuscular disorders, sepsis, organ failure, and metabolic dysfunction.[3] Hips positioned in external rotation or in a "frog-leg" position in the term newborn indicates abnormal muscle tone. *Hypotonia*, low muscle tone, most commonly presents in the newborn or infant as *"floppy infant syndrome,"* which includes limited muscle tone and strength in the extremities, arms often straight at the infant's side, and hips are abducted with lower extremities abducted on the exam table. When placed in ventral suspension, the infant's head and extremities will hang or drape over the examiner's hand with inability to maintain or move to a horizontal position due to hypotonia of trunk muscles. Infants with *hypotonia* can actively move all extremities through normal range of motion, but spontaneous movements may be less frequent than in infants with normal muscle tone.[35]

In older children and adolescents, tone can be a challenge to evaluate, since it is gauging the muscles' resistance to passive movement. It is essential that the person is relaxed; distraction by conversation or task such as counting backward should be provided throughout the exam. Each movement should be repeated at different speeds since clinical findings are velocity dependent. Tone can be assessed at the arm by pronating and supinating the forearm, rolling the hand around at the wrist, and flexing the arm through full range of motion while holding the forearm and elbow. Legs can be assessed while the patient is supine. With the patient's legs extended straight, roll the knee from side to side, then put your hand under the knee and lift it rapidly. Next, hold the ankle and flex and dorsiflex the foot. A child with normal tone will exhibit slight resistance through all these movements, with minimal lift of heel off the surface. This exam may find areas of decreased tone, where heel does not lift off the bed; if weakness is severe it can be termed *"flaccid."*

Increased tone can result in varied findings. *Spasticity* presents as resistance to movement and is elicited with faster movements. The clinician varies the speed of movements throughout the exam to evaluate for *spasticity*. *Paratonia* is the resistance to movement throughout a maneuver.[35]

Preterm infants may have *hypertonia*, or increased extensor tone in their lower extremities, during the first year of life, as well as decreased truncal tone. Infants who have *hypotonia* initially may later develop *hypertonia* or *spasticity* as the cerebral cortex matures. Asymmetry in muscle tone may not be identified early in infancy due to the primitive reflexes and lack of voluntary control of the musculoskeletal system from the cerebral cortex. Transient *hypertonia* may be noted in drug-exposed infants in the neonatal period. It generally diminishes during the first year of life and disappears by 2 years of age. If the infant exhibits opisthotonos, a persistent arching of the back and extension of the neck, this indicates serious neurologic compromise and needs urgent referral.[3]

Sensory Function

Touch, deep pressure, pain, temperature, and vibration are all characteristics assessed in sensory function. Tactile sensation can be tested in the verbal child by gently touching different areas of the body with a cotton swab when the eyes are closed. The child should be able to identify the spot by pointing to the area of the body. Pain sensation can be tested similarly in the verbal child by touching the body with the sharp and dull ends of a reflex hammer. Temperature and vibration are sensations not usually elicited in early childhood, but either can be tested using a tuning fork. Discrimination sensation can be assessed in children older than 5 to 6 years of age using the following tests:

- **Stereognosis:** The ability to recognize an object by its feel. With eyes closed, ask the child to identify small familiar objects placed in the palm, such as a key or a coin. If you are not testing expressive language, have the child point to the correct object when eyes are open. Children with CP are generally unable to identify the object.
- **Graphesthesia:** The ability to identify shapes traced on the palm. Younger children are usually tested with shapes and older children with numbers. May be repeated

in each palm to ensure accuracy in testing. Children with spatial and proprioceptive dysfunction will not be able to discriminate shapes or numbers.

- **Two-point discrimination:** A test of spatial discrimination of the body. With the child's eyes closed, touch lightly on the skin with two points in close proximity on the body, and then follow with touching the child with one point. Ask whether the child felt one or two points.

Loss of sensation can reflect impairment in the peripheral nervous system, spinal column, brainstem, or cerebral cortex. Children under 5 years of age often have difficulty with sensory testing and comparing touch points.

Cranial Nerves

Cooperative young children and school-age children usually delight in the activity of testing the cranial nerves. Tables 19.2 and 19.3

TABLE 19.2 CRANIAL NERVE TESTING IN THE NEWBORN AND INFANT

Cranial Nerve	Test	Response
Cranial nerve I, olfactory	Pass strong-smelling substance (e.g., cloves, peppermint, anise oil) under nose (not often tested in newborns)	Observe for startle response, grimace, sniffing
Cranial nerve II, optic	Light source/ophthalmoscope on medium/large aperture	Pupils constrict in response to light, able to fix on object and follow for 60–90 degrees, blink to light
Cranial nerve III, oculomotor Cranial nerve IV, trochlear Cranial nerve VI, abducens	Elicit pupillary response to test optic nerve by shining pen light toward pupil, track and follow light "Doll's eye" or oculovestibular — rotate head and body from side to side, observe eyes moving away from direction of rotation	Evaluate shape, size, symmetry of extraocular movements of pupil Eyes should deviate left when turning head right; if eyes remain fixed or do not track in opposite direction, suspect brainstem dysfunction
Cranial nerve V, trigeminal	Touch infant's cheek area Test jaw muscles by placing gloved finger in infant's mouth	Infant turns cheek toward touch stimulus Infant should bite down on gloved finger and begin sucking
Cranial nerve VII, facial	Observe infant's face for symmetry of facial movements and observe when crying	Asymmetrical nasolabial folds/asymmetrical facial expression may indicate nerve palsy
Cranial nerve VIII, acoustic	With infant lying supine, ring bell sharply within a few inches of infant's ears	Observe for response to sound stimulus, such as mild startle/blink reflex NOTE: Auditory-evoked response is a more objective assessment of acoustic nerve, mandated by most states
Cranial nerve IX, glossopharyngeal	Use tongue blade to apply pressure on midtongue area to overcome tongue thrust	Elicit gag reflex; observe tongue movement, strength

Continued

TABLE 19.2 CRANIAL NERVE TESTING IN THE NEWBORN AND INFANT—CONT'D

Cranial Nerve	Test	Response
Cranial nerve X, vagus	Observe infant while crying	Evaluate pitch of cry and assess for hoarseness, stridor; normal cry is loud and angry; shrill, penetrating cry indicates intracranial hemorrhage; whiny, high-pitched cry indicates central nervous system dysfunction
Cranial nerve XI, accessory	With infant lying supine, turn infant's head to one side	Infant should work to bring head to midline
Cranial nerve XII, hypoglossal	Observe infant when feeding	Sucking, swallowing should be efficient, coordinated

Data from Thureen PJ, Deacon J, Hernandez J, et al. *Assessment and Care of the Well Newborn.* 2nd ed. Philadelphia, PA: Saunders; 2005.

TABLE 19.3 CRANIAL NERVE TESTING IN EARLY TO MIDDLE CHILDHOOD

Cranial Nerve	Test
Cranial nerve I, olfactory	• Block one nare at a time and allow patient to smell substances such as hand sanitizer, herbal oils, or gum
Cranial nerve II, optic	• Visual acuity testing as indicated by developmental level
Cranial nerve III, oculomotor Cranial nerve IV, trochlear Cranial nerve VI, abducens	• Use ophthalmoscope or light source to test direct and consensual pupillary response to light • With examiner's hand under chin, have child follow toy, light source, or index finger through six cardinal fields of gaze to test eye movement
Cranial nerve V, trigeminal	• Observe child chewing and swallowing to test normal jaw strength • Touch facial area with cotton swab and observe child move away from stimulus
Cranial nerve VII, facial	• Ask child to smile, frown, and puff cheeks, observe for symmetrical facial expressions
Cranial nerve VIII, acoustic	• Perform audiometric testing to evaluate range of hearing • Test vestibular balance with eyes closed
Cranial nerve IX, glossopharyngeal Cranial nerve X, vagus	• Observe tongue strength and movement • Observe uvula and palate rise • Child is able to swallow without difficulty • Voice quality and sound is normal and intact
Cranial nerve XI, accessory Cranial nerve XII, hypoglossal	• Have child stick tongue against interior cheek wall while examiner palpates external cheek • Shrug shoulders to assess trapezius muscle strength • Turn head from side to side against resistance to test sternocleidomastoid muscle strength

summarize the assessment of cranial nerves in infancy and early and middle childhood. Cranial nerve testing may be difficult to assess in infants if they are drowsy, crying, or satiated after feeding and in young children if they are fearful or irritable during the physical examination.

Reflexes

The *primitive reflexes* appear as early as 25 weeks' gestation. They are involuntary and controlled at birth by the brainstem. The *primitive reflexes* should always be symmetrical and are considered abnormal if asymmetrical or absent at birth (Table 19.4; Figs. 19.15 through

TABLE 19.4 PRIMITIVE REFLEXES

Reflex	How Initiated	Response
Asymmetrical tonic neck	With infant on flat surface turn head 90 degrees to surface	Arm and leg extend on same side infant is turned toward, arm and leg on opposite side flex
Moro	Support infant at 30-degree angle above flat surface with examiner's hand; allow head and trunk to drop back to surface supported by examiner's hand; or pull infant up by hands to 30-degree angle above examining table; gently drop infant back to surface quickly and release arms	Arms extend and abduct, hands open, fingers fan out, thumb and forefinger form a C; then arms flex and adduct, knees clench, hips flex, eyes open, infant may cry
Palmar grasp	With infant's head midline, touch palm of infant's hand on ulnar surface with examiner's thumb	Fingers clasp examiner's thumb
Placing	Hold infant upright under arms over edge of table; touch dorsal surface of foot to table edge	Flexion of knees/hips, foot lifts as if stepping up on table
Plantar grasp	Touch infant on plantar surface of foot at base of toes	Toes curl downward
Rooting	Touch or stroke cheek	Infant's head turns toward stimulus and mouth should open
Stepping	Hold infant upright under the arms above exam table; palmar surface of feet should be allowed to just touch table surface	Stepping-like motion with alternate flexion and extension of legs
Sucking	Gently stroke the lips	Infant's mouth opens, sucking begins; gloved finger inserted into mouth evaluates strength of suck reflex
Truncal incurvation or Galant reflex	Hold infant firmly suspended in prone position with examiner's hand supporting chest; with opposite hand, stroke along spine lightly with fingernail just adjacent to vertebrae from shoulders to coccyx	Hips and buttocks curve/turn toward stimulus side

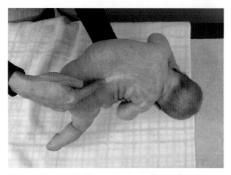

FIGURE 19.15 Truncal incurvation reflex.

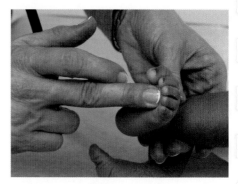

FIGURE 19.18 Plantar grasp reflex.

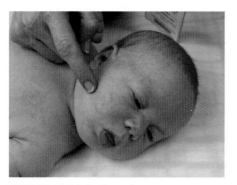

FIGURE 19.16 Rooting reflex.

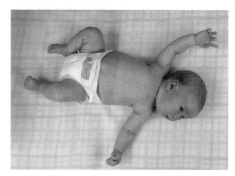

FIGURE 19.19 Asymmetrical tonic neck reflex.

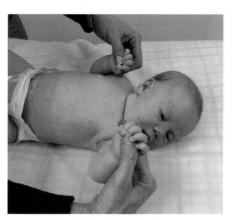

FIGURE 19.17 Palmar grasp reflex.

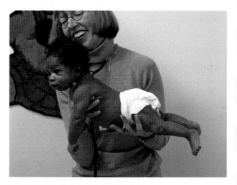

FIGURE 19.20 Landau reflex.

19.19). The *primitive reflexes* normally diminish by 3 to 4 months of age as the cerebral cortex matures during the first year of life. They disappear altogether in the typical full-term newborn by 4 to 6 months of age and are considered abnormal if persistent after 6 months of age. The *primitive reflexes* provide the earliest indication of CNS dysfunction. If an infant is very sleepy, irritable, or satiated after feeds, the *primitive reflexes* will be diminished and should be reevaluated when the infant is alert.

The appearance of the *postural reflexes* predicts normal development (Table 19.5; Figs. 19.20, 19.21). The *postural reflexes* appear between 5 and 6 months in the term infant and

TABLE 19.5 POSTURAL REFLEXES

Reflex	How Initiated	Response
Neck righting	Infant's head is turned to the right or left from the midline 90 degrees to the examination table	Rotation of the trunk in the direction in which the head of the supine infant is turned; this reflex is absent or decreased in infants with spasticity
Landau	Hold infant firmly suspended in prone position with examiner's hand supporting abdomen and head; legs should extend over hand	Infant should lift head, extend spine/lower extremities
Lateral parachute	Assessed at 5–7 months of age in term infant. Hold infant prone and firmly supported; slowly lower infant toward flat surface	Observe symmetry of hand opening; infant should try to protect self by extending arms/legs
Forward parachute	Assessed at 7–9 months of age in term infant. Suspend infant in prone position with arms/legs extended, support with both hands over flat surface	Observe symmetry of hand opening; infant will lift head and extend spine along horizontal plane
Positive support	Hold infant upright and firmly supported under arms while over exam table; touch infant's feet to surface	Infant should extend legs and bear some weight

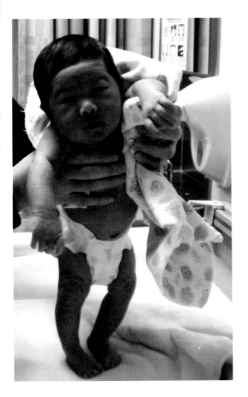

FIGURE 19.21 Positive support reflex. (From Gerber RJ, Wilks T, Erdie-Lalena C. Developmental milestones: motor development. *Pediatr Rev.* 2010;31(7):267–277.)

progress in a cephalocaudal direction beginning with head control. Typical development of the *postural reflexes* supports upper body posture. If *postural reflexes* do not appear by 8 to 9 months of age, it is considered an abnormal finding. Remnants of the *postural reflexes* persist throughout life.[6]

Deep tendon reflexes are a product of the "*reflex arc*," a complex function of the musculoskeletal and nervous systems. Each reflex requires an intact sensory neuron, a functional synapse in the spinal cord, an intact motor neuron, a functional neuromuscular junction, and a competent muscle (Table 19.6; Figs. 19.22 through 19.28). Reflex testing is useful

TABLE 19.6 DEEP TENDON AND SUPERFICIAL REFLEXES

Reflex	Test	Response
Deep Tendon Reflexes		
Biceps reflex	With examiner's thumb pressed against biceps tendon in antecubital space, support arm with palm prone; tap thumb briskly; tendon should respond by tightening	Flexion of forearm
Triceps reflex	Hold arm in flexed position slightly forward toward chest with forearm dangling downward, tap directly behind elbow on triceps tendon	Contraction of triceps and elbow should extend slightly
Brachioradialis reflex	Support child's forearm with palm resting down; tap briskly on radius approximately 2 inches above wrist	Flexion of elbow and pronation of forearm
Patellar reflex	Palpate patellar tendon just below patella and tap briskly with leg dangling; having child lock fingers and pull hard in outward direction can help elicit reflex	Contraction of quadriceps and extension of knee
Achilles tendon reflex	Support foot with ankle slightly flexed and leg relaxed, tap above heel; vary degree of flexion of foot to assist in eliciting reflex	Observe plantar flexion
Clonus	In infant, knee should be slightly flexed with infant in supine position; apply pressure to sole of foot to bring ankle into dorsiflexion	In newborn, rapid tonic-clonic movement of 4–5 beats is normal response; beyond newborn period, no rhythmic movements are expected, sustained clonus at any age is abnormal.
Superficial Reflexes		
Plantar reflex	Stroke sole of foot from heel to ball of foot curving medially with flat object	Movement of toes downward (in infancy toes will dorsiflex or "up-toeing")
Abdominal reflex	Stroke briskly above and below umbilicus	Abdominal muscles contract and umbilicus deviates toward the stimulus
Cremasteric reflex	In male, lightly scratch upper inner thigh	Testicle will elevate slightly on stimulated side
Anal reflex	Gently stroke anal area to test sphincter tone	Quick contraction of sphincter

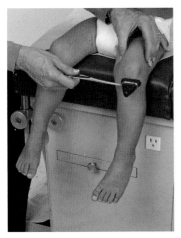

FIGURE 19.22 Patellar reflex.

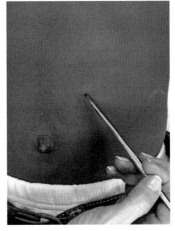

FIGURE 19.25 Abdominal reflex.

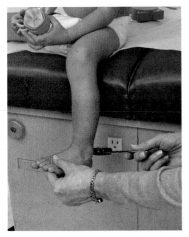

FIGURE 19.23 Achilles tendon reflex.

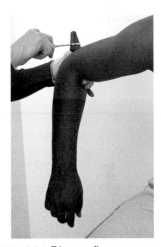

FIGURE 19.26 Triceps reflex.

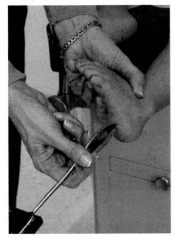

FIGURE 19.24 Plantar reflex.

in young children because it provides information on the normal development and maturation of the neuromuscular system. Assessment of the deep tendon reflexes may help to distinguish between upper and lower motor neuron lesions. Abnormally brisk reflexes with *clonus* may suggest upper motor tract involvement. Absent reflexes are consistent with a neuropathic lesion, an inflammatory demyelinating disorder such as Guillain Barre syndrome, or severe myopathy.[4] Box 19.3 shows the scale used to grade responsiveness to the deep tendon reflex examination.

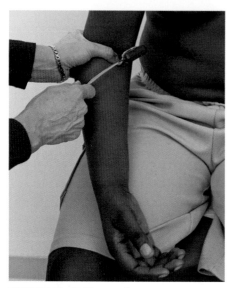

FIGURE 19.27 Biceps reflex.

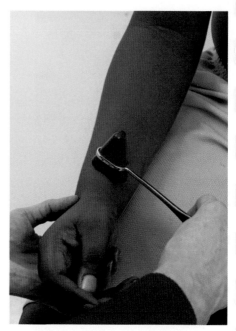

FIGURE 19.28 Brachioradialis reflex.

BOX 19.3	GRADING SCALE FOR RESPONSE TO DEEP TENDON REFLEX EXAMINATION

- 4+: Brisk, markedly hyperactive with clonus
- 3+: Active, brisker than normal
- 2+: Normal response
- 1+: Diminished response, low normal
- 0: Absent or no response

DIAGNOSTIC PROCEDURES

The Pediatric Emergency Care Applied Research Network (PECARN) Pediatric Head Injury/Trauma Algorithm[46] provides a guide for many neurological clinical imaging decisions. Both computed tomography (CT) and MRI are sensitive enough to identify concussion injuries. MRI can assess for secondary headache disorders, neurologic injury, or a cerebral abnormality. MRI is advantageous because it does not involve radiation exposure; however, it takes longer to scan the child and may require sedation if the child does not have the developmental skill to stay still for the duration of the scan. The advent of the rapid MRI has allowed even young children or urgent presentations to be evaluated. Some clinical settings can also attempt swaddling or other calming measures to perform MRI on infants without sedation. Ultrasound may be used in evaluating neonates and infants with an open *anterior fontanel* for hydrocephalus or intraventricular hemorrhages.[47] Clinical assessment is key in influencing provider choice to image, as well as access to timely imaging and need for conscious sedation for the young child.[46]

Electroencephalogram (EEG) is used as a diagnostic tool to evaluate infants or children presenting with history of spasms or seizures. There are several different settings and durations for obtaining EEG; the most common is outpatient sleep-deprived EEG to capture both wakefulness and sleep in children with concerns for seizure. Overnight EEG and ambulatory EEG may provide further information if initial EEG does not capture the event of concern.[48] It is important to remember that an EEG may not capture seizure activity, and the diagnosis of seizures remains a clinical diagnosis.

NEUROLOGIC CONDITIONS

Neurologic disorders are the largest proportion of Disability Adjusted Life Years (DALYs), a measure of healthy life lost as a result of disability.[2] This health impact is greater than cancer, pulmonary disease, or heart disease. Disparities in diagnosis and treatment of neurologic disorders exist locally and globally, largely due to inequities in access to neurologic care. The WHO has found that most countries have "inadequate resources for neurologic disorders," including lack of diagnostic equipment and in-country manufacturing of medications that contribute to increasing disparities in care.[2] Table 19.7 presents the most common neurologic conditions occurring in infants, children, and adolescents.

Headache

Headache is one of the five most common pediatric diseases and the most common neurologic disorder in children.[52] It is essential for the clinician to differentiate between primary headaches and secondary headaches. *Primary headaches* are "intrinsic to the brain" and a result of both genetic and environmental risk factors. Primary headaches are termed *migraine headache* when they are episodic and recurrent. *Secondary headaches* are caused by

TABLE 19.7	NEUROLOGIC CONDITIONS IN INFANTS, CHILDREN, AND ADOLESCENTS
Condition	**Description**
Abusive head trauma	Characterized by severe trauma or shaking in small infants causing acceleration and deceleration of the delicate brain tissue within the periosteum. Additional clinical findings include: retinal hemorrhages (bruising or bleeding in the retinal region, visible by fundoscopy), skull fractures, fractures to other bones, and within the brain, subdural hematomas, subarachnoid hemorrhage, and shearing of axons.[49]
Seizure disorders	Episodic events caused by abnormal neuronal activity in the brain.[50] Can range from acute and short-limited, as with febrile seizures, to chronic, as with epilepsy. Signs range from very subtle behaviors to tonic-clonic movements of the entire body.
Prader-Willi syndrome	A rare chromosomal disorder characterized by hypotonia, insatiable appetite, obesity and uncontrolled appetite, hypogonadism, incomplete sexual development, and developmental delay.
Neurofibromatosis Type 1 and 2	Characterized by any two of the following: six or more café au lait macules over 5 mm in diameter, axillary or inguinal freckling (typically appears between ages 3 and 5 years), subcutaneous neurofibromas, Lisch nodules on the iris (typically develop in adolescence), optic nerve gliomas (usually appear by age 6), bone deformities, or a first-degree relative with NF1. Requires annual ophthalmology, dermatology, and neurology assessments.[51]
Migraine headache	Characterized by pulsating pain and high pain intensity. Episodic and recurrent. May be preceded by aura.
Tension-type headaches	Characterized by pressing, mild pain and described as less intense than migraine headaches.

BOX 19.4   SNOOP7 Pneumonic for Headache Red Flag Findings

Systemic symptoms including fever
  Neurologic deficits
  Onset is abrupt
  Occipital Headache
  P-(seven P's)- Positional headache, Precipitated by sneezing, coughing or exercise, Papilledema, Progressive headache, Painful eye, Post-traumatic onset of headache, Pathology of the immune system
  Your headache changes from usual headache

---

a variety of clinically significant findings that cause increased intracranial pressure including the following: head trauma, brain tumors, infection, and inflammatory diseases. Secondary headaches may also be caused by medication overuse that alters *nociceptor activity*. *Nociceptor activity* is the neural process of encoding and processing noxious stimuli. The many types and symptoms of primary headaches can be classified using the International Classification of Headache Disorders (ICHD).[52]

Clinicians differentiate primary versus secondary headache using a detailed headache history including a screening for red flags, a complete physical, and a neurologic exam. Red flags in the history or focal deficits in the neurologic exam are the key elements that determine if neuroimaging is indicated. Red flag screening can be conducted using the mnemonic SNOOP7 to triage the need for emergent care or imaging[53] (see Box 19.4).

Movement Disorders and Seizures

Tics are a common movement disorder characterized by sudden, involuntary, rapid, abrupt, repetitive, recurrent, and nonrhythmic movements or vocalizations.[43] If tics last more than 12 months, the condition is termed chronic tic disorder. The more severe form of *tics* is defined as Tourette syndrome and includes two or more motor *tics* and at least one vocal *tic* for over a year. Children with *tics* are more likely

to have comorbid psychiatric conditions and difficulty with sleep.[43] Pediatric Autoimmune Neuropsychiatric Disorders Associated with Streptococcal Infections (PANDAS) is a condition where, among other symptoms, the child has a sudden onset of disabling *tics*.[54] History, impact on daily function, and complete physical and neurologic exam are necessary clinical tools for evaluation of *tic* disorders.

Seizures are "transient events emanating from abnormal excessive neuronal activity in the brain."[50] Symptoms of seizures vary widely, and the seismology (description) of a seizure is critical to identification of seizure type. Similar to headaches, a primary care clinician's detailed history and exam can allow the specialty to triage the referral accurately. Many other disorders mimic seizures, such as pallid syncope, tic disorders, and paroxysmal disorders including sleep walking.[55] Seizures can range from very subtle behavioral arrest to tonic-clonic movements of the entire body. The International League Against Epilepsy (ILAE) defines seizure types and epilepsy diagnostic criterion.[56] There are three types of seizures, four types of epilepsy, and six etiological causes of seizure syndromes. The most common seizure type in children is *febrile seizures*, defined for children older than 1 month of age as "associated with a febrile illness, in the absence of a central nervous system infection or acute electrolyte imbalance."[57] Typically, *febrile seizures* occur between ages 3 months to 5 years, with a peak at 18 months.[55] Worldwide incidence of febrile seizures varies with genetic ancestry and ranges between 2% and 14% of children.[57] Only 2% to 10% of children with febrile seizures will go on to develop *epilepsy*. Numerous studies have tested various cognitive outcomes in children with febrile seizures, finding no differences in a variety of academic and intellectual measures.[57]

Unprovoked seizures require an evaluation by a neurology team. A comprehensive history of the events, including before and after the episode, should be recorded by caregivers. The Epilepsy Foundation Website (www.epilepsy.com) has extensive patient education materials and tools available in several languages, including a useful seizure observation tool using pictures to describe the event.[58] Smartphone apps for seizure tracking are also available. Children with epilepsy are at risk of comorbid conditions that impact learning; close monitoring of school performance should also be included in assessment.

Interprofessional collaboration is paramount for children and adolescents with neurological disorders. It is important for pediatric health care providers to provide team-based collaborative care with pediatric neurological and developmental specialists, occupational and physical therapists, behavioral health, and learning specialists to assess cognitive and intellectual function, and gross and fine motor skills. Connection to pediatric social supports such as regional centers, children's services, and supplemental social security is essential. Clear communication with schools in support of individual education plans (IEP), seizure action plans, and migraine action plans should be assessed at every visit.[52]

MALTREATMENT

Screening and detection of trauma in infants and children is part of every clinician's role, and the report of suspected maltreatment is mandated by law. Early detection may prevent re-abuse and can allow for intervention and support for the caregiver and the child.[59] It is estimated that up to 3% of children presenting to the emergency department have experienced child maltreatment. Screening tools such as the Escape Questionnaire use standardized validated screening questions to detect risk for maltreatment (see Box 19.5).[60]

Abusive Head Trauma (AHT), previously termed "shaken baby syndrome," can cause lifelong health consequences; over 60% of children who have experienced *abusive head trauma* have significant disability from physical, neurologic, and behavioral impairments. It is the number one cause of mortality due to nonaccidental trauma in children under the age of 2 years.[49] Infants have brains with

---

> **BOX 19.5 ESCAPE QUESTIONNAIRE TO SCREEN FOR CHILD MALTREATMENT**
>
> 1. Is the history consistent?
> 2. Was seeking medical help unnecessarily delayed?
> 3. Does the onset of the injury fit the developmental level of the child?
> 4. Is the behavior of the child and their caregiver's interaction appropriate?
> 5. Are the findings of the head-to-toe examination in accordance with the history?
> 6. Are there signals that make you doubt the safety of the child or other family members?

---

greater water content, more space due to larger subarachnoid spaces, and immature neurons and are more vulnerable to damage when they experience "acceleration-deceleration and rotational forces."[49] Neuroimaging is essential in the examination of a child with suspected AHT. Additional clinical findings include: retinal hemorrhages (bruising or bleeding in the retinal region, visible by fundoscopy), skull fractures, fractures to other bones, and within the brain, subdural hematomas, subarachnoid hemorrhage, and shearing of axons.[49] Studies have found that neurologic anatomy can be impacted by maltreatment, leading to lifelong changes including differences in gray and white matter, the amygdala, hippocampus, and corpus callosum.[60] These anatomical changes impact function, as evidenced by decreased executive function and motor skills.[16,49,59,60]

TELEHEALTH TIPS

Much of the head and neurological system can be examined via video in a telehealth visit. All areas of observation including facies and head shape can be assessed. Developmental milestones may be more easily observed when the child is in their home setting, since there is reduced stranger anxiety and improved comfort. The following elements of the neurological exam can be appropriately examined via telehealth: mental status, cranial nerves, some motor (gait, coordination, and balance) and some sensory status (patient or caregiver can be instructed to touch various areas and report sensation as same or different). Deep tendon reflexes and bulk cannot be assessed. Some observations of tone may be completed but are limited since a full tone assessment is reliant on examiner interaction. *Primitive* and *postural reflexes* may be examined by giving the caregiver clear instructions. Involuntary movements may also be noted via a telehealth visit.

SUMMARY OF EXAMINATION

- Observe the infant for head control. Head lag is normal until 3 to 4 months of age when pulling the infant to the sitting position.
- Observe shape and size of the head in the infant and young child. Monitor head circumference for abnormal growth. Note any misshapen skull or masses, nodules, or lesions on scalp.
- Fontanels should be palpated for size, pulsations, level of tenseness, or depression of fontanel.
- Evaluating developmental milestones and understanding the range of expected ages of developmental milestones across all domains is an essential component of the neurologic exam.
- The neurologic exam includes the assessment of mental status, cranial nerves, reflexes, and motor and sensory function. Each element is adjusted for the developmental stage of the child.
- Delays in preterm and term infants can occur in any area of gross motor, fine motor, language, social/emotional, or cognitive skills, but delays are usually first noted in gross motor skills and abilities.
- Elements of the pediatric neurological examination can be evaluated via telehealth including mental status, cranial nerves, some motor (gait, coordination, and balance) and sensory status as well as developmental milestones.

DOCUMENTATION

18-Month-Old
Neurologic: Alert, active, follows simple directions; gait, balance, and coordination typical for age, DTRs intact +2 bilaterally, muscle strength equal and symmetrical, cranial nerves II–XII grossly intact, developmental screening results appropriate for age.

DTR, Deep tendon reflex.

REFERENCES

1. World Health Organization. Social determinants of health. https://www.who.int/health-topics/social-determinants-of-health#tab=tab_1. Accessed April 2, 2022.
2. Noble JM. *Global burden of neurologic disease*. In: *Merritt's Neurology*. Philadelphia, PA: Wolters Kluwer; 2022.
3. Louis ED, Mayer SA, Noble JM. In: *Merritt's Neurology*. Philadelphia, PA: Wolters Kluwer; 2022.
4. Ouyang M, Dubois J, Yu Q, Mukherjee P, Huang H. Delineation of early brain development from fetuses to infants with diffusion MRI and beyond. *Neuroimage*. 2019; 185:836–850.
5. Sechi A, Neri I, Patrizi A, et al. Scalp hair whorl patterns in patients affected by Neurofibromatosis Type 1: a case-control study. *Int J Trichology*. 2020;12:56–61.
6. Swaiman KF, Phillips J. Neurological examination after the newborn period until 2 years of age. In: Swaiman KF Ashwal S Ferriero DF Schor NF et al. editors, *Swaiman's Pediatric Neurology: Principles and Practice*. 6th ed. Edinburgh: Elsevier; 2018: 14–19.
7. Gilmore JH, Knickmeyer RC, Gao W. Imaging structural and functional brain development in early childhood. *Nat Rev Neurosci*. 2018;19:123–137.
8. Weernink MG, van Wijk RM, Groothuis-Oudshoorn CG, et al. Insufficient vitamin D supplement use during pregnancy and early childhood: a risk factor for positional skull deformation. *Matern Child Nutr*. 2016;12:177–188.
9. Yokota S, Takeuchi H, Hashimoto T, et al. Individual differences in cognitive performance and brain structure in typically developing children. *Dev Cogn Neurosci*. 2015;14:1–7.
10. Bach CC, Henriksen TB, Larsen RT, Aagaard K, Matthiesen NB. Head circumference at birth and school performance: a nationwide cohort study of 536,921 children. *Pediatr Res*. 2020;87:1112–1118.
11. Harris SR. Measuring head circumference: Update on infant microcephaly. *Can Fam Physician*. 2015;61: 680–684.

12. Ross EJ, Graham DL, Money KM, Stanwood GD. Developmental consequences of fetal exposure to drugs: what we know and what we still must learn. *Neuropsychopharmacology*. 2015;40:61–87.

13. Wade M, Browne DT, Plamondon A, Daniel E, Jenkins JM. Cumulative risk disparities in children's neurocognitive functioning: a developmental cascade model. *Dev Sci*. 2016;19:179–194.

14. Zee, E. Wu Tsai Neurosciences Institute Stanford University. Stanford study shows wood smoke can harm the brain. https://neuroscience.stanford.edu/news/stanford-study-shows-wood-smoke-can-harm-brain. Accessed April 1, 2022.

15. United States Department of Health and Human Services. Adverse childhood experiences. https://www.childwelfare.gov/topics/preventing/overview/framework/. Accessed April 1, 2022.

16. Cabrera C, Torres H, Harcourt S. The neurological and neuropsychological effects of child maltreatment. *Aggress Violent Behav*. 2020;54:101408.

17. Zitelli BJ, McIntire SC, Nowalk AJ, Garrison J, Davis HW. *Neurology. Zitelli and Davis' Atlas of Pediatric Physical Diagnosis*. Amsterdam: Elsevier; 2022:585–616.

18. Hersh DS, Bookland MJ, Hughes CD. Diagnosis and management of suture-related concerns of the infant skull. *Pediatr Clin North Am*. 2021;68:727–742.

19. Gupta M. Fetal face and neck anomalies. In: Kumar B, Alfirevic Z, eds. *Fetal Medicine. Royal College of Obstetricians and Gynaecologists Advanced Skills*. Cambridge: Cambridge University Press; 2016:96–101.

20. Rosch KS, Mostofsky S. Development of the frontal lobe. *Handb Clin Neurol*. 2019;163:351–367.

21. Dieterich M, Brandt T. The parietal lobe and the vestibular system. *Handb Clin Neurol*. 2018;151:119–140.

22. Patel A, Biso GMNR, Fowler JB. Neuroanatomy, temporal lobe. [Updated 2021 Jul 31]. StatPearls [Internet]. Treasure Island, FL: StatPearls Publishing; 2022. Available from: https://www.ncbi.nlm.nih.gov/books/NBK519512/ Accessed March 30, 2022.

23. Rehman A, Al Khalili Y. Neuroanatomy, occipital lobe. [Updated 2021 Jul 31]. StatPearls [Internet]. Treasure Island, FL: StatPearls Publishing; 2022. Available from: https://www.ncbi.nlm.nih.gov/books/NBK544320/ Accessed March 30, 2022.

24. Young CB, Reddy V, Sonne J. Neuroanatomy, basal ganglia. [Updated 2021 Jul 31]. StatPearls [Internet]. Treasure Island, FL: StatPearls Publishing; 2022. Available from: https://www.ncbi.nlm.nih.gov/books/NBK537141/ Accessed March 30, 2022.

25. Stoodley CJ. The cerebellum and neurodevelopmental disorders. *Cerebellum*. 2016;15:34–37.

26. Piña-Garza JE and James KC. Lower brainstem and cranial nerve dysfunction. In: Piña-Garza JE and James KC. Fenichel's Clinical Pediatric Neurology 8th ed. Philadelpia: Elsivier; 2019: 326–345.

27. Sherr E, Hahn J, et al. Disorders of Forebrain Development. In: Swaiman KF Ashwal S Ferriero DF Schor NF et al. editors, *Swaiman's Pediatric Neurology: Principles and Practice* 6th ed. Edinburgh: Elsevier; 2018: 192–198.

28. Torrico TJ, Munakomi S. Neuroanatomy, thalamus. [Updated 2021 Jul 31]. StatPearls [Internet]. Treasure Island, FL: StatPearls Publishing; 2022. Available from: https://www.ncbi.nlm.nih.gov/books/NBK542184/.

29. Long RK and Rosenthal SM. Endocrine Disorders of the Hypothalamus and Pituitary in Childhood and Adolescence. In: Swaiman KF Ashwal S Ferriero DF Schor NF et al. editors, *Swaiman's Pediatric Neurology: Principles and Practice* 6th ed. Edinburgh: Elsevier; 2018: 1165–1172.

30. Ono D, Yamanaka A. Hypothalamic regulation of the sleep/wake cycle. *Neurosci Res*. 2017;118:74–81.

31. Burdakov D, Peleg-Raibstein D. The hypothalamus as a primary coordinator of memory updating. *Physiol Behav*. 2020;223:112988.

32. Michaelson, DJ. Spinal Fluid Examination. In: Piña-Garza JE and James KC. *Fenichel's Clinical Pediatric Neurology* 8th ed. Philadelpia: Elsivier; 2019: 73–77.

33. Kaiser JT, Lugo-Pico JG. Neuroanatomy, spinal nerves. [Updated 2021 Jul 31]. StatPearls [Internet]. Treasure Island, FL: StatPearls Publishing; 2022. Available from: https://www.ncbi.nlm.nih.gov/books/NBK542218/ Accessed March 15, 2022.

34. Stanford Medicine 25. Deep tendon reflexes. Stanford Medicine 25. https://stanfordmedicine25.stanford.edu/the25/tendon.html. Accessed April 7, 2022.

35. Fuller, G. Neurological Examination Made Easy. In: Fuller G, *Neurological Examination made Easy*. 6th ed. Edinburgh: Elsevier; 2020.

36. Sport Concussion Assessment Tool—5th edition. *Br J Sports Med*. 2017;51:851–858.

37. Pujalte GGA, Dekker TM, Abadin AA, Jethwa TE. *Concussion Management for Primary Care*. Cham: Springer; 2020.

38. McCrory P, Meeuwisse W, Dvorak J, et al. Consensus statement on concussion in sport—The 5th International Conference on Concussion in Sport held in Berlin, October 2016. *Br J Sports Med*. 2017;51:838–847.

39. McClain R. Concussion and trauma in young athletes: prevention, treatment, and return-to-play. *Prim Care*. 2015;42:77–83.

40. Moreland G, Barkley L. Concussion in sport. *Curr Sports Med Rep*. 2021;20:181–182.

41. Holmes JF, Palchak MJ, MacFarlane T, Kuppermann N. Performance of the pediatric glasgow coma scale in children with blunt head trauma. *Acad Emerg Med*. 2005;12:814–819.

42. Harper-Shankie M, Little H. Child with Gait Disturbances. In: Kamat, D.M., Sivaswamy, L. (eds) *Symptom-Based Approach to Pediatric Neurology*. Switzerland; Springer, 2022: 501–511.

43. Ueda K and Black KJ. Child with Tics and Other Common Disorders. In: Swaiman KF Ashwal S Ferriero DF Schor NF et al. editors, *Swaiman's Pediatric Neurology: Principles and Practice* 6th ed. Edinburgh: Elsevier; 2018: 519–523.

44. Ueda K, Black KJ. A comprehensive review of tic disorders in children. *J Clin Med*. 2021;10:2479.

45. Kelley SA, Knupp KG. Infantile spasms-Have we made progress? *Curr Neurol Neurosci Rep*. 2018;18:27.

46. Runde D, Beiner J. Calculated decisions: PECARN pediatric head injury/trauma algorithm. *Pediatr Emerg Med Pract*. 2018;15(Suppl 6):CD3–CD4.

47. Sandhu PK, Banker H, Cohen HL. Neurosonography assessment, protocols, and interpretation. [Updated 2021 Jul 21]. StatPearls [Internet]. Treasure Island, FL: StatPearls

Publishing;2022.Availablefrom:https://www.ncbi.nlm.nih.gov/books/NBK573073/ Accessed March 22, 2022.

48. Rayi A, Murr N. Electroencephalogram. [Updated 2021 Oct 9]. StatPearls [Internet]. Treasure Island, FL: StatPearls Publishing; 2022. Available from: https://www.ncbi.nlm.nih.gov/books/NBK563295/ Accessed March 20, 2022.

49. Kabbouche, M, Kacperski, J, OBrien, H, Powers, S, and Hershey, A. Headache Disorder in Children and Adolescents. In: Swaiman KF Ashwal S Ferriero DF Schor NF et al. editors, *Swaiman's Pediatric Neurology: Principles and Practice* 6th ed. Edinburgh; Elsevier: 2018: 647–655.

50. Do TP, Remmers A, Schytz HW, et al. Red and orange flags for secondary headaches in clinical practice. *Neurology.* 2018;92:134–144.

51. Pandas Physicians Network: What is PANS/PANDAS? https://www.pandasppn.org/what-are-pans-pandas/. Accessed April 2, 2022.

52. Pearl, P. Overview of Seizures and Epilepsy in Children. In: Swaiman KF Ashwal S Ferriero DF Schor NF et al. editors, *Swaiman's Pediatric Neurology: Principles and Practice* 6th ed. Edinburgh: Elsevier; 2018: 497–500.

53. Katyayan A, Diaz-Medina G. Epilepsy: epileptic syndromes and treatment. *Neurol Clin.* 2021;39:779–795.

54. Fisher RS, Cross JH, French JA, et al. Operational classification of seizure types by the International League Against Epilepsy: Position Paper of the ILAE Commission for Classification and Terminology. *Epilepsia.* 2017; 58:522–530.

55. Seinfield, S and Shinmar, S. Febrile Seizures. In: Swaiman KF Ashwal S Ferriero DF Schor NF et al. editors, *Swaiman's Pediatric Neurology: Principles and Practice* 6th ed. Edinburgh: Elsevier; 2018.

56. Seizure Description Form. Epilepsy Foundation. Accessed June 12, 2022. https://www.epilepsy.com/sites/default/files/atoms/files/Seizure-Description-Form-English-Spanish_0.pdf

57. Bennett CE, Wood JN, Scribano PV. Health care utilization for children in foster care. *Acad Pediatr.* 2020:20341–20347.

58. Dinpanah H, Akbarzadeh Pasha A. Potential child abuse screening in emergency department; a diagnostic accuracy study. *Emerg (Tehran).* 2017;5(1):e8.

59. Cartocci G, Fineschi V, Padovano M, Scopetti M, Rossi-Espagnet MC, Giannì C. Shaken baby syndrome: magnetic resonance imaging features in abusive head trauma. *Brain Sci.* 2021;11:179.

60. Neurofibromatosis Fact Sheet for patient-caregiver education. National Institutes of Health. Accessed June 13, 2022. https://www.ninds.nih.gov/health-information/patient-caregiver-education/fact-sheets/neurofibromatosis-fact-sheet

Note: Page numbers followed by "*f*" indicate figures, "*t*" indicate tables, and "*b*" indicate boxes.